Treating Childhood Depression with Contextual Emotion Regulation Therapy

Treating Childhood Depression with Contextual Emotion Regulation Therapy

Maria Kovacs

THE GUILFORD PRESS
New York London

A Division of Guilford Publications, Inc.
370 Seventh Avenue, Suite 1200, New York, NY 10001
www.guilford.com

Printed in the United States of America

This book is printed on acid-free paper.

Last digit is print number: 9 8 7 6 5 4 3 2 1

Library of Congress Cataloging-in-Publication Data

Names: Kovacs, Maria (Professor of psychiatry), author.
Title: Treating childhood depression with contextual emotion regulation therapy / Maria Kovacs.
Description: New York : The Guilford Press, [2023] | Includes bibliographical references and index.
Identifiers: LCCN 2023015835 | ISBN 9781462552375 (paperback ; alk. paper) | ISBN 9781462552382 (hardcover ; alk. paper)
Subjects: MESH: Depressive Disorder—therapy | Child | Emotional Regulation | Psychotherapy—methods | BISAC: PSYCHOLOGY / Psychotherapy / Child & Adolescent | PSYCHOLOGY / Psychopathology / Depression
Classification: LCC RJ506.D4 | NLM WM 171.5 | DDC 618.92/8527—dc23/eng/20230523
LC record available at *https://lccn.loc.gov/2023015835*

About the Author

Maria Kovacs, PhD, is Distinguished Professor of Psychiatry at the University of Pittsburgh School of Medicine. Dr. Kovacs has been internationally recognized for her expertise in childhood depression. Since the 1980s, her research and clinical work have focused on ways to understand, prevent, or mitigate childhood-onset depression and its sequelae later in life. She led an international team that studied the early development of the self-regulation of sadness and distress in young children, the role of emotion regulation problems as risk factors that enable the emergence of clinical depression, and ways in which family context, physiology, genetics, and personal characteristics can enable or counteract these risk factors. She developed many research tools, including the Children's Depression Inventory and the Feelings and Me Questionnaires, the latter discussed in depth in this book. Dr. Kovacs has lectured extensively on her work, both internationally and nationally, and has published more than 200 articles in scientific journals.

Preface

Professional views of childhood depression have changed substantially across the years. Prior to the late 1960s, mental health professionals believed that children were psychologically incapable of experiencing depression. The study of childhood depression took a new direction during the mid- to late 1970s as some investigators in child psychiatry turned to a then novel research paradigm promulgated in adult psychiatry. Within the framework of this paradigm, patients had to be assessed in a uniform and standardized manner; diagnoses were defined operationally via specific criteria (rather than based on clinical judgment); and establishing the validity of psychiatric diagnoses was a research priority (Feighner et al., 1972).

Embracing these innovations and modifying them for younger patients, Dr. Joaquim Puig-Antich and his associates were the first to apply operational diagnostic criteria to identify depressed children for a clinical trial of antidepressant medication (Puig-Antich et al., 1979). Paralleling this work, my research group investigated the phenomenology of pediatric depression and demonstrated the validity of the diagnoses of depressive disorders in childhood. We documented, for example, that the various depressive disorders in clinic-referred children were more serious than had been believed, that depressed children often had other psychiatric disorders that contributed to a multitude of problems, and that children with major depressive disorder were likely to have recurrent episodes as time went by (e.g., Kovacs et al., 1984a, 1984b, 1988, 1989; Kovacs, Akiskal, et al., 1994; Kovacs, Gatsonis, et al., 1994; Kovacs, Obrosky, et al., 1997). These findings underscored the need for effective therapies for children suffering from depression.

Contextual emotion regulation therapy (or CERT) for pediatric depression was conceived in response to the need for a developmentally sensitive, nonpharmacological intervention for the younger ages. The central thesis of CERT is that the inability to appropriately modulate (i.e., attenuate) sadness, distress, and dysphoria is a key risk factor for clinical depression and also plays a crucial role in its maintenance. This idea was prompted years ago by the accounts of parents in my longitudinal study of depressed children (see Kovacs et al., 1984a, 1984b). Parents often told us that when their children were well (i.e., free of depression), even ordinary stressful events (e.g., being assigned to a new class, having a playmate move away) could elicit prolonged sadness, irritability, or upset. It was notable in many accounts that, while the children's *initial* reactions of sadness or upset to trigger events were generally appropriate (although at times more intense than warranted), the distress or dysphoria eventually "got the upper hand" and not infrequently segued into a new episode of clinical depression. Once in a depressive episode, it became very evident that these same children had trouble attenuating their negative mood even in the face of positive events and regardless of their particular circumstances. In these regards, depressed children were very reminiscent of depressed adults.

The processes that the parents of depressed children described eventually came to be known in the field as *emotion dysregulation* and to form the basis of CERT.

CERT was developed and pilot-tested in an academic clinical research environment. This book is a greatly expanded version of the CERT treatment manual that was used in research studies (at the University of Pittsburgh; Kovacs, 2009); it also addresses the clinical symptoms and course of childhood depression and covers some issues likely to arise in nonacademic clinical settings. An attempt also has been made to summarize the most up-to-date research findings that buttress the various components of CERT.

This expanded version of the original manual also includes changes that reflect the evolution of my own thinking about emotions and their self-regulation. For example, while I have retained the phrase *emotion regulation* as the central construct of interest in CERT and continue to use it when the intervention is explained to young patients and their parents, I now prefer the phrase *mood repair* as a more faithful reflection of the target of CERT. The reason is this: *Emotion regulation* applies to any emotion and refers either to intensifying and maintaining the emotion of interest or to decreasing and attenuating it, while *mood repair* has come to refer specifically to attempts to decrease sadness and dysphoria (Isen, 1985; Josephson et al., 1996).

The long process of developing CERT has involved many enthusiastic colleagues. Special thanks are due to members of the treatment development team who helped to gather pilot data during the 1990s for various ideas in this book, participated in discussions, and were involved in CERT's initial testing with depressed children: namely, Vincent Ho, MD; Rebecca Krol, LSW; Myrna Pollock, MSW; Andrew Renouf, PhD; Joel Sherrill, PhD; Rameshwari V. Tumuluru, MD; and Melina Young, MSW. Appreciation also is due to Dr. Stephen Shirk for his very helpful comments on an earlier version of this book and Barbara Watkins, now retired Senior Editor, The Guilford Press, for her thoughtful feedback and far-reaching editorial assistance, which have reshaped this book in many important ways. Additional thanks are due to Kristen Nicholls for her competent assistance, particularly in the management of the extensive list of references and citations in this book. I would also like to acknowledge my mentor of many, many decades ago, the late Dr. Aaron T. Beck, under whose guidance I came to appreciate the importance of treatment manuals, and who has remained an inspiration for his unfailing commitment to psychotherapy as the route to alleviate the suffering caused by depression.

Finally, I owe particular gratitude to the many children, adolescents, young adults, and their families who participated in our various research studies of childhood depression. They graciously allowed repeated probes into their lives and patiently endured often very lengthy and emotionally demanding interviews. This book, and CERT itself, would not have been possible without them and is a testimony to their willingness to share their inner experiences and life stories. It is my hope that this new treatment will find a place in the armamentarium of approaches that therapists can use to help youngsters recover from depression.

Contents

Purchasers of this book can download and print enlarged versions of select materials from the appendices at *www.guilford.com/kovacs-forms* for personal use or use with clients (see copyright page for details).

Treating Childhood Depression with Contextual Emotion Regulation Therapy

Introduction

This book introduces to professionally trained and licensed child psychotherapists a new treatment for pediatric depression—contextual emotion regulation therapy—or CERT. This intervention was originally designed for children in the 7- to 13-year-age group, but it is applicable to older adolescents as well. CERT targets youngsters who suffer from clinical depression. *Clinical depression* signifies at a minimum the following: (1) that the child is experiencing not only depressed, dysphoric mood but also several other symptoms such as sleep problems, fatigue, inability to concentrate on schoolwork, or social withdrawal, (2) that the collection of depressive symptoms impairs the child's functioning within the family, with peers, in school, or in other settings, and/or has been very distressing to the child, and (3) that given the specific triggers or presumed causes, the overall symptom presentation is out of the norm for that youth's age, circumstance, and cultural context.

Some mental health professionals conceptualize clinical depression in terms of the overall severity of depressive symptoms (i.e., by using a quantitative approach). Thus, children would be classified as clinically depressed if they achieved a predefined score on some symptom checklist or questionnaire (for related information, see Chapter 5). However, the term *clinical depression* is used here to signify any of the various types of depressive disorders (not due to a drug of abuse, medication, or a medical condition) that meet diagnostic criteria.

The content of this book covers two broad areas: first, research-based information about pediatric depression and emotion regulation (Chapters 1–2), and second, a detailed description of the conceptual underpinnings of CERT, its clinical targets and goals, and how its key components can be implemented (Chapters 3–10). The latter chapters constitute a treatment manual (e.g., Carroll & Rounsaville, 2008). The manual component of this book contains specific *dos, how tos,* and *whens* as well as *don'ts.* But I want to emphasize that CERT is a not a paint-by-numbers intervention. On the contrary, one of CERT's guiding principles is that the content of the sessions should be tailored to the developmental phase, needs, and context of the given young patient. The therapist should also take advantage of the dynamic nature of the therapeutic process.

One of the most striking features of clinically depressed youngsters (and adults) is that they tend to be sad, miserable, unhappy, despondent, and cranky much of the time and that even the most well-meaning efforts to cheer them up have only transient (if any) effects. The depressed, dysphoric mood is not only a constant companion, but also affects how such children relate to others and their environment. For example, depressed children typically view other people as not sufficiently loving. Others, in turn, can perceive them as depressing; hence, friends may stay away, parents may prefer to spend time with other offspring. Indeed, a great many of the problems that finally push parents to seek help for their depressed children can be traced back to the direct effects of despondent dysphoric mood on parent–child, child–siblings, and child–peer relations.

It is precisely this aspect of pediatric depression—persistent dysphoria—that constitutes the main target of CERT. CERT's central thesis is that difficulty in appropriately modulating (regulating) sadness, dysphoria, and distress predates and is a key risk factor for clinical depression and also plays a crucial role in maintaining it. It is not unusual for children to react to depressogenic triggers of daily life with sadness or distress. While most children bounce back from such reactions in a fairly short time and with relative ease, some other children find it difficult to do so and experience a more protracted or complicated emotional reaction. There is compelling evidence that whether the initial dysphoric reaction resolves or lingers reflects in large measure the person's emotion self-regulation skills, namely the person's (usually automatic) responses to the emotion being experienced in the given context. If the dysphoric emotion persists, it segues into dysphoric mood, which is more persistent, and which can then initiate a cascade of further depressive symptoms (such as sleep problems, worthlessness, fatigue). The resultant clinical depression is maintained by reactions that inadvertently prolong or worsen the sad, dysphoric mood.

Therefore, a central goal of CERT is to correct children's ineffective or faulty sadness regulation, which involves helping the child and parent to recognize regulatory efforts that unwittingly maintain the sad affect, along with those that help to alleviate it. At the same time, CERT also addresses the contextual and environmental factors that can help or hinder a child's ability to effectively regulate sadness and distress. Because emotion regulation skills are acquired developmentally and in the social context of the family, CERT requires active parental participation in the child's treatment. The treatment is implemented in individual sessions, where both the child and at least one parent are present. During the earlier phase, the focus is on symptom reduction (accomplished in large measure by attenuating dysphoric mood), while during the later phase, the focus turns to coping skills training to decrease the likelihood of depression recurrence. CERT is delivered at a gradually reducing dose, starting with two sessions per week and eventually tapering to one session every 2–4 weeks. Each of these features of CERT is addressed in more detail in the various chapters that follow.

To anchor CERT in the clinical phenomena it targets, Chapter 1 presents an overview of childhood depression, starting with the various psychiatric diagnoses that are covered by the term, as well as key clinical and demographic features that are particularly relevant to treatment. I also review briefly evidence-based treatments for pediatric depression and explain how CERT differs from them. Chapter 2 focuses on what research has revealed about emotion regulation and mood repair and their developmental unfolding through childhood and adolescence. The material summarized in Chapter 2 provides the developmental scaffolding and empirical basis for CERT. In that chapter, I also explain CERT's unique approach to emotion regulatory responses.

Chapter 3 includes an overview of CERT: its distinguishing features, treatment goals, intervention strategies, and approach to symptom reduction. Chapter 4 covers practical issues in preparing to deliver CERT, such as the therapist's basic therapeutic stance, session structure, the role of homework, and use of visual and behavioral aids. Chapter 5 provides guidelines about diagnostic assessment, case formulation, and treatment planning. Chapter 6 outlines key elements of the initial sessions. Chapter 7 introduces case examples (followed throughout the book) to illustrate CERT's approach; in this chapter the goal is to reduce sadness and dysphoria by strengthening adaptive mood repair responses. (Case examples in this book are composites.) Chapter 8 addresses CERT's approach to nonaffective symptoms of depression, such as self-deprecation and suicidal ideation or behavior. Subsequent to symptom reduction, CERT focuses on ways to reduce the risk of depression recurrence by teaching affect-specific coping skills: Chapters 9 and 10 explain the strategies for achieving this goal.

CERT employs a broad array of teaching aids, including didactic posters that illustrate aspects of emotion regulation as well as a parent manual. These teaching aids are presented in Appendices B and D, respectively. Application of these aids is illustrated throughout the treatment manual segments of this book.

Chapter 1

Childhood Depression

Key Features and the Need for Treatment

The past several decades have witnessed an explosion of research on clinical, physiological, and psychosocial aspects of childhood depression, along with new conceptual perspectives. In this chapter, I focus on topics that are relevant to the psychosocial treatment of depressed youngsters. I also briefly comment on evidence-based interventions for pediatric depression and highlight that contextual emotion regulation therapy (CERT) is the only treatment for younger, school-age children that is grounded in the developmental literature.

The alert reader will notice that a substantial portion of the studies I cite in this chapter were published before 2000. Indeed, the late 1970s, the 1980s, and the 1990s were the years during which the validity of operationally defined depression diagnoses in childhood were confirmed and key features of these disorders (e.g., rates, clinical characteristics, familiality) were established. Building on this body of knowledge, subsequent studies have focused on uncovering variables that moderate features of pediatric depression and variables that mediate a variety of outcomes. Later in this chapter, I provide a few examples from the literature on moderation and mediation effects in pediatric depression.

Types, Rates, and Developmental Aspects

The psychiatric diagnostic system used in the United States (American Psychiatric Association, 1980, 1994, 2013, 2022) and the system used in Europe and other parts of the world (World Health Organization [WHO], 1992, 2019) uniformly recognize various types of clinical depression. These diagnostic categories (described in the section that follows) have been embraced in research and clinical practice and have been shown to be generally valid in the younger ages. However, the fact that the diagnostic criteria make few accommodations for children's developmental levels continues to be a source of some concern and criticism.

While some professionals prefer to think of depression as existing on a continuum of severity of symptoms (dimensional approach), diagnoses (categorical approach) serve several useful goals. For example, diagnoses convey information about course, outcome, and familiality, which can be important components of patients' psychoeducation. Diagnoses also help clinicians to communicate about their patients. Although CERT was developed with (and for) children suffering from major depression and/or dysthymia, it can be implemented to counter other depression diagnoses as well.

The Diagnostic Categories

There are four diagnostic categories of depression: major depression, persistent depressive disorder (dysthymia), unspecified depressive disorder, and adjustment disorder with depressed mood. Their defining features (also known as *operational criteria*) were first articulated in the third revision of the *Diagnostic and Statistical Manual of Mental Disorders* (DSM-III) of the American Psychiatric Association (APA; 1980), were changed somewhat in the fourth revision (APA, 1994), and are essentially the same in the fifth and fifth text revision (APA, 2013, 2022). The Mental and Behavioral Disorders section of the International Classification of Diseases (WHO, 1992, 2019) had been designed to parallel in important ways the DSM system, which is evident in the diagnoses of the various depressions.

Major depressive disorder (MDD) is the most common form of clinical depression. The criteria for an episode of MDD in children and adolescents include prominent and persistent depressed mood or loss of pleasure, or irritability, along with other symptoms such as fatigue and difficulty with schoolwork. The symptoms need to be present for a while and interfere with the child's functioning either at home, in school, or in other contexts.

Clinicians typically distinguish unipolar depression (single or multiple episodes of major depression) and bipolar depression (an episode of major depression as part of a bipolar disorder diagnosis). The symptomatic diagnostic criteria for an episode of major depression have remained essentially the same since they were first introduced in the DSM-III (APA, 1980) and highlight the centrality of dysregulated, dysphoric mood.

Persistent depressive disorder (dysthymia) is another form of clinical depression. It has a more protracted course but is less common than major depression. The symptom criteria for dysthymic disorder have undergone substantial changes in the various revisions of the DSM. It is notable that, in addition to the core mood symptom required for this diagnosis in DSM-IV, DSM-5, and DSM-5-TR, 3 out of the 6 criterion symptoms are physical or so-called neurovegetative in nature. In contrast, only 2 (sleep disturbance, low energy) out of 13 symptoms in the DSM-III version were neurovegetative in nature, with the rest representing psychological complaints. It is not known which definition of dysthymia is more valid in the juvenile years: the DSM-III definition, with its stronger emphasis on psychological symptoms, or the later DSM definitions, with their emphasis on neurovegetative symptoms? Owing to a lack of research, we don't know the answer: But at least one study reported that the clinical picture of dysthymia among 7- to 18-year-old patients was not fully consistent with DSM-IV criteria (Masi et al., 2003).

Unspecified depressive disorder and **adjustment disorder with depressed mood** are the two other categories of depression. The former diagnosis is used for a variety of presentations that do not meet the criteria for major depression or dysthymia. In adjustment disorders (including with depressed mood), symptoms develop in response to a stressor (other than bereavement), and cause significant functional impairment (APA, 2013, 2022).

Rates of Depressive Disorders and the Effect of Sex and Age

How frequent is childhood depression? While clinical depression has been identified as early as between ages 3 and 6 (Luby et al., 2002, 2003), it is infrequent in children younger than 10: However, its rate increases with the onset of adolescence.

According to earlier studies, between 0.4 and 2.5% of youngsters suffer from depression (major depression, dysthymia, unspecified depression) (Birmaher et al., 1996). But according to a later overview, the 12-month prevalence of pediatric depression is more likely between 2.8 and 5.9% up to age 18, depending on the age and sex of the respondents (Costello et al., 2006). In a community-based pediatric sample (mean age = 6 years), 5.7% reportedly had significant symptoms of depression (Fuhrmann et al., 2014). But in a nationwide health insurance database, less than 0.01% of primary school–age children (6–10 years old) had depressive episode diagnoses consistent with the *International Classification of Diseases, 10th Revision* (ICD-10; World Health Organization, 1992; Frey et al., 2020). Even among 15- to 19-year-old adolescents, who are easier to diagnose than children, variable lifetime rates of major depressive disorder have been reported, including 9.4% in a sample residing in the U.S. Northeast (Reinherz et al., 1993), 13.5% in a nationwide U.S. sample (Kessler & Walters, 1998), and 24% in a sample recruited in the state of Oregon (Lewinsohn et al., 1998). The variable rates of child and adolescent depression in the literature most likely reflect differences in assessment tools, definitions, and sample characteristics typical of various regions.

Although the prevalence of pediatric depression in the population has yet to be confirmed, there is considerable information about its various forms and the impact of sex and age on depression rates. We know that, just as is the case among adults, major depression is far more frequent among youngsters than dysthymia, both in community and clinical settings (Kessler & Walters, 1998; Kovacs et al., 1984a; Lewinsohn et al., 1998). (Adjustment disorder with depressed mood is rarely studied.) As noted previously, it also is well known that depression rates are low during childhood but rise dramatically around mid- and late adolescence (Costello et al., 2006). It is well established that young boys and girls either have similar rates of depression, or depressed boys tend to outnumber girls, but around adolescence, the rates of depression among girls suddenly become at least twice as high as the rates among boys (e.g., Wesselhoeft et al., 2015). The emergence of sex differences in depression rates around age 15 has been reported as far back as the 1990s (Nolen-Hoeksema & Girgus, 1994): The differential rates were confirmed in a later sample of U.S. adolescents, but beginning earlier at age 13 (Salk et al., 2016).

A meta-analysis of sex differences in nationally representative samples reported its emergence even earlier at age 12, with a peak rate among girls in mid-adolescence (Salk et al., 2017). No particular explanation has yet garnered unequivocal support about why girls and boys have different rates of depression only after the onset of adolescence (Angold & Worthman, 1993; Cyranowski et al., 2000; Eid et al., 2019; Kendler et al., 2001; Nolen-Hoeksema & Girgus, 1994).

Developmental Stage and the Expression of Depression

How does development affect the expression of depression? In the DSM systems, the diagnostic criteria for major depressive episode and dysthymic disorder include only two accommodations for age: (1) For children and adolescents, irritability qualifies as a manifestation of dysphoric mood for both diagnoses and (2) the minimum duration required to diagnose dysthymic disorder in youngsters is 1 year (rather than the 2 years required for adults) (APA, 1994, 2013, 2022).

Given such minor accommodations, the DSM system has been criticized for fostering adult-based depression criteria regardless of age (for a review, see Weiss & Garber, 2003) and for disregarding how development may influence the symptoms of depression. As one example, because abstract thinking does not fully emerge until late adolescence or young adulthood, it is believed that worthlessness, which presupposes abstract thinking, should not be a criterion symptom among children. As another example, the stage of pubertal development, which is known to influence the rates of depression (Angold & Worthman, 1993), may constrain the type of neurovegetative symptoms children have. Thus, it could be argued that symptom criteria should differ by pubertal status. However, in the first published report of how cognitive and pubertal development relate to young, depressed patients' symptoms, we found that more advanced development did not signal more severe depression or more sophisticated cognitive symptoms (Kovacs & Paulauskas, 1984).

Over the years, most studies of development and depression symptoms have used chronologic age as the index of developmental stage. The findings have been equivocal (for an overview, see Kovacs, 1996). In their review of this area, Weiss and Garber (2003) could only conclude that neurovegetative symptoms (e.g., fatigue) were more likely to occur among depressed adolescents than among depressed children. In one of our studies of 559 depressed young patients (ages 7–14), we likewise found that the clinical picture of major depression becomes somewhat more neurovegetative as children get older; that is, symptoms such as hypersomnia, fatigue, or psychomotor retardation are more likely among older rather than younger depressed children (Baji et al., 2009). However, neither the developmental factors responsible for this presentation nor their clinical significance is well understood.

A child's *ability to report* on her own emotional well-being and symptoms is another factor that is influenced by developmental stage (Kovacs, 1986). For example, because time perspective, autobiographical memory, and metacognition are not yet fully developed in the younger years, 7- or 8-year-olds are unlikely to provide reliable and valid accounts of how long they had felt cranky and irritable on any given day and whether persistent dysphoria had lasted as long as 1 year (one of the criteria for dysthymia) or the extent to which they were bothered by feelings of worthlessness (a symptom of major depression).

Relatedly, it is helpful to be aware that young children are more likely to express some depression symptoms behaviorally than via verbalized complaints. For example, given constraints on the ability to conceptualize and report on the experience of anhedonia, this symptom can manifest as attenuated play activity, marked reduction in smiling, or complaints of being bored. As another example, difficulties concentrating are likely to present as the child repeatedly failing to finish projects or having problems with school tasks.

All in all, the effects of development on the experience and expression of pediatric depression are an area that remains underexplored and only partially understood. Nevertheless, it is important to keep in mind that development involves multiple processes and functional domains and its effects on psychopathology may vary across young patients of the same age.

Clinical Characteristics

Research on major depressive and dysthymic disorders in various pediatric samples has unequivocally shown that these conditions are neither mild nor transient. While youngsters in community-based samples tend to have shorter and less severe episodes of depression than do clinically referred young patients (e.g., Dunn & Goodyer, 2006; Kovacs et al., 1984a; Lewinsohn et al., 1998), depressive episodes are invariably associated with functional impairment and other subsequent problems. In this section, I focus on diagnosed depression among treatment-seeking (rather than community-based) pediatric cases because they are the targets of CERT.

As documented in the three sections that follow, rates of recovery, recurrence, comorbidity, and other clinical features of pediatric depression had been established by a series of now classic studies conducted mostly in the 1980s and 1990s.

Subsequent investigations then focused to a great degree on the relations between some clinical characteristics and treatment response or other outcomes (see Rao & Chen, 2009, for an overview).

Recovery and Recurrence

The first detailed study of the course of *major depressive disorder* among child psychiatric outpatients (8- to 13-year-olds) found that the average episode length is about 9 months, starting when the child meets diagnostic criteria and ending when the child becomes essentially asymptomatic (and remains so for at least 2 months); however, close to 20% of young patients have episodes longer than 1½ years (Kovacs et al., 1984a; Kovacs, Obrosky, et al., 1997). A study of 7- to 17-year-old inpatients and outpatients similarly found that, on average, a major depressive episode lasts about 9 months (McCauley et al., 1993), although lengthy episodes of major depression may be increasingly common among youth. In a subsequent study, the average MDD episode lasted for 15 months among patients 8–13 years old and for 18 months among those 12–16 years old (Birmaher et al., 2004). Thus, major depression during childhood and adolescence kidnaps a significant portion of a youngster's life.

Pediatric MDD episodes also are associated with high recovery rates. In our naturalistic follow-up study, 92% of young patients had recovered by 1½ years after the onset of their first major depressive episode (Kovacs et al., 1984a; Kovacs, Obrosky, et al., 1997). Similarly high recovery rates have been reported for other samples of depressed youth (McCauley et al., 1993) including more recent birth cohorts (Birmaher et al., 2004). The high recovery rate associated with pediatric major depression parallels the course of depression among adults (e.g., Solomon et al., 1997): Given a sufficiently long time period, almost all depressed children, adolescents, and adults recover from their depression (irrespective of whether or not they receive treatment).

Unfortunately, as time goes by, about 40–70% of clinically referred young patients with MDD will have one or more further episodes. In our study, which involved long-term follow-up, after young patients recovered from their prior depression episode, the risk of a next major depression ranged from .55 to .69 (Kovacs et al., 2016). In other samples of depressed children and adolescents, from about 40–54% had a recurrent major depressive episode across 3- to 5-year follow-up intervals (Birmaher et al., 2004; McCauley et al., 1993), whereas across a 7-year period, 69% of depressed adolescents had recurrent MDD episodes (Rao et al., 1995). Notably, a 5-year follow-up of adolescents who received state-of-the-art depression treatment in a randomized clinical trial found that close to 50% experienced a recurrent major depression (Curry et al., 2011). A review of clinical trials with depressed adolescents likewise reported a 52% recurrence rate across a 5.7-year follow-up (Melvin et al., 2013). Although earlier studies that followed depressed youngsters into adulthood have reported varying rates of eventual recurrence (e.g., Dunn & Goodyer, 2006; Weissman et al., 1999a, 1999b), they uniformly found that only a minority of cases remain fully well into the youth's adult years.

Indeed, there is now no question that pediatric major depression signals recurrent episodes across adolescence and adulthood. Especially when persistent, such early onset also predicts functional impairment in multiple areas in adulthood (Copeland et al., 2021). Recurrent MDD during adolescence may be particularly impairing in young adulthood (Wilson et al., 2015), and depression that dates back to the juvenile years is more recurrent, severe, and functionally impairing than depression that onsets during young or older adulthood (Zisook et al., 2007).

Comparatively little effort has been expanded on the study of *dysthymic disorder* in childhood. This is most unfortunate because there is evidence that pediatric dysthymic disorder is extremely chronic. For example, among clinically referred youngsters, dysthymic disorder persisted for more than 3 years, on average (Kovacs et al., 1984a; Kovacs, Akiskal, et al., 1994). The chronicity of dysthymic disorder also has been documented among adolescents in the community (Lewinsohn et al., 1993).

Unspecified depressive disorder is a diagnostic label that is used when the child's clinical picture does not satisfy the criteria for the specific depressions. Very often, such children have a major-depression-like history with various noncriterion depressive symptoms such as low self-esteem or pessimism but are one symptom short of those needed for MDD. Less commonly, children with unspecified depression have a dysthymia-like presentation for less than 12 months or may have fewer symptoms than needed. This diagnostic category has not garnered much research interest.

Finally, there has been comparatively little research interest in the diagnosis of *adjustment disorder with depressed mood*. The available information typically concerns all types of adjustment disorders (i.e., with depressed mood, with anxiety, with disturbance of conduct) lumped into one group. Furthermore, most reports have been based on diagnoses in medical records that were not derived through standardized assessments (e.g., Andreasen & Wasek, 1980; Jones et al., 2002). Not surprisingly, while some researchers report favorable outcomes for adjustment disorders, others do not (for a review, see Newcorn & Strain, 1992). However, there is consensus that adjustment disorders typically last longer than the 6 months specified in the DSM system. Using a standardized psychiatric interview and requiring at least three symptoms (in addition to the existing DSM criteria), we found that adjustment disorders in children last typically about 7 months (Kovacs, Gatsonis, et al., 1994).

Comorbid Psychiatric Disorders

According to the DSM (APA, 1994, 2013, 2022), a patient can be diagnosed with multiple psychiatric disorders, a practice that had sparked considerable debate (e.g., Frances et al., 1990) and has been strongly criticized in child psychiatry (Rutter, 2011). The presence of multiple mental disorders in the same person is known as *psychiatric comorbidity*. Comorbidity can signify disorders other than depression any time during the child's life (lifetime comorbidity) or having depression and some other disorder contemporaneously (concurrent comorbidity).

It has long been established that psychiatric comorbidity is the rule, rather than the exception, in pediatric depression (for reviews, see Birmaher et al., 1996; Rao & Chen, 2009), particularly in connection with major depressive and dysthymic disorders (e.g., Kovacs et al., 1984a, 2016; Masi et al., 2003). An anxiety disorder is the most common comorbid condition (for a review, see Cummings et al., 2014): Around 40% of depressed youth have comorbid anxiety disorders, and the onset of the anxiety disorder usually antedates the onset of the first episode of depression (Avenevoli et al., 2001; Birmaher et al., 2004; Goodyer et al., 1997; Kovacs et al., 1984a, 1989). It is worth noting that an anxiety disorder also is the most common comorbid psychiatric diagnosis among adults suffering from mood disorders (Maser & Cloninger, 1990). Cummings et al. (2014) have proposed pathways to anxiety–depression comorbidity, which differ as a function of the type of anxiety disorder. Comorbid anxiety disorder prognosticated less favorable recovery in a state-of-the-art clinical trial with depressed adolescents (Brent et al., 1998) and increased rate of posttreatment depression recurrence in another trial (Curry et al., 2011).

A behavior disorder, typically conduct or oppositional defiant disorder, is the second most common comorbid psychiatric diagnosis among depressed children (for an overview, see Rao & Chen, 2009). Up to about 35–40% of depressed youngsters have such comorbid diagnoses (e.g., Avenevoli et al., 2001; Birmaher et al., 2004; Goodyer et al., 1997; Hammen et al., 1999). Reconfirming previous reports, Kovacs and colleagues (1988) found that conduct disorders in depressed children typically emerge as complications of the depression but often persist after the depression has remitted and signal later functional problems. While the comorbidity of conduct problems and depression was established quite a while ago, attempts continue to explain its etiology and development (e.g., Burke & Loeber, 2010; McDonough-Caplan et al., 2018; Wolff & Ollendick, 2006).

Suicidal Behavior and Bipolar Outcome

Although suicidal behavior is one symptom of major depression, it warrants separate attention as a clinical characteristic because of the associated risk of mortality. Suicidal behavior in youngsters almost always occurs in the context of some depressive episode. However, that episode can be an adjustment disorder with depressed mood as well as major depression (Kovacs et al., 1993). Suicidal behaviors have been described in children ages 6 and younger (Luby et al., 2019). However, given the cognitive immaturity of young children and their lack of understanding of the finality of death, Nock and colleagues (2008) have proposed that the actionable risk period for suicidal behaviors onsets around age 12.

According to the DSM system, suicidal behavior can manifest in four ways, namely as: recurrent thoughts of death, recurrent suicidal ideation, specific suicide plans, and suicide attempts. Repeatedly thinking about one's own death is the most common form, and attempting suicide is the least common form of suicidal behaviors. In a clinical sample of more than five hundred fifty 7- to 14-year-olds suffering from major depression, about 68% had recurrent thoughts of death, 48% had suicidal ideation, 30% had a suicide plan, and 12% had attempted suicide (Liu et al., 2006). In a follow-up study of 159 children who had major depression, 7 were found to have died by suicide by early adulthood, yielding a high mortality rate of 4.4% across approximately 10 years (Rao et al., 1993). Reviewers of the field have confirmed that affective disorders, such as major depression, are significantly associated with suicide attempts in young people (Gili et al., 2019). Conversely, suicidal ideation was found to predict the increased risk of recurrent major depression among adolescents treated with state-of-the-art methods (Curry et al., 2011).

Finally, a high rate of switching from unipolar to bipolar disorder was one of the most surprising early clinical findings about pediatric depression (for a review, see Kovacs, 1996). In a 2- to 5-year follow-up of 6- to 12-year-old patients with major depression, close to 32% had developed bipolar disorder (Geller et al., 1994). In a clinical sample of youngsters with dysthymic disorder, 13% converted to bipolar illness during naturalistic follow-up (Kovacs, Akiskal, et al., 1994). And according to another follow-up study (Rao et al., 1995), 19% of a group of depressed adolescents converted to bipolar disorder across a 7-year period.

Treatment Implications

The literature on the clinical characteristics of pediatric depression can be very useful to the therapist. For example, we know the typical length of an episode of major depression, and also that recovery is most likely during the earlier phases of the episode and becomes gradually less likely the longer the child has been depressed (Kovacs et al., 1984a). Having ascertained during the initial assessment the date of onset of the child's current depression episode, the therapist can set their own expectations about the pace of recovery for that youth. For example, if the young patient has been depressed for close to a year (longer than the average duration), recovery will likely be slower than if the depression had onset only a few months earlier.

The high rate of psychiatric comorbidity in pediatric depression underscores the need for a comprehensive diagnostic evaluation: The therapist must be confident that depression is the child's sole or most pressing problem. Depressed young patients with concurrent nonaffective psychiatric disorders may pose a treatment challenge. For example, in a study of depressed adolescents (Brent et al., 1998), patients with comorbid anxiety disorder were likely to be still depressed at the end of treatment. Furthermore, interventions recommended for some comorbid disorders are the opposite of the strategies used in CERT to alleviate depression (this is discussed in Chapter 5).

Based on the literature, the therapist can anticipate a high likelihood that the depressed child will manifest some form of suicidal behavior. The risk of suicidal ideation or a suicide attempt is magnified about twofold if the child has been (or will be) receiving antidepressant medication (Maalouf & Brent, 2012). The presence of suicide plans or a suicide attempt warrants various targeted management approaches (addressed in Chapters 5 and 8) for which the therapist needs to be prepared.

Recognition that depression in children can segue into bipolar disorder has multiple treatment implications. For example, the therapist ought to monitor if the young patient has subsyndromal manic symptoms because they have been associated with a poor response to depression treatment (Maalouf & Brent, 2012). Furthermore, a child who quickly or unexpectedly "recovers" should give pause, especially if the recovery is accompanied by elated or irritable mood and a sudden increase in energy and goal-directed activities. Such signs, possibly indicating that the child is converting to bipolar disorder, should prompt an immediate psychiatric evaluation and plans for antimanic pharmacotherapy.

Finally, some families may want to know what to expect after the child has ended treatment. I suggest full transparency and the sharing of published and valid empirical information about the course of depression. The fact is that most children who are treated for depression are highly likely to experience one or more further episodes. Indeed, as I commented in an article (Kovacs et al., 2016), the posttreatment rates of recurrence of major depression in several randomized state-of-the-art clinical trials with depressed adolescents were like the rates observed during naturalistic follow-ups (noted earlier). That is one of the reasons why the final phase of CERT focuses on preventing depression recurrence.

When sharing information with families about the clinical features of pediatric depression, it is important to emphasize that outcomes are probabilistic, and that even high-probability outcomes do not signify certainty. Therefore, the high probability of a recurrent depression episode, for example, should be framed as providing opportunities for prevention and proactive intervention (the goal of CERT's final phase) rather than a reason for pessimism.

Environmental and Family Correlates

To develop more effective interventions, researchers have scrutinized how environmental events, family interactions, and family history of depression may contribute to the onset and course of depression (for extensive reviews, see Kaslow et al., 1994; Rao & Chen, 2009; Sheeber et al., 2001). The usual conclusions have been that depressed youngsters have greater exposure to stressful events, less supportive and more conflictual family environments, and more extensive family histories of depression than do typically developing peers. There has been particular interest in the role of early parenting in depression risk. However, a meta-analysis found that the association between parenting behavior and childhood depression is "modest" at best: Parenting accounted only for 8% of the variance in predicting childhood depression, with parental hostility and rejection being the strongest correlates (McLeod et al., 2007).

Stressful Life Events

There is a compelling body of literature showing that adults who suffer from depressive symptoms or disorders have been exposed to higher levels or a greater number of stressful events than nondepressed peers (for an overview, see LeMoult, 2020). These findings hold up regardless of whether the stressors are discrete events such as divorce or loss of a job, or chronic difficulties such as having a child with a disabling medical condition (Kessler, 1997).

The association between stress early in life and depression during childhood and adolescence also has been confirmed (for a meta-analysis, see LeMoult et al., 2020). Clinically depressed children experience a greater number of negative life events than do children with other psychiatric disorders or normal peers (e.g., Luby et al., 2006; Mayer et al., 2009; Williamson et al., 2005) and appear to have been exposed earlier in their development. According to our study of more than 400 young patients with major depression (Mayer et al., 2009), these youngsters had accumulated multiple stressors by the time they were 7–9 years old, after which the rate of negative life events leveled off and stabilized. In contrast, comparison peers experienced a gradually increasing (and smaller) number of stressful events from childhood to mid-adolescence. We also found that parental health-related events, death of close relatives, and intrafamilial stressful events (e.g., family arguments, parental divorce) were significantly associated with having major depression (Mayer et al., 2009). Consistent with our findings, a meta-analysis of early life stress and risk of pediatric major depression likewise found that intrafamilial stressful events like emotional and physical abuse, domestic violence, and death of a family member were more strongly associated with MDD than stressors like poverty (LeMoult et al., 2020).

However, it is unclear if the association of stress and depression remains the same across multiple episodes of MDD in childhood. In a seminal article, Post (1992) proposed that owing to a "kindling effect" (neurobiological sensitization) in the brain, less and less stress is required to trigger each recurrence of a mood disorder episode; this phenomenon has been verified among adults (Tennant, 2002). Research has clearly shown that in the context of depression, certain stressors have measurable effects on biological systems, including the brain, and that the associations between stress and biological changes may be bidirectional (reviewed by Hammen, 2015; Park et al., 2019). Research also has shown that stress may lead to depression by facilitating epigenetic changes (e.g., triggering gene expression) that impact behavior (reviewed by Park et al., 2019). Thus, the clinician should be aware that, for children with recurrent depressive episodes, even seemingly minor (or questionable) stressors may trigger a new bout of depression.

It is also known, however, that not everyone who is exposed to a given stressor becomes clinically depressed (Averill et al., 2018). For example, among 5- to 12-year-old children mourning the loss of a parent, only 37% developed a major depressive disorder (Weller et al., 1991). And among adolescents who were exposed to the suicide of a peer, 30% had major depression (Brent et al., 1993). There is some evidence that stress is more likely to lead to depression if the youngster has negative cognitive characteristics such as dysfunctional attitudes or low self-esteem (Hammen, 2005; LeMoult, 2020). And because a child's temperament can influence stress reactivity (Compas et al., 2004), it also may play a role in whether she becomes depressed subsequent to a stressor.

Family History of Depression

It has long been recognized that depression among adults "runs in the family" (for a meta-analysis, see Sullivan et al., 2000). Studies eventually revealed that the same is true of depression among children (for a review, see Tompson et al., 2015). Although the findings differ somewhat depending on the comparison group, depressed youngsters have generally higher rates of depression among their first- and second-degree relatives than psychologically well comparison children or children with nonaffective psychiatric disorders (Klein et al., 2001; Kovacs, Devlin, et al., 1997; Puig-Antich et al., 1989; Todd et al., 1993; Tompson et al., 2015; Wickramaratne et al., 2000). In fact, children with a mood disorder may have higher rates of relatives affected with mood disorder than the relatives of adults with a mood disorder (Neuman et al., 1997).

Research that established the familiality of pediatric depression eventually gave rise to high-risk family studies, which have emphasized the prospective investigation of premorbid vulnerability factors and potential mechanisms of depression transmission (Avenevoli & Merikangas, 2006). For example, high-risk children and adolescents (owing to parental depression) have been found to be less successful than low-risk peers on several dimensions of behavioral emotion regulation (Daches et al., 2019). According to another study, children in a large normative cohort with histories of parental depression evidenced reduced volumes of several brain regions that have been implicated in reward responding (Pagliaccio et al., 2020). One review has concurred that children of parents with major depression have altered volumes and thickness in various brain regions (Kemp et al., 2022).

How is depression transmitted within families? While some experts believe that familial transmission of major depression reflects mostly genetic influences

(Sullivan et al., 2000), both psychosocial and genetic mechanisms are likely to contribute to pediatric depression. Modeling (social learning) is one avenue of psychosocial transmission (reviewed by Goodman, 2020). By observing and interacting with depressed relatives, children and youth may learn certain context-specific responses and behaviors (e.g., undue self-criticism) that facilitate the emergence of depressive symptoms and disorders. Depressed parents also may transmit depression to children by differentially reinforcing responses, which initiate or maintain depressive-like behaviors (e.g., intensifying sad feelings) and not reinforcing responses that counter depression risk (e.g., positive affect). The specific ways in which depressed mothers parent their young offspring have been shown to be one route of psychosocial transmission of depression (for a review and meta-analysis, see Goodman et al., 2020).

The notion that pediatric depression may have genetic bases is relatively recent (Todd et al., 1993), and the full range of genes that are involved has yet to be identified. Our research group has reported initial findings that implicate genes related to synaptic plasticity and those involved in the regulation of the hypothalamic–pituitary–adrenal axis, which orchestrates stress reactivity (e.g., Dempster et al., 2007; Strauss et al., 2005). Work on the genetics of depression continues (for reviews, see McIntosh et al., 2019). However, it is important to be aware that there is no such thing as a "depression gene." Instead, many different genes (most of which remain to be identified) are likely to act in concert to increase a youth's vulnerability to depression.

Treatment Implications

The therapist can use the information just summarized in many ways. Explaining to families what we know about the link between stress and depression may help family members to view the depressed child's behavior in a new light and make it easier for them to accept the child's symptoms. Explaining what is known about the possibility of sensitization to stress may help families to understand how even relatively mild or innocuous negative events might trigger depression in a child with prior depression. And families may benefit from knowing that one way in which stressful events cause depression is through their detrimental effects on daily life (Kessler, 1997).

Evidence that relatives, especially parents and/or siblings, have had depression is valuable information for the therapist because it suggests that the child may have been subject to multiple avenues of psychosocial depression transmission. Given that several studies of clinic-referred, depressed children reported high rates of parental depression (see Gladstone et al., 2019, for a review), it is more than likely that the young patient's caregiving parent (probably the mother) will be depressed. This is relevant because, as the Gladstone review noted, it is current parental depression (rather than a history of depression) that appears to compromise a child's response to treatment. In Chapter 5, I address what to do if parental depression exists and list self-rated questionnaires that can serve to assess it (along with other psychopathological symptoms).

Depression as Chemical Imbalance

The idea that depression reflects some form of "chemical imbalance" in the brain is a somewhat dated view but has become widely quoted, often leading to the conclusion that depression is solely biological in nature. Consequently, it has been argued that successful depression prevention and treatment must likewise be biologically or physiologically based. Parents may therefore ask questions such as "Does my son's depression mean that he has a brain disorder?" And "If childhood depression is due to a chemical imbalance in the brain, how can psychotherapy possibly help my daughter?"

In response, the therapist can point out that thinking, wishing, or hoping—indeed all behaviors and actions—derive from and are the outcomes of physiological and biochemical processes in the brain. It is therefore not surprising that clinical depression, which signals abnormal functioning, is associated with abnormal brain physiology when it comes to neurotransmitter availability (for an overview, see aan het Rot et al., 2009) as well as atypical brain structure and function (for a review, see Anderson et al., 2020). However, it is not currently known if atypical brain features are consistently present before the onset of a depression episode (rather than being caused by it) and whether they are causally related to the symptoms and functional impairment that characterize depression.

The chain of reasoning may continue that, for example, if depression is due to a chemical imbalance in the brain, then treatments should target that aspect of the brain's faulty physiology. However, this proposition incorrectly implies that brain and behavior are separable and that physiological phenomena can only be altered by physiological means or tools. Quite the contrary, research in the neurosciences is revealing the plasticity of the brain and its sensitivity to diverse inputs (e.g., Xin & Chan, 2020) and that a variety of training can alter brain structure and function in youth (Tymofiyeva & Gaschler, 2021). Thus, if parents question whether psychological processes can impact dysfunctional physiology, they can be advised of research evidence that brain processes and brain structural components can be affected by nonphysiological means (e.g., via changing one's behavior, learning, skill acquisition).

Existing Treatments and the Need for CERT

During the past several decades, randomized treatment–outcome research on pediatric depression has focused mostly on cognitive-behavioral therapy and interpersonal psychotherapy (e.g., Maalouf & Brent, 2012). Results show that these interventions are generally more effective at relieving depression than no treatment, being on a wait list, or receiving some form of placebo. However, because the clinical trials have been mostly confined to adolescents, there is scant systematic evidence about effective ways to help depressed school-age children younger than 10.

But new treatment directions are being pursued as exemplified by a modified form of parent–child psychotherapy for depressed 3- to 6-year-olds (Luby et al., 2018), and family-focused treatment for depressed 7- to 14-year-olds (Tompson et al., 2017, 2020). Recent overviews of psychosocial interventions for youth depression, which range from the modestly hopeful (Eckshtain et al., 2020) to the somewhat pessimistic (Weisz et al., 2019), support the need for new treatments especially for the pre-adolescent ages (Weersing et al., 2017).

Cognitive-Behavioral Therapies

Some form of *cognitive-behavioral therapy* (CBT) has been the most extensively examined psychotherapy for pediatric depression (for reviews and meta-analyses, see Weersing et al., 2017; Zhou et al., 2015, 2020). The various versions of CBT for youth originated as "downward" adaptations of interventions that were designed for depressed adults (e.g., see Stark et al., 1987). While the pediatric adaptations have several novel features, their cores represent some combination of elements from three models of adult depression: Aaron T. Beck's cognitive model that highlights the importance of negative cognitive schemata and distorted interpretations of events (Beck, 1967; Beck et al., 1979); Peter Lewinsohn's behavioral model that focuses on the importance of positive reinforcers (Lewinsohn & Graf, 1973; Lewinsohn et al., 1980); and Lynn Rehm's model that centers on behavioral self-control, self-reinforcement, and attributions (Rehm, 1977).

CBT interventions "target cognitive distortions and behavioral skill deficits" (Weersing et al., 2009, p. 29). The various versions differ in whether behaviors or cognitions are emphasized, the amount of structure (i.e., mandatory treatment elements), and the preferred delivery modality (group vs. individual; see Weersing et al., 2009, 2017). A wide variety of therapeutic techniques are allowed that address cognitive restructuring, behavioral activation, and adaptive problem solving. In their updated analyses of the treatment outcome literature, Weersing et al. (2017) concluded that CBT is a "well established" intervention for depressed *adolescents;* but for depressed *children,* CBT merits the classification of being "possibly efficacious." The latter conclusion is echoed by a meta-analysis of CBT for depressed 8- to 12-year-olds (Arnberg & Öst, 2014).

Interpersonal Psychotherapy

Interpersonal psychotherapy (IPT) for depressed adults (Klerman et al., 1984) combined elements of psychodynamic and social psychiatry perspectives and focused on the interpersonal context that contributes to and maintains depression. According to IPT, four interpersonal problem areas are associated with clinical depression: grief, role disputes, role transitions, and interpersonal deficits. Its modification for teenagers, called *interpersonal psychotherapy for depressed adolescents* (IPT-A; Moreau et al., 1991; Mufson et al., 1994), includes one further problem area, single-parent families. With a variety of intervention techniques used, the goal of IPT-A is to help young patients resolve the interpersonal problem area(s) associated with their depression. In randomized clinical trials, IPT-A was shown to have positive effects on adolescents' depressive symptoms (for an overview, see Zhou et al., 2020) and has been judged to be a "well established" treatment for depressed *adolescents* (Weersing et al., 2017). According to a meta-analysis, the effects of IPT were larger than the effects of CBT (Eckshtain et al., 2020). IPT-A has been revised for use with depressed 9- to 12-year-olds and reframed as a family-based intervention (Dietz, Mufson, et al., 2008; Dietz et al., 2015).

The Need for a Larger Armamentarium of Psychotherapies

Treatment outcome studies with youth have revealed that, even with evidence-based interventions for depression, overall treatment effects are modest, and many young patients continue to have residual symptoms (Brent & Maalouf, 2009). The treatment of younger school-aged, depressed children continues to be a particular challenge. Notably, a meta-analysis of CBT for children age 13 and younger found questionable evidence of effectiveness (Yang et al., 2017). An earlier meta-analysis reported that psychotherapy had no measurable advantage for depressed children in the 6- to 12-year age group (Watanabe et al., 2007). And Weersing et al. (2017) have noted that the evidentiary base for the successful treatment of depressed children is "notably weaker" than for depressed adolescents. Indeed, every review and meta-analysis of the field has underscored the need for more treatment development initiatives focusing on younger school-age children. As a hopeful sign, there have been trials of other interventions with diagnosed, 12-year-old and younger school-aged patients with depression (e.g., Tompson et al., 2020; Trowell et al., 2007), which are yet to be replicated by groups other than the treatment developers.

The less-than-hoped-for benefits of CBTs and IPT for younger depressed patients are likely to reflect (at least in part) the fact that they are downward extensions of treatments originally designed for adults. Thus, CBTs for depressed youngsters are not conceptually anchored in the developmental literature on cognition, and neither are IPT-A and its version for younger ages anchored in the developmental literature on social cognition and interpersonal behaviors. There consequently is a lack of synchrony between key treatment targets, components of CBT or IPT-A, and children's developmentally constrained competencies such as cognitive or interpersonal reasoning skills, respectively. Additionally, except in family-based interventions, parents seem to play secondary roles in CBTs or

IPT-A. If parents do participate, they generally do so in separate parent groups, or in a limited number of sessions that are not closely tied to the main thrust of the intervention.

CERT enriches the armamentarium of psychotherapeutic interventions for pediatric depression in various regards. It differs from other interventions because of its developmental foundation: The developmental antecedents of treatment targets are clear; the particular role CERT assigns to parents in the treatment of their children also is developmentally justified. Because it focuses on individual differences (which is a hallmark of a developmental approach), CERT makes it possible to match the content and pace of the treatment with the needs of the given patient—hence, it can be delivered in a personalized manner, which should improve treatment outcome (Brent & Maalouf, 2009). Because it focuses on younger school-age children, it represents a much needed tool in the treatment of that age group.

CERT: A Brief Overview

One vital component of human development is learning how to handle the various emotions that are part and parcel of daily life; this process is called *emotion regulation.* Emotion regulation encompasses both the inner experience (i.e., feeling, physiological reaction) and the external, visible display of an emotion after it has been triggered; it can result in the maintenance, amplification, attenuation, or termination of the emotion. Appropriate or adaptive regulation is culturally defined and often tied to the context in which the emotion was triggered. For example, every culture acknowledges the appropriateness and importance of grieving after the death of a close relative. However, some cultures encourage intense and public expressions of grief for a specific duration, while other cultures view bereavement as primarily a private experience of variable duration.

CERT targets the emotions of sadness, dysphoria, and distress, and focuses on how children's responses to their own emotions shape the subsequent course of those emotions. CERT's basic premise is that children with clinical depression do not have the requisite regulatory responses to adaptively manage sadness and dysphoria. On the contrary, when faced with stressors (triggers) that elicit sadness, dysphoria, and distress, their attempts to feel better are either unsuccessful or worsen how they feel. As a result, these emotions segue into protracted negative mood, which then progresses to a full-blown clinical depression. Once clinical depression is present, dysfunctional regulatory responding to even small perturbations in daily affect maintains or exacerbates the depressed child's negative mood and associated symptoms.

The process of attenuating or alleviating sadness and dysphoria has also been called *mood repair.* CERT seeks to help children experience mood repair success and overcome mood repair failure, and thereby recover from sadness and dysphoria. Mood repair success is made possible by building up a repertoire of adaptive regulatory responses and decreasing the use of maladaptive responses. To accomplish this goal, CERT uses a sports team model and enlists the active help of the depressed child's parent(s). The parent facilitates the child's recovery from depression by acting as the assistant coach in reaching treatment targets, while the therapist is the main coach and the child is the player. It is mostly through teaching the parent and child adaptive mood repair responding that CERT accomplishes its primary target of depressive symptom reduction.

To implement CERT, the therapist can draw on a broad range of empirically based techniques, problem-focused strategies, and approaches to environmental manipulation. The successful treatment of sad and dysphoric affect through adaptive mood repair is typically accompanied by remission of other depression symptoms. However, CERT also accommodates the treatment of nonaffective depression symptoms (e.g., sleep disturbance, negative self-evaluation) as warranted.

CERT's additional goal is to reduce the risk of future episodes of depression. This is accomplished by helping the child to cope better with stressors and events that are likely to elicit sadness and dysphoria. Learning proactive coping involves the continuous practice of adaptive mood repair responses and being able to anticipate, prepare for, and, if possible, modify potential depressogenic situations.

Considering all the features just noted, CERT offers various conceptual and practical advantages over existing treatments for depressed children, especially for younger age groups. CERT is based on current understanding of the normative development of emotion regulation and mood repair. CERT's developmental foundation accommodates individual differences and makes it comparatively easy to tailor the intervention to the regulatory needs and abilities of a given child. Thus, the therapist's approach can (and will) be different in treating a 7-year-old as compared to a 12-year-old. CERT therefore represents a crucial step toward personalized intervention (Brent & Maalouf, 2009). Furthermore, parental involvement in CERT echoes the important roles they played in the early development of their offspring's emotion self-regulation attempts.

The results of a small open trial with chronically depressed children, ranging in age from 7 to 12 years old, revealed preliminary evidence of CERT's potential effectiveness (Kovacs et al., 2006). The young patients were diagnosed with DSM-IV dysthymic disorder (with an average duration of 24.4 months at study entry). In this sample of 20 children (35% of whom were girls), up to 40% had psychiatric comorbidity, including major depression, anxiety disorder, or oppositional defiant disorder. CERT was delivered as a 30-session, four-phase intervention across a 10-month period, with two follow-up assessments. At the end of treatment, 80% of the children who entered the study with major depression were fully remitted from that disorder. Of the treatment completers (75%), 53% were fully remitted and 13% were partially remitted from their dysthymic disorder. Importantly, by the 6-month and 12-month follow-ups, 79% and 92% of the cases, respectively, had completely recovered from their dysthymia. There also were indications that CERT may have more beneficial effects on comorbid anxiety disorders than comorbid oppositional defiant disorder. However, given its limitations (e.g., lack of a control group), an open trial cannot prove or disprove CERT's effectiveness. It is hoped that the publication of this book will facilitate the conduct of larger-scale randomized treatment trials of CERT addressing various forms of depression in younger children.

Chapter 2

Emotion Regulation and Mood Repair

What the Research Shows

This chapter focuses on research findings that support the basic tenets of contextual emotion regulation therapy (CERT) and its approach to the self-regulation of sadness and dysphoria. The topics include the normative development of emotion regulation and mood repair responses and some skills that underpin them, the processes that appear to account for how mood repair works (potential mechanisms), and ways in which mood repair goes awry in depressed youngsters. To conclude, I address the practical implications of the research literature.

Some Basic Definitions

The words *emotion*, *feeling*, and *mood* that repeatedly appear in this book are commonly used in everyday language, readily understood by most people, and refer to familiar human experiences. However, one is hard-pressed to find definitions of these terms, or of the word *affect*, that are universally accepted by scientists. A similar problem characterizes the term *emotion regulation*, which also appears repeatedly in this book. So, let me begin by defining these terms as used in this book.

Emotion, Feeling, Mood, and Affect

Experts agree that the ability to experience and appropriately display a wide range of emotions is an integral component of human development and social adjustment (see, e.g., Eisenberg & Morris, 2002). But the word *emotion* has been defined in various ways and from significantly different conceptual perspectives (e.g., Campos et al., 1994; Ekman, 1992; Izard & Ackerman, 2000; Sroufe, 1995). The definition favored in this book is that an *emotion* is a reaction with physiological and psychological (experiential or subjective) components, which represents an individual's response to a valenced stimulus and signals some action tendency toward a goal (e.g., Cicchetti et al., 1995; Ekman, 1992; Gross, 1999; Thompson, 1994).

The subjective component of emotion is generally called a *feeling:* It is the inner experience conveyed by statements such as "I am feeling happy" or "I am feeling sad." Thus, for example, seeing a bear about to attack will elicit the emotion of fear, which entails the subjective experience of feeling afraid, as well as increased heart rate and rapid breathing (strong physiological arousal), along with running away from the bear (action tendency).

Scholars distinguish emotion from *mood* based on duration (and sometimes intensity), time course, and the presence of a specific cause or object of reference. It is generally believed that emotions are brief and fleeting, while moods are longer-lasting, persistent, and "nagging"; that emotions are typically elicited by specific triggers, while moods appear to sneak up, often without warning; that emotions usually are associated with distinct behavioral goals, while moods have nonspecific and pervasive effects; and that emotions are presumably more intense than moods (e.g., Larsen, 2000; Morris & Reilly, 1987; Rottenberg & Gross, 2007). In brief, emotions presumably are "about something in particular," with a clear cause and/or a specific target, whereas moods lack causal specificity and focus (Berkowitz & Harmon-Jones, 2004).

However, the just noted distinctions are not universally accepted (e.g., Berkowitz & Harmon-Jones, 2004; Morris, 2000). For example, one is hard-pressed to find agreed on rules as to how long an emotion can last before it is called a mood—does it have to last 1 minute, 5 minutes, 30 minutes, an hour, longer than an hour? Furthermore, emotions, but not moods, are supposed to have causes, although people often can identify why they are in a bad mood. In this book, therefore, the words emotion and mood are used interchangeably with the understanding that emotions do not last as long as moods.

The word *affect* also is used repeatedly in this book as a super-ordinate category label or umbrella term, which includes both emotion and mood, without regard to causal or temporal characteristics (Hemenover et al., 2008; Rottenberg & Gross, 2007). Gross (2014) has proposed a similar definition, also noting that past definitions of affect have been wide-ranging (e.g., Carver & Scheier, 1990; Larsen, 2000; Westen, 1994).

Emotion Regulation

The overall process whereby individuals respond to and manage their emotions is usually called *emotion regulation* (ER), although the terms *mood regulation* or *affect regulation* also have been used (e.g., Larsen, 2000). Emotion regulation is critical to adaptive human functioning and a key developmental achievement (Eisenberg & Morris, 2002; Thompson, 1994).

Emotion regulation is a key component of self-regulation (Cole et al., 2019), and competent self-regulation in childhood predicts good academic achievement, successful social behavior, aspects of mental health, and healthy living later in life (for a meta-analytic review, see Robson et al., 2020). Adaptive emotion regulation in early childhood is specifically associated with school readiness (reviewed by Harrington et al., 2020) and predicts better social and academic functioning in elementary school (e.g., Eisenberg, Fabes, et al., 1995, 2000; Graziano et al., 2007).

Emotion regulation is learned and practiced in a social context. And every culture that has been studied has rules as to what is (and what is not) normative emotion experience and display (e.g., Eisenberg & Morris, 2002; Izard & Ackerman, 2000; Trommsdorff & Cole, 2011). Notably, as early as the first 3 months of life, there are culture-specific pathways whereby mothers shape aspects of their infants' emotion regulation skills (Lavelli et al., 2019). Cross-cultural differences have also been documented in regulatory response use later in life (e.g., Joshanloo & Weijers, 2014; Matsumoto et al., 2008). And across various cultures, the greatest emphasis typically is on the regulation of negative emotions (Barrett et al., 2001).

As used in this book, the term *emotion regulation* refers to the processes that alter the strength and duration of an already activated emotion by magnifying or prolonging it, or conversely, by decreasing and attenuating it. This definition separates the emotion generation phase (elicitation of an emotion) from the subsequent regulatory phase and is similar (although not identical) to the one proposed by Cole et al. (2004).

Most scholars believe that the regulatory process impacts all the components of an emotion, namely its experiential-subjective, behavioral-expressive, and physiological aspects (e.g., Gross, 2014). In CERT, the goal is to help the depressed child feel better and less dysphoric; thus, the primary emphasis is on *regulating the experiential component of sadness, dysphoria, and distress.* Depending on the child's clinical state, however, the behavioral-expressive dimension of emotion also may be targeted.

Here are several snapshots of children and adults in various contexts in everyday life as they engage in emotion regulation. Note the differences in what triggered the affective reaction, the regulatory responses, and the regulatory outcomes:

- A mother asks her young son to put away his toys in preparation for sitting down for family dinner, which he is reluctant to do. The boy wants to keep playing and becomes tearful when his mother takes the toys. When he fails to get her to return the toys, he works himself up into a full tantrum, making his father angry, which, in turn, exacerbates the boy's distress.

- At school, an adolescent girl learns that she has won a coveted scholarship. While she is overjoyed, she tries to contain her sense of pleasure and downplays its overt expression, knowing that several of her friends sitting close by did not win.

- A man returns a piece of high-priced but faulty merchandise to an electronics store. The salesperson is not very helpful and is, in fact, somewhat rude: The buyer becomes increasingly annoyed and then angry and finally asks to speak to a manager, who resolves the issue.

- Several young teenagers have been glued to the internet seeking information about the recent tragic death of an idol. As they consider the incoming news and keep discussing the event, they become increasingly downcast and several of them start to cry.

- A young boy steps outside the house and sees a mouse. He has always been terrified of them. He starts shaking, lets out a sharp yell, and then passes out.

- A father becomes very angry when he finds out that his teenage son took the family car for a drive without permission and had an accident. Before continuing the conversation, the father decides to step outside the home for about 15 minutes and vigorously walk around to calm himself.

- A young girl has become increasingly sad since her parents announced their decision to divorce. Whenever she sees a peer with both parents in tow, she becomes tearful and keeps telling herself that if her parents really loved her, they wouldn't be divorcing; she then feels worse than before and wants to hide.

- An elderly man lost his wife more than a year ago. But he is continuously enveloped by his sadness: He has not yet removed her clothes from their bedroom, spends hours looking at her picture, is no longer interested in socializing with his neighbors, repeatedly envisions his wife's face, and remains profoundly dejected.

- A girl finds out that her boyfriend is planning to break up with her. She is upset and sad, and finds it difficult to stop crying. She decides to text her two best friends to ask them to come over to help her feel better.

- A young boy is upset because his schoolmates do not want to include him in their games. When this happens several times, he becomes increasingly sad, which is noticed by his father. Having figured out the reason for the boy's sadness, the father decides to set up a basketball hoop near their garage and encourages the child to practice, rather than worry about the other kids.

As these examples illustrate, a wide range of behaviors can function as responses to one's own emotions; some responses are seemingly automatic, while others are deliberate and planned; and both positive and negative emotions trigger regulatory responses. If we envision these scenarios continuing to unfold, it is clear that some responses are likely to result in the *perpetuation, up-regulation,* or *intensification* of the given affect, whereas other responses are likely to lead to the *down-regulation, attenuation,* or *termination* of the triggering affect. It could be argued that some of the vignettes exemplify *emotion* regulation (e.g., the mouse vignette), while others mirror *mood* regulation (loss of the idol and boyfriend examples). However, paralleling the fact that no clear demarcation exists between emotion and mood, there is no body of evidence that human beings rely on different regulatory responses to manage a specific emotion and its mood counterpart.

Mood Repair

As the previous snapshots illustrate, the phrase *emotion regulation* refers to regulating any emotion in ways that can result in maintaining, attenuating, or strengthening the given emotion. In contrast, the phrase *mood repair* (Isen, 1985; Josephson et al., 1996) or *negative mood repair* (Parrott, 1993) refers specifically and narrowly to attenuating sadness or dysphoria. The term implies that when a person feels sad, dysphoric, or is in a bad mood, there is a natural inclination to behave in ways that will result in feeling better (e.g., Morris & Reilly, 1987). Thus, mood repair involves a subset of the processes and responses that comprise emotion regulation.

Some scholars believe that the goal of mood repair is not merely to attenuate sadness but also to increase happiness (e.g., for a discussion, see Parrott, 1993). The stance taken in this book is simpler: It is assumed that feeling sad or dysphoric generally is unpleasant (both psychologically and physiologically) and therefore the individual is motivated to return to an earlier, more homeostatic affective state. Such a homeostatic perspective on the regulatory process has been proposed in the past (e.g., Bonanno, 2001; Larsen, 2000) and does not presuppose that the prior mood state was one of happiness.

While the use of CERT assumes that depressed children and youth want to repair their dysphoric mood, it has been argued that in some contexts (e.g., at the funeral of a friend), a person may want to maintain or intensify feelings of sadness and dysphoria (Aldao, 2013; Erber & Erber, 2000; Parrott, 1993; Tamir, 2009, 2016). However, depressed children do not want to stay depressed and families of depressed children seek treatment to reduce and ameliorate the offspring's dysfunctional mood, not to increase it. This is why, in CERT, the goal is clearly and unambiguously defined as teaching skills and responses that allow the young depressed patient to attenuate or down-regulate sadness, dysphoria, and distress.

Mood Repair Responses

To repeat, the term *mood repair* means specifically that the affect being regulated is sadness, dysphoria, or distress and that the goal is to attenuate, reduce, or shorten that affect experience. It is important to note that attenuating dysphoria does *not* mean suppressing or denying it. Rather, adaptive regulation of dysphoria means that the child is not disabled or incapacitated by the mood and is able to function as required.

What sort of responses attenuate sadness and dysphoria? Classical surveys with adults have identified 200–300 self-regulatory responses (Parkinson & Totterdell,

1999; Rippere, 1977; Thayer et al., 1994). However, there probably are even more than that because, as Koole (2009) noted, any activity that can alter a person's emotion can potentially be recruited to serve regulatory goals. Therefore, one challenge has been how to organize or classify regulatory responses. Although various multidimensional organizational schemas have been proposed (e.g., Braunstein et al., 2017; Tamir, 2016), there has been scant recent discussion about the key dimensions on which emotion regulatory responses should be defined.

There is no doubt that one important dimension is the emotional outcome of the response for the person who is regulating. Did the response help the person feel better? In a study of adults on the interpersonal regulation of affect, this dimension was defined as "affect improving versus affect worsening" (Niven et al., 2009), while in a study of 10- to 13-year-olds (Reijntjes et al., 2007), emotional outcome was defined in terms of "mood enhancement." Another plausible dimension is some characteristic of the responses themselves. Koole (2009), for example, distinguished between automatic and deliberate responses, which subsequently has been labeled implicit versus explicit regulation (e.g., Koole et al., 2015). Other response dimensions include engagement versus disengagement with the target emotion (Larsen, 2000; Niven et al., 2009; Parkinson & Totterdell, 1999; Reijntjes et al., 2007), active versus passive mood management (Thayer et al., 1994), and seeking to change the person who is experiencing the mood versus seeking to change the situation (Larsen, 2000). Investigators also have distinguished between behavioral and cognitive mood repair responses (Larsen, 2000; Niven et al., 2009; Parkinson & Totterdell, 1999; Reijntjes et al., 2007; Thayer et al., 1994).

In CERT, mood repair responses are defined and organized along three dimensions: **outcome**, namely adaptive responses that attenuate versus maladaptive responses that maintain or exacerbate dysphoria; **process**, namely conscious versus automatic responses; and the **domain of functioning** through which the response is instantiated, namely whether it is a behavioral, cognitive, or interpersonal response.

The Outcome: Adaptive versus Maladaptive

The notion that adaptive regulation is one that helps to diminish negative affect, whereas maladaptive regulation maintains or increases it, can be traced back to research with toddlers. Specifically, an important early developmental achievement is the ability to contain negative emotions such as distress, anger, and frustration. Thus, responses that help children to lower the intensity of the negative affect (or bring it to a manageable level) have been labeled as appropriate, constructive, desirable, or adaptive (Calkins et al., 1999; Calkins & Johnson, 1998; Silk et al., 2003). Likewise, in CERT, attempts that diminish, lessen, attenuate, or terminate sadness and dysphoria are defined as *adaptive mood repair responses,* but only if the responses are functionally helpful both in the short and long run.

Adaptive mood repair responses include self-soothing, reaching out to a caregiver for emotional relief, refocusing attention away from one's dysphoria, engaging in problem solving, or getting involved in physical activity, among others. Mood repair responses that attenuate sadness in the short run but are dysfunctional in the long run are not considered to be adaptive. For example, binge eating, which has been documented even among 8- to 13-year-olds (Czaja et al., 2009), can help some youth to feel better but is certainly not an adaptive way to repair mood in the long run (e.g., Whiteside et al., 2007; for a review, see Leehr et al., 2015). As a further example, adolescent psychiatric inpatients report that deliberate self-harm without suicidal intent (e.g., burning or scratching oneself) leads to significant attenuation of dysphoric mood (Sim et al., 2009), a phenomenon that also has been reported among community dwelling adolescents (Robinson et al., 2021), but is clearly not functionally adaptive.

Studies of normally developing, very young children and adolescents also have described regulatory responses to distress that were not adaptive or were counter-effective because they maintained, prolonged, or exacerbated negative affect (Calkins et al., 1999; Silk et al., 2003). In CERT, these are called *maladaptive mood repair responses.* (The definition does not apply in the context of mourning or other significant loss, except if the mourning process is protracted.) Nonadaptive or counter-effective emotion regulation responses include physical "venting" such as aggression (e.g., banging, hitting, kicking), behavioral passivity, social withdrawal or avoidance, and in older children rumination, self-disparagement, and expressive suppression (Calkins & Johnson, 1998; Calkins et al., 1999; Cracco et al., 2017; Czaja et al., 2009; Schafer et al., 2017).

There has been growing acceptance in the field that emotion regulation attempts can be regarded as adaptive versus maladaptive (e.g., Aldao et al., 2010; Cracco et al., 2017; Schafer et al., 2017). Acceptance of this classification dimension can be traced to the meta-analysis of Aldao and colleagues (2010), subsequently replicated by others (e.g., Schafer et al., 2017), which found that regulatory responses labeled maladaptive (e.g., rumination) are associated with high levels of psychopathology, while responses labeled adaptive (e.g., cognitive reappraisal, problem solving) are generally associated with low levels of psychopathology.

The Process: Automatic versus Deliberate

Whether a response is automatic versus deliberate is another important feature of mood repair (e.g., Davidson et al., 2000). *Automatic responses* can be conscious or nonconscious, whereas *deliberate responses,* also called *volitional* or *planned responses,* are fully conscious; this distinction also has been labeled as *explicit versus implicit emotion regulation* (e.g., Koole et al., 2015). A basic tenet of CERT is that mood repair responses typically are automatic and are deployed without deliberation, and that adaptive responses that are deliberate are most likely to be deployed if the initial, automatic "default" response failed to lessen the person's dysphoric mood. However, as Mauss et al. (2007) have noted, research has focused on deliberate, volitional, and conscious forms of affect regulation and has paid scant attention to regulation that occurs automatically or without deliberation.

From a developmental perspective, several factors underscore that the initial emotion regulatory responses of an individual to a depressogenic trigger are likely to be automatic. It is evident that very early in life, regulatory responding is neither planned nor deliberate. As discussed in detail later in this chapter, several mood repair responses originate as reflexive actions (e.g., gaze aversion, self-soothing). Such responses probably are maintained via operant conditioning and continue to be deployed without deliberation in their original versions, and then in some developmentally more suitable form as children become older. Other responses that children learn during the first several years of life by modeling or being taught such responses by their parents are likely to become automatic as a function of practice and experience (Davidson et al., 2000).

Research on older age groups also supports the automaticity of some emotion regulatory responses. One study of youth's emotions in daily life found that "involuntary" or automatic regulatory strategies (that could be conscious or not) were a regular component of emotional responding: Importantly, involuntary responses (such as ruminating or acting impulsively) had the most marked adverse effects on negative mood (Silk et al., 2003). In studies with college students, experimentally induced distress set into motion an adaptive regulatory process that was both automatic and nonconscious (DeWall et al., 2011).

Studies of various areas of human behavior have documented the automaticity of many forms of higher-level goal pursuits in daily life (Bargh & Chartrand, 1999). For example, there is compelling evidence that many evaluations of one's environment are automatic (i.e., rapid and with a lack of intention) and that even when one is aware of some stimulus, behavior responses can be without awareness (for a brief review, see Ferguson & Zayas, 2009). Research on various information processing, attitude formation, behavioral preferences, or biases likewise found that human beings can display response tendencies totally without awareness (e.g., Murray, 2007; Stein & Peelen, 2021; Sweldens et al., 2014).

If responses to one's own dysphoria can occur automatically, does that mean that children or adults are unable to report on them or alter them? Not at all. Given some rudimentary ability to self-reflect, children as well as adults often can report on their automatic regulatory responses when asked to do so. This is similar to the situation of a practiced driver of a car with standard transmission who changes gears automatically and without reflection. But if prompted to do so, this very same driver can describe the actions that he deployed while shifting gears.

The Substance: Three Functional Regulatory Domains

Mood repair responses also can be organized according to the domains of functioning that are being primarily utilized. If one examines the developmental literature, it becomes evident that the responses to distress that emerge in rapid succession from about the age of 6–8 months mirror four areas of functioning: the somatic-sensory, cognitive, social–interpersonal, and behavioral domains (Kovacs et al., 2008). Chronologically, the earliest somatic-sensory response is self-soothing, the earliest cognitive response is gaze aversion (attention refocusing), the earliest interpersonal response is caregiver-directed distress vocalization, and the earliest behavioral response is leaving the scene.

When we pilot-tested CERT and discussed with families the four domains of functioning, which can be used in the service of mood repair, we found that it was often challenging for them to distinguish somatic-sensory and behavioral responses; this was understandable because the former always involves some type of behavior or action. To make it easier for parents and children to implement CERT, we therefore conceptually merged the somatic-sensory and the behavioral response domains into one category, resulting in a threefold grouping. The following grouping reflects the substance of mood repair responses:

- The *behavioral response domain* includes responses that reflect action-oriented and instrumental behaviors, and self-focused, body- and sensory-oriented behaviors not involving others.
- The *cognitive response domain* includes responses that primarily rely on attention refocusing, thinking, information processing, and visual imagery.
- The *social–interpersonal response domain* includes responses that rely on social and interpersonal processes involving other people to alter one's own affect experience.

This threefold grouping is a heuristic, which helps children, parents, and the therapist to communicate about regulatory responses and to identify the child's preferred approach(es) to mood repair. However, it should be clear that the three domains of regulatory responding overlap and have "fuzzy" boundaries. For example, if a child attempts to reduce her sadness by playing with her dollhouse, which refocuses her attention away from the dysphoric affect, the behavioral response (playing with the dollhouse) crosses boundaries with the cognitive response (attention refocusing). Later in this book, I give examples of how to decide which regulatory domain is more important whenever a response involves multiple domains or has fuzzy boundaries.

Developmental Aspects of Emotion Regulation and Mood Repair

Emotion regulation unfolds in a social context, as I describe in the section that follows. Then I summarize general age-related trends in emotion regulation and various basic skills that undergird the regulatory process. I follow with an overview of the development of mood repair responses in the behavioral, cognitive, and interpersonal regulatory domains. I conclude this discussion with notes on some personal traits that affect regulatory success.

The Role of Social Context

The unfolding of emotion regulation skills takes place in the child's social context, which includes the immediate and extended family, the family's wider social network, and the larger community. The various social contexts themselves change over time along with the participants who populate them.

It has long been recognized that the child's immediate familial environment is *the* crucible in which emotion regulation unfolds: This process starts around the age of 3–6 months and parents or primary caregivers have central roles (e.g., Calkins, 1994; Hofer, 1994; Kopp, 1989; Thompson, 1994). While parental input into the emotion regulation of offspring continues throughout adolescence (e.g., Waller et al., 2014; for a brief review, see Morris et al., 2017), as children transition into their teens, extrafamilial social contexts are believed to play increasing roles in shaping regulatory responses.

As proposed by Morris et al. (2007, 2017), family context impacts on children's developing regulatory competence in several ways. It provides opportunities for the child to learn and emulate regulatory responses by observing emotion-related behaviors and interactions: This is called *modeling*. Parenting practices related to emotions, such as so-called emotion coaching, shape the child's developing emotion regulation repertoire on several fronts. For example, a mother who has good emotion coaching skills may respond to her child's sadness by accepting (rather than ignoring or rejecting) it and simultaneously engage in emotion naming ("Yes—it's OK to be sad—you are sad because your puppy is very sick") and also suggest a way to feel better ("Let's go and organize all Rusty's toys while we wait for the medicine to work"). And finally, the emotional climate of the family, which includes maternal and paternal parenting styles (e.g., being harsh and punitive vs. supportive), also shapes children's emerging regulatory repertoire. For example, a parent who is responsive to and supportive of the offspring's emotions creates a favorable environment for the unfolding of social/interpersonal mood repair responses. However, a meta-analysis of studies of parenting styles (e.g., positive control) of preschoolers and categories of self-regulation failed to find such a relationship between them (Karreman et al., 2006).

As part of the family context, sibling relationships are also believed to be important crucibles for developing emotion relevant skills: For example, older siblings may model or teach emotion identification and empathy and ways to regulate emotions (Kramer, 2014). In one of our studies of 11- to 19-year-olds, self-reports of youngsters and their siblings regarding cognitive and behavioral adaptive mood repair response repertoires were significantly correlated (Bylsma et al., 2016). However, given the scant information in this area, the roles of siblings are not yet well understood in children's emotion regulation development (briefly reviewed by Barthel et al., 2018).

In social contexts other than the family, friendships are likely to contribute to a child's unfolding emotion regulation competence (e.g., Barthel et al., 2018). Although it is not yet known at what age peers start to have enduring effects, studies of friendship dyads found that among sixth-graders, or around age 13, friends clearly influence each other's use of some emotion regulation responses (Reindl et al., 2016; von Salisch & Zeman, 2018). And peer influence can be dysfunctional, as evidenced by co-rumination among friends in their mid-adolescence (Waller et al., 2014).

Children's wider social contexts, such as schools and neighborhoods, also have ramifications for the development of emotion regulation and mood repair. For example, preschool teachers' emotion coaching and regulatory behavior facilitate emotion regulation competence among 4- to 6-year-olds (Silkenbeumer et al., 2018). On the other hand, exposure to neighborhood violence has adverse effects on children's and adolescents' regulation of sadness and anger (Criss et al., 2016). While the wider social milieu thus can affect emotion regulation competence, the mechanisms are not yet understood.

General Age-Related Trends in Regulatory Responding

Age-related changes that have been documented include the manner in which a response is initiated, the level of sophistication of a response, the size of the response repertoire, and response effectiveness (for a brief overview, see Ratcliff et al., 2021). One of the most dramatic developmental changes in emotion regulatory responding that occurs during the first decade of life involves the initiation of the response: There is a shift from extrinsic to mostly intrinsic modes of regulation, or from reactive responding to voluntary or effortful control (Eisenberg & Morris, 2002; Fox & Calkins, 2003). This developmental shift occurs around ages 3–4 in Western societies. In other words, while emotion regulation among infants and very young children typically is reflexive or guided by caregivers, the regulatory responses of older children become increasingly planful and self-initiated.

A more gradual developmental shift is the progression from rudimentary to increasingly sophisticated regulatory responses. For example, as noted in Kopp's (1989) classic article, up to the preschool years, children's emotion self-regulation mostly involves simple approaches including responses that help to regulate sensory intake, leaving the distressing scene, or engaging in reassuring self-talk. But just prior to or around the start of elementary school, children begin to deploy more complex responses such as strategically shifting attention away from an upsetting stimulus, systematically engaging the help of another person for distress relief, or thinking differently about the cause of distress to minimize its importance. The progression toward increasingly sophisticated regulatory responses is believed to continue across adolescence (Bariola et al., 2011).

Development is also believed to involve a growing repertoire of regulatory responses (e.g., Thompson, 1991), which then enables children to tailor their reactions to the context of the emotion (Davis et al., 2010; Garber et al., 1995). While the rapid expansion of regulatory repertoires is evident during early childhood, it is not clear if this expansion continues in a linear fashion or for how long. Furthermore, different pictures emerge when children report about their own responses, when parents report on their offspring, and when children's responses are experimentally elicited. For example, contrary to expectations, in one of our studies of 7- to 14-year-olds, younger children reported larger adaptive regulatory response repertoires than older children (Kovacs et al., 2019). Another study of respondents from 11 years to adulthood likewise found that younger respondents reported larger regulatory repertoires than older ones, but this trend eventually reversed (Zimmerman & Iwanski, 2014). However, parental reports of their children's adaptive mood repair response repertoires showed no age-related trends (Kovacs et al., 2019).

Experimental studies of age and response use have failed to clarify the relations of development and response repertoire size. In a study of how 3- and 4-year-olds reduce distress, older children deployed fewer emotion regulation responses than younger children (Stansbury & Sigman, 2000). However, using a story completion task with 3- to 6-year-olds, older children endorsed a greater number of responses than younger children (Sala et al., 2014). On the other hand, among 10- to 23-year-olds, the number of reappraisal strategies used to decrease the impact of negative visual stimuli was unrelated to age (Nook et al., 2020).

Possibly, the number of regulatory responses actually deployed in any mood repair effort is not a valid index of development. Indeed, 5- and 6-year-olds reportedly used only two regulatory responses per upsetting event, on average, with a maximum of five different responses per event (Davis et al., 2010). In a study of 12- to 17-year-olds that surveyed eight regulatory responses, respondents reported 1.2 strategies, on average: Almost 90% of the events elicited only a single regulatory strategy and less than 1% involved more than five strategies (Lennarz et al., 2019). But in another sample of 15- to 25-year-olds, a single regulatory response was reported only for 1.9% of the stimulus events and 70% of the events were associated with five or more regulatory responses (Hiekkaranta et al., 2021).

Emotion regulation is also believed to become more effective with age as regulatory systems undergo reorganization and responses become more sophisticated (Steinberg, 2005). Indeed, evidence exists that younger children are not as good at mood repair as older ones. For example, 6-year-old children are more likely than 9-year-olds (Waters & Thompson, 2014) and 8-year-olds are more likely than 10-year-olds to select ineffective (maladaptive) ways to repair sadness such as venting (López-Pérez & Pacella, 2021). And 13-year-olds use reappraisal less effectively than 15-year-olds, although this was not the case for distraction (Theurel & Gentaz, 2018).

However, it is unclear whether regulatory effectiveness continues to improve up to about age 16 and then plateaus (Silvers et al., 2012) *or* if mid-adolescence signals a maladaptive shift in mood repair (for a review, see Schweizer et al., 2020). For example, among 8- to 18-year-olds, those ages 12–15 were less likely to deploy adaptive responses and more likely to deploy maladaptive regulatory responses than the younger and older subjects (Cracco et al., 2017). A study of 11- to 50-year-olds likewise found that mid-adolescence (ages 13–15) was associated with the smallest adaptive response repertoires in general, and the least adaptive responses to sadness in particular (Zimmermann & Iwanski, 2014). But a longitudinal study of a small sample of 13- to 14-year-olds reported continued positive change in emotion regulation across a 4-year interval, subject to family context and social class (Herd et al., 2020). Overall, therefore, the relations of response effectiveness and age have yet to be clarified.

Basic Skills Supporting the Regulatory Process

In this section, I focus on the development of attention, executive function skills, language skills, and emotion knowledge as some of the presumed building blocks of the ability to manage one's own emotions. Much of the descriptive developmental research in these areas was carried out in the late 1990s and early 2000s. The major takeaways from the vast literature on these topics are that each of these skills has multiple components, that developmental trends may differ depending on the complexity of the task used to assess the skill, and that much of development is not linear, with the effects of age on the unfolding of skills being more pronounced prior to age 10 than at later ages (Best et al., 2009; Korkman, 2001; Korkman et al., 2013).

Let us consider *attention skills,* which include the ability to focus, switch attention, and resist distracters: Overall, these skills increase dramatically after the first year of life (Ruff & Lawson, 1990), show significant gains around ages 5–8, level off between ages 9–12, and then may exhibit a further "spurt" around age 15 (Klenberg et al., 2001; Korkman et al., 2001; Manly et al., 2001).

However, visual and auditory attention follow different trajectories. Auditory attention matures quite early, with impressive gains by age 7, whereas visual attention continues to develop into early adolescence and possibly even later (for a review, see Hendry et al., 2019; Korkman et al., 2001). According to developmental neuroimaging work, the brain regions subserving visual attention are quite mature by age 12 (Booth et al., 2003), which suggests that performance improvements across subsequent years are a function of learning and practice. But visual attention itself, which has been studied the most extensively (Amso & Scerif, 2015; Hendry et al., 2019), includes separable attention systems (e.g., Petersen & Posner, 2012), and those systems have independent developmental trajectories.

For example, according to a longitudinal study of 6- to 11-year-olds (Lewis et al., 2018), the "alerting" attention system, which is involved in maintaining vigilance, continues to improve between the ages of 6 and 11; the "orienting" attention network, which is involved in focusing on sensory input, is already developed by age 6; while the executive attention network, which is mobilized while focusing on and pursuing a task, seems well developed by age 7. Other work suggests continued development during adolescence with a possible asymptote around age 16 (Kramer et al., 2005).

Executive function skills concern the use of mental processes to plan and carry out goal-directed behavior (e.g., Hsu et al., 2014). Although there are varying perspectives on the best way to conceptualize executive function development (e.g., Best & Miller, 2010; Perone et al., 2021), and this skill appears to be undifferentiated in very young children (e.g., Visu-Petra et al., 2012), it is generally believed to include the ability to inhibit or suppress undesirable responses (e.g., resist temptation), update working memory, and shift attention or task, each of which develops at different rates (for reviews, see Best & Miller, 2010; Diamond, 2013; Zelazo & Carlson, 2020).

As Best and colleagues (2009) noted, the ability to inhibit unwanted responses shows striking gains during preschool, further significant improvements between ages 5 and 8, and little additional improvement during adolescence and later; however, some forms of inhibition level off by age 12 (Zamora et al., 2020). Developmental trends in working memory differ as a function of the complexity of the task used to assess it: Performance increases linearly until about age 16 or 17 on difficult tasks, while remembering visual patterns (a simple task) levels off by around age 11 (Best et al., 2009). Switching or shifting between mental sets or tasks can be accomplished by 3- and 4-year-olds if only one switch is involved; for more complex tasks, performance improves until early adolescence (Best et al., 2009). The ongoing development of various executive function skills as late as age 17 or older is not surprising since they have been linked to the prefrontal cortex, the late-maturing part of the brain (for a review, see Bahmani et al., 2019). Indeed, there is increasing evidence of relationships between the development of executive functions and changes in brain structure and resting state neural connectivity (e.g., Shanmugan & Satterthwaite, 2016).

The gradual development of other higher-order cognitive skills, including operations implicated in problem solving (e.g., if–then reasoning, reasoning by analogy) as well as metacognition, has been extensively documented (for selective overviews, see Kuhn, 2000; Muijs & Bokhove, 2020). It is notable that a study of children from grade 3 to adolescence found that early executive function skills predicted analogical reasoning development across the follow-up years (Richland & Burchinal, 2013). There is some disagreement as to whether metacognition in general or some of its components are accessible to children younger than 6 or mostly after children reach age 8, and whether development involves quantitative or qualitative changes (Muijs & Bokhove, 2020). But the adolescent years are uniformly believed to herald marked improvements in deductive reasoning, efficient problem solving and planning, and social reasoning (Steinberg, 2005).

Language development, the neural basis of which is beginning to be understood (Olulade et al., 2020), is another crucial building block of emotion regulation. As with the other traits just discussed, language development is a multicomponent process and includes expressive and receptive language and fluency (e.g., Kuhl, 2000), as well as language modalities such as semantics and syntax (Luinge et al., 2006). As evidence of early linguistic development, 9-month-old infants already show a marked preference for patterns of their native language (Kuhl, 2000). By around age 2, there is a rapid expansion of vocabulary, language comprehension, and related language skills (Courage & Howe, 2002) that are essential for various emotion regulation responses, and by age 6, children are sufficiently fluent to tell stories, use the correct word order in language production, and understand tasks that involve multiword sentences (Luinge et al., 2006). Aspects of verbal and semantic fluency continue to develop during adolescence (Klenberg et al., 2001; Korkman et al., 2001).

According to a classical perspective on language acquisition (Vygotsky, 1962), a language development phase of great importance is the transition from language used only as a social signal to others (generally prior to age 3) to its use as a means of self-regulation. The transition is bridged by the advent of "private speech" (Vygotsky, 1962; Winsler & Naglieri, 2003). Private speech is overt vocalization directed to the self as opposed to others and, in childhood, it serves to self-guide and self-regulate behavior (Alderson-Day & Fernyhough, 2015). It emerges between ages 2–5, has its own developmental trajectory, and culminates in covert verbal thinking (e.g., Alderson-Day & Fernyhough, 2015; Frauenglass & Diaz, 1985; Kronk, 1994; Vygotsky, 1962; Winsler & Naglieri, 2003; Winsler et al., 2000). Although private speech or overt verbal thinking (also called verbal problem solving) is believed to "go underground" around age 5, some reports suggest that it may continue even in adulthood (Alderson-Day & Fernyhough, 2015). Because many of the ways in which youngsters manage their own affect involve overt verbal thinking, it is not surprising that 6- to 13-year-olds with language impairment (particularly boys) have more difficulties regulating negative emotion than typically developing peers (Fujiki et al., 2002).

While language as overt verbal thinking can facilitate general self-regulation early on, with development language can serve as a specific emotion regulation tool by establishing psychological distance (e.g., Orvell et al., 2019). For example, shifting from "I" to using one's name or the third-person singular provides a more distant perspective when relating an emotion experience or personal narrative. Among typically developing 4- and 6-year-olds, self-distancing via the use of the third-person singular helped to reduce experimentally induced frustration (Grenell et al., 2019). According to Nook et al. (2020), by late childhood (around age 10), linguistic distancing seems to be used spontaneously to facilitate affect regulation and stronger distancing predicted better regulation in the sample of 10- to 23-year-olds. Self-distancing by shifting from "I" to "we" pronouns also predicted better affective outcome among college students (Seah et al., 2021).

Finally, *knowledge and understanding of emotions* also are believed to be foundational to the unfolding of regulatory competence. Early work in this area sought to characterize the components of emotion knowledge and their developmental trajectories, which include the evolution of emotion naming and self-referent skills such as knowing what you are feeling (e.g., Barrett et al., 2001; Stegge & Terwogt, 2007). The components of emotion knowledge emerge sequentially (e.g., Pons et al., 2004). As a general trend, children initially understand emotions in terms of external causes and observable expression (by around age 5), which segues into a more mentalistic understanding (by about age 7), leading to an appreciation (by around age 11) of the interface of cognition and emotion and the existence of mixed emotional states (Pons et al., 2004). On the other hand, it also has been reported that even 3- and 4-year-olds (Dennis & Kelemen, 2009) as well as 5- to 6-year-olds (Davis et al., 2010) appear to understand that emotions have inner experiential components, that negative emotions can be changed or regulated, and that strategies for changing emotions can be mentalistic or cognitive.

Importantly, there are impressive individual differences in emotion knowledge at every age: For example, the level of emotion understanding of some 4- to 5-year-olds has been found to rival that of some 10- to 11-year-olds (Pons et al., 2003). The wide range of individual differences could reflect variable language skills as well as the impact of families' emotional expressiveness and family discussions about emotions (Ogren & Johnson, 2020; Pons et al., 2003).

To what extent is the successful regulation of dysphoria dependent on the child's emotion knowledge? The relation of competent mood repair and emotion knowledge has been explored among 4- to 7-year-olds with equivocal results: Although the two constructs are related, it is unclear if regulatory responding facilitates the acquisition of emotion knowledge, or if emotion knowledge has to precede regulatory responding (DiMaggio et al., 2016; Lucas-Molina et al., 2020). Furthermore, in a study of 8- to 10-year-olds, accurate knowledge and recognition of sadness did not play a role in its adaptive regulation (López-Pérez & Pacella, 2021), whereas among 8- to 15-year-olds, low emotional awareness had unfavorable effects on the use of adaptive regulatory strategies (Van Beveren, Goossens, et al., 2019). Therefore, more research is needed to clarify the relation of emotion knowledge and successful affect regulation.

Unfolding of Responses in the Three Mood Repair Domains

The literature on the unfolding of normative emotion regulation is dominated by short-term follow-up studies and cross-sectional studies targeting mostly infants, toddlers, and young children. That body of work reveals that there is a rapid emergence of regulatory responses during the first 2–3 years of life: Some responses debut as reflexive acts (e.g., self-soothing), others as operants (e.g., gaze aversion), while still others mirror social learning (e.g., recruiting caregivers). However, after the early years of childhood, the developmental trajectories of regulatory responses can only be inferred from cross-sectional studies conducted with various (often discontinuous) age groups: Such literature suggests that with age, some regulatory responses become less evident (e.g., self-soothing), some responses take increasingly sophisticated forms (e.g., attention deployment), while some responses emerge only in late childhood (e.g., cognitive reappraisal).

Behavioral Response Domain

Recall that the *behavioral response domain* includes two groups of responses: ways to feel better that involve somatic-sensory modalities, and instrumental or goal-directed responses.

Physical self-soothing or self-comforting is the developmentally earliest somatic-sensory behavioral regulatory response to distress. It has been extensively documented in infants, toddlers, and 2-year-olds: Adaptive forms include sucking of the toes, fingers, and other body parts, fingering parts of the body, hair twisting, and rocking, and maladaptive forms include high-intensity motor behaviors (Calkins et al., 1999; Ekas et al., 2013; Grolnick et al., 1996; Jean et al., 2014; Manian & Bornstein, 2009; Ratcliff et al., 2021; Stifter & Braungart, 1995; for a succinct overview of early work, see Stansbury & Sigman, 2000).

In a rare follow-up study involving 2-year-olds, assessed at yearly lab visits until age 5, self-soothing to overcome frustration and distress declined in frequency (but not in average duration); although it was still evident at age 5, it was used less often than other regulatory responses that were monitored (Ratcliff et al., 2021). However, there is scant information about self-soothing for mood repair in middle childhood and later. Furthermore, it appears that somatic-sensory responses take different forms (undergo transformations) across development, while new ones emerge with age. For example, anecdotal accounts indicate that taking a relaxing bath or being exposed to certain scents can counter dysphoric affect. Ratcliff et al. (2021) likewise proposed that self-soothing is likely to take "different forms" after age 5 and mention the breathing component of mindfulness training. (Receiving affectionate touch and caress also exemplifies a somatic-sensory route to mood repair; I discuss it in the section on social–interpersonal emotion regulation that follows.)

Engaging in vigorous physical and sports activities also takes advantage of the somatic-sensory route to mood repair: Indeed, there is no question that physical activity can attenuate momentary negative affect (for an overview of the neuroscience of exercise, see Portugal et al., 2013). The salubrious effects of physical activity on dysphoric mood have been extensively documented, although mostly among adults (for reviews, see Chan et al., 2019; Shafir, 2015); physical exercise is one of the three most effective ways to alter one's mood according to an early meta-analysis (Augustine & Hemenover, 2009). Importantly, a meta-analysis of the effects of physical activity on executive functions among 6- to 12-year-olds found that acute physical activity facilitated attention skills, while regular recurrent physical activity bolstered executive functions (de Greeff et al., 2017). (I discussed attention and executive functions in the section "Basic Skills Supporting the Regulatory Process," above.)

The unfolding of somatic-sensory regulatory responses also includes those that exacerbate rather than attenuate the distressed child's affect. Maladaptive somatic-sensory responses to dysphoria include binge eating (e.g., Czaja et al., 2009), the use of alcohol, drugs, and tobacco (e.g., Weiss et al., 2016; for a meta-analysis, see Weiss et al., 2022), and some forms of intentional self-harm. However, there is scant information about the developmental trajectories of such responses in typically developing children.

Instrumental and goal-directed behaviors constitute much of the behavior response domain. The developmentally earliest instrumental behavior appears among toddlers: When exposed to a distressing stimulus in the laboratory, they manage to feel better by crawling away from it ("leaving the scene") or by manipulating the environment (e.g., moving around furniture or toys; see Thompson, 1994, for further examples). However, a story completion task with young children revealed that only the 5- and 6-year-olds (but not the 3- to 4-year-olds) proposed purposefully engaging in some behavior to alter emotion experience (Sala et al., 2014). Younger as well as older children may attempt to recover from feeling sad and dysphoric through activities such as making art (e.g., Drake & Winner, 2013), the benefits of which were confirmed among older youth as well (Genuth & Drake, 2021).

Indeed, as early surveys in the field have long documented, any instrumental behavior, such as doing chores, starting a project, taking care of a pet, putting one's room in order, cooking, gardening, building model airplanes, dancing, singing, writing, or washing the car, can serve the goal of mood repair (e.g., Rippere, 1977, 1979). However, empirical information about behavioral mood repair responses across middle or later childhood and adolescence had been elusive possibly because most of these responses cannot be performed in the laboratory under controlled conditions. But newer approaches, such as surveying respondents about the experience and regulation of emotion during daily life, have been used with adolescents. Results reveal that engaging in some activity to keep busy was the second most frequent strategy to regulate negative affect among college students (Heiy & Cheavens, 2014). Trying to do something to modify a depressogenic *event* was the fourth most often reported response (from among seven) by 15- to 25-year-old respondents, including the 15- to 18-year-old subset (Hiekkaranta et al., 2021).

Maladaptive behavioral responses to distress are most evident in the younger years. For example, aggression was one of the primary responses of 1.9-year-olds to laboratory-induced frustration (Susa et al., 2014). When 4.5-year-old children faced negative emotions, aggression was the most common response and behavioral avoidance the least common response observed by teachers (Smith & Walden, 2001). The dysregulated responses of 8- to 12-year-olds to negative affect likewise included aggression, along with self-injury (Uhl et al., 2019). Behavioral passivity in response to a depressogenic stressor, which is another maladaptive response, was associated with worsening mood among 10- to 13-year-olds who were subjected to peer rejection (Reijntjes et al., 2006a, 2006b). However, maladaptive behavioral responses become less common with age. For example, among 12- to 17-year-olds, behavioral avoidance of a situation that caused distress was a low-frequency emotion regulation response and was used by fewer than 5% of the sample (Lennarz et al., 2019).

The Cognitive Response Domain

The *cognitive response domain* includes the use of attention and thinking (including visual imagery) as the path to decreasing dysphoria.

As far back as 1990, Morrow and Nolen-Hoeksema reported that depressed mood could be lifted by having participants engage in a cognitively distracting activity, a finding that has been extensively replicated among adults (e.g., Erber & Tesser, 1992; Joormann et al., 2007; Trask & Sigmon, 1999; Van Dillen & Koole, 2007). Furthermore, a meta-analysis found that distraction or refocusing attention was one of the three most effective ways to change mood states (Augustine & Hemenover, 2009).

Refocusing of attention is a cognitive process (e.g., Eisenberg et al., 2000; Posner & Rothbart, 2000), and as Kopp (1989) noted in her classic paper, gaze aversion is one of its developmentally earliest manifestations. When young infants are presented with a distressing visual stimulus (such as a still and unexpressive face), they "catch on" that by looking away, they are no longer subjected to the unwanted stimulus (e.g., Ekas et al., 2013; Jean et al., 2014; Manian & Bornstein, 2009). By the age of 3–6 months, upset infants can be predictably distracted by both visual and auditory stimuli, and their distress is measurably reduced as long as the distracter is present (Harman et al., 1997). As infants mature, the ability to respond to distracters segues into the purposeful refocusing of attention for mood repair.

With the advent of toddlerhood, attention refocusing is used increasingly for distress relief (e.g., Diener & Mangelsdorf, 1999). By about age 2, attention refocusing is the most frequent mood repair strategy to manage distress in laboratory settings (Grolnick et al., 1996) and remains so among older children (Silk et al., 2006). About two-thirds of 3- to 4-year-olds cited attention refocusing as the way to improve the affect of another person (López-Pérez et al., 2016). Importantly, the previously noted study, which followed 2-year-olds until age 5, found that as children grew older, they were increasingly likely to use distraction to manage dysphoria, with developmental spurts in frequency and duration of use between ages 2–3 and 4–5; furthermore, mood repair via distraction predominated over the other two strategies that were monitored (Ratcliff et al., 2021). Likewise, among 4- to 11-year-olds, distraction was reported more often than cognitive reappraisal to reduce experimentally induced distress (Parsafar et al., 2019). Notably, however, in the latter study, when children did not receive regulatory instructions, only about 20% reported the spontaneous use of distraction.

There is evidence that as early as age 4, children's use of attention focusing away from a distressing scenario does reduce levels of sadness (Morris et al., 2011). Studies of children ranging in age from 9 years to early adolescence confirmed that by those ages, attention refocusing (distraction) for mood repair can be easily implemented and is effective at attenuating dysphoric affect in the laboratory (Reijntjes et al., 2006a, 2006b; Volkaert et al., 2020; Wante et al., 2018), but its effectiveness appears to level off by about age 15 (Theurel & Gentaz, 2018).

The cognitive response domain also includes strategies like changing one's thoughts about one's situation or affective state, among which neutral reappraisal has received the most attention. Neutral reappraisal means to reinterpret or reframe the cause, nature, and implication of the dysphoria in ways that are counter-depressogenic (reviewed in Augustine & Hemenover, 2009). It is around the age of 6 or 7 that children start to deploy cognitive reappraisal for mood repair, but there is scant information about its subsequent developmental trajectory. In one study, cognitive reappraisal for mood repair was endorsed by 5- to 6-year-olds but not by 3- to 4-year-olds (Sala et al., 2014). Davis et al. (2010) reported that 69% of 5- to 6-year-olds claimed to have used a cognitive strategy to lift sad mood and that reappraising goals was the most common response: For example, if sadness was caused by not being able to play baseball because of an injured leg, the response could be to watch such games on TV. In the study of 3- to 8-year-olds, having the distressed person evaluate the situation differently as the way to feel better was offered as the response by less than 10% of the youngest group, but by about one-third of the 7- to 8-year-olds (López-Pérez et al., 2016). In the study of 10- to 23-year-olds, some forms of reappraisal increased, while other forms decreased as a function of age (e.g., changing the circumstance and changing consequences, respectively): By young adulthood, reframing the circumstances of a distressing event was the most used form of reappraisal (evident in 70% of affective events), while other ways of reappraisal, such as reinterpreting consequences, were employed less than 10% of the time (Nook et al., 2020).

The fact that the use of cognitive reappraisal to reduce distress is mediated by development was confirmed in a sample of 4- to 11-year-olds (Parsafar et al., 2019). But a 2-year follow-up of 9- to 15-year-olds failed to find an age-related increase in use and, in fact, found decreased use among the older students (Gullone et al., 2010). Thus, if frequency of response use is an index of development, then the Gullone et al. (2010) and Theurel and Gentaz (2018) studies suggest that the developmental unfolding of cognitive reappraisal plateaus around age 12 or shortly thereafter. Interestingly, however, rumination, a well-known maladaptive cognitive regulatory response, increases in use across the 12- to 15-year-old age span (Theurel & Gentaz, 2018).

There is evidence that reappraisal helps to attenuate dysphoria. Reappraisal decreased negative affect in the laboratory among 10- to 23-year-olds irrespective of age (Nook et al., 2020). In a similar vein, a neuroimaging study of 4- to 10-year-olds reported that guided cognitive reappraisal decreased the subjective experience of negative affect (Dougherty et al., 2015). Laboratory studies of 9- to 13-year-olds and those in early adolescence likewise found that cognitive reappraisal was readily implemented by those ages and was effective in reducing experimentally induced dysphoria (Volkaert et al., 2020; Wante et al., 2018). And although in another study, 12-, 13-, and 15-year-olds were similarly likely to use reappraisal to change mood, the two older groups used it more effectively than the 12-year-olds (Theurel & Gentaz, 2018).

Other cognitive mood repair responses for managing distress that have been studied among youth, ranging in age from 9 to 18 years, include putting things in perspective, positive reappraisal, planning, and problem solving. Paralleling the findings on neutral reappraisal, the general trends are that these cognitive strategies are significantly more likely to be deployed by older than younger respondents (Garnefski & Kraaij, 2006; Garnefski et al., 2007; Lennarz et al., 2019).

Observations of typically developing children as well as clinical experience suggest that visual imagery (another form of cognitive activity) also can serve the goal of mood repair. Visual imagery has received attention mostly as one way to improve performance in sports and the performing arts (Cumming & Williams, 2013), although it also has been proposed as one pathway to reduce unwanted mental images in bipolar disorder (Steel et al., 2020). Notably, self-reported imagery ability and emotion regulation via reappraisals are positively correlated (Anuar et al., 2016). Of import for CERT, the training of 11- to 16-year-old boys in picture–word mental imagery impacted their mood and cognition (Heyes et al., 2017).

The Social-Interpersonal Response Domain

Discussions and studies of interpersonal emotion regulation typically focus on the person who is tasked to influence the affect experience of another individual (e.g., Gummerum & López-Pérez, 2020; Zaki & Williams, 2013). In CERT, however, the focus is on the child whose dysphoria is being regulated via responses in the *social–interpersonal domain.*

It has long been established that turning to and receiving intervention from others are consistent features of emotion regulatory repertoires across the life span (e.g., Parkinson & Totterdell, 1999; Rippere, 1977; Thayer et al., 1994). The ubiquity of social–interpersonal emotion regulation regardless of age probably reflects the many ways in which one person can intervene in the affective experience of another (Niven et al., 2009; Urano et al., 2022; Williams et al., 2018).

During infancy and very early childhood, emotion regulation is primarily social–interpersonal in nature because regulatory responses typically are initiated and facilitated by parents or other caregivers (reviewed by Bariola et al., 2011, and Morris et al., 2017; see also Kopp, 1989). Importantly, parents who recognize and fulfill the infant's emotion regulatory needs and help her to regain emotional homeostasis also exemplify that adults can be a source of comfort in the face of distress. Indeed, iconic scholars in the field have emphasized that as they continue to develop, children who have had positive early experiences with caregivers in managing negative emotions will feel comfortable turning to others for help when distressed (e.g., Bretherton, 1985; Hofer, 1994; Kobak & Sceery, 1988). It is therefore noteworthy that by the fifth grade, companionship is the preferred way to resolve distress provoked by rejection or failure and remains so among seventh- and ninth-graders (Clark et al., 2008).

During the early years of development, caregivers typically regulate offspring's distress by gentle touching, caressing, and hugging (physical comforting), smiling, or reassuring vocalizations. However, even during early development, infants have rudimentary skills, which enable them to recruit regulators for distress relief. The earliest example of infant-initiated interpersonal regulation is caregiver-directed distress vocalization, which is evident by the age of 6 months; as established by several classic studies, seeking the help of caregivers when distressed then becomes increasingly frequent and strategic with age (Braungart & Stifter, 1991; Diener & Mangelsdorf, 1999; Grolnick et al., 1996; Mangelsdorf et al., 1995; Rothbart et al., 1992; Stifter & Braungart, 1995). Turning to others to overcome sadness is recognized by 3-year-olds and is increasingly deployed by 6-year-olds (Sala et al., 2014). In the previously noted follow-up study of 2-year-olds, the frequency of "bids" to caregivers while frustrated had an inverted U-shape curve, with a peak at age 3 (Ratcliff et al., 2021). Notably, both 6- and 9-year-olds judge the intervention of adults as particularly effective to counter sadness (Waters & Thompson, 2014). Consistent with developmental expectations, a study of 8- to 10-year-olds found that younger subjects were more likely than older ones to select ineffective or maladaptive interpersonal regulatory responses (López-Pérez & Pacella, 2021).

From the vantage point of the distressed child, a key developmental change in the social–interpersonal emotion regulatory domain is the progression from recruiting caregivers for distress relief via nonverbal communication (e.g., eye contact, caregiver-oriented crying) to using simple verbal requests for help and then relying on more complex language and oral discourse (e.g., Ratcliff et al., 2021; Thompson, 1994). Another developmental progression, which has received scant research attention, is children's growing ability to identify and recruit nonfamilial adults (e.g., teachers) as well as peers for distress relief.

There also are developmental changes in the modalities through which social–interpersonal regulation is received. As already noted, distressed infants and young children typically receive touch-based comforting (Weller & Feldman, 2003). With older children, the parent also may reinforce some instrumental behavior that provides distress relief (e.g., Hofer, 1994), help focus the child's attention away from the dysphoria (e.g., Jean et al., 2014), or alter the aspect of the environment that may have triggered the dysphoria (e.g., remove a sibling who contributes to the upset of the child). As children transit into the school-age years, interpersonal regulatory responses increasingly involve receiving verbal reassurance or advice, getting help in solving the problem, sharing feelings and reassuring autobiographical memories, and seeking emotional support (e.g., Clark et al., 2008; Kraaij & Garnefski, 2019; Maswood et al., 2018; Niven et al., 2009).

Children's ability to implement specific regulatory responses also is developmentally mediated. While 3- to 8-year-olds recognize that there are multiple ways to help a distressed person to feel better (López-Pérez et al., 2016), in a study of 3- to 4-year-olds' actual reactions to a distressed peer in natural settings, 22% of the responses involved offering comfort such as hugging or verbal/physical assistance, while 40% involved just watching the distressed peer (Farver & Branstetter, 1994). Extending the latter observations, a study of 3- to 8-year-olds found that younger children were more likely than older ones to try to distract a distressed child, while older children were more likely to help a distressed child to view the situation from multiple perspectives (López-Pérez et al., 2016). There also is some intriguing evidence that by adulthood individuals recruit different confidants to regulate different affects (Cheung et al., 2015).

We have limited understanding of the processes or mechanisms whereby the various interpersonal regulatory responses attenuate dysphoria and distress. Undoubtedly, the effects are mediated through what the regulator does, how he does it, the sensory modality that is employed, and the contribution of the child being regulated. In the "Key Mood Repair Response Mechanisms" section below, I address attention refocusing, activation of positive affect, and cognitive reprocessing—three plausible mechanisms that are likely to be responsible for the effects of many mood repair responses. When a parent reinforces a child's instrumental behavior in the service of mood repair, the mood-altering effect may be due to having refocused the child's attention away from the experience of distress. When a parent engages a distressed child in play activity, its mood repair affects may reflect a combination of attention refocusing and activation of positive affect. A reassuring conversation with a distressed youngster may calm him perhaps because it can alter the form or content of the youngster's cognitions, that is, help to reprocess the salient emotional information in a nondepressogenic manner (Lepore, 1997; Luminet et al., 2000). Because affective touch is one of the developmentally earliest routes through which distress is regulated interpersonally, I now review in more detail what is known about its mechanism.

Touch is the first sensorial experience prenatally (for an overview, see Crucianelli & Filippetti, 2020) and is an efficient vehicle for communicating positive affect like love and sympathy (Hertenstein et al., 2006). The importance of gentle and affectionate maternal touch in infants' emotion regulation has been confirmed among 5.5-month-olds (Jean et al., 2014) and 12-month-olds (Hertenstein & Campos, 2001) and continues to serve a regulatory function throughout the life span (Crucianelli & Filippetti, 2020). Early research has focused on neurochemical (e.g., neuropeptide) and neuroendocrine (e.g., cortisol) pathways whereby affective touch has salubrious effects on mood (e.g., Field et al., 1998; Jones & Field, 1999; Olausson et al., 2002). It was proposed that the antidepressant effects of pleasant touch may be due to its impact on physiological arousal: Namely, affective touch decreases cortisol secretion and decelerates heart rate and by ascending (bottom-up) pathways blocks excitatory circuits in various brain regions (e.g., Field et al., 1998; Jones & Field, 1999). More contemporary work has established that gentle and affective touch activates specialized unmyelinated nerve fibers, or afferents called *C-tactile* (CT) fibers, which also have been implicated in the development of the social brain (Björnsdotter et al., 2014; Crucianelli & Filippetti, 2020). The brain mechanisms for processing affective touch are present already in early infancy, have a distinct developmental trajectory across the first year of life, become increasingly adultlike by age 2 (Björnsdotter et al., 2014; Jönsson et al., 2018; Maria et al., 2022; Miguel et al., 2019a; Tuulari et al., 2019), and may be modified by individual differences in affective reactions to being touched (Miguel et al., 2019b, 2019c). Affectionate touch has its beneficial effects by virtue of the fact that the CT fibers project to the posterior insular and anterior cingulate cortices and eventually to prefrontal and orbitofrontal brain regions that have regulatory functions (for an overview, see Burleson & Quigley, 2021).

Sensory modalities other than touch also can be vehicles for interpersonal emotion regulation. For example, a regulator's visual emotion signals such as reassuring smiles are processed more easily than linguistic emotion-relevant information conveyed via prosody (e.g., a reassuring tone) (for an overview, see Adolphs, 2002; Wild et al., 2001). Relatedly, the importance of maternal smiles in infants' emotion regulation was confirmed among 5.5-month-olds (Jean et al., 2014). Thus, these studies suggest that a parent may more easily comfort a young distressed child by smiling than by soothing vocalizations.

Affect-Related Personal Characteristics and Mood Repair

Among the various personal characteristics that can influence a child's mood repair success, I briefly address four dispositions: temperament, emotion-related self-efficacy, emotional intelligence, and attachment style. *Temperament,* especially excessive negative emotional reactivity, has received much attention (e.g., Calkins et al., 2019; Fox & Calkins, 2003). Temperament refers to innate individual differences in physiological reactivity (arousability) and overall self-regulation (e.g., Calkins, 1994; Eisenberg et al., 2000; Posner & Rothbart, 2000): It is believed to affect the threshold and speed at which a dysphoric episode is triggered and its felt intensity. In turn, how strongly a person experiences dysphoria will influence how easily it can be regulated (Calkins et al., 1999; Larsen & Diener, 1987) and possibly the type of emotion regulation strategy that is deployed (e.g., Zimmermann & Stansbury, 2003). As early as 6 months old, infants with temperamental negativity use fewer adaptive attention regulation strategies and more avoidance responses to manage distress than comparison infants (Thomas et al., 2017). In middle childhood, negative emotionality likewise predicts poor emotion regulation (Santucci et al., 2008; Uhl et al., 2019). And in later childhood and adolescence (ages 9–17), having a negative predisposition is related to rumination, a maladaptive regulatory response (Van Beveren, Kuppens, et al., 2019).

Emotion-related self-efficacy and *emotional intelligence* are two further personal traits with broad implications for emotion regulation. Not surprisingly, adults who believe that they can successfully manage their own negative moods are indeed able to do so, and the ability to self-monitor, clearly identify, and accurately label emotions, which constitute emotional intelligence (Salovey & Grewal, 2005), presages successful emotion regulation and adaptive coping (for a review, see Heimpel et al., 2002; Hemenover et al., 2008; Peña-Sarrionandia et al., 2015; Salovey et al., 2002). It has been reported that children who lack confidence in their own regulatory skills are likely to have suboptimal emotion regulation (Garber et al., 1995). However, little is known about how emotional intelligence may bear on mood repair success in middle or later childhood because the construct has been studied mostly among adolescents (e.g., Mikolajczak et al., 2009).

Attachment style, as a dispositional characteristic, may impact mostly on the social–interpersonal regulatory mood repair domain. Attachment style, which is believed to affect psychotherapy outcome (Levy et al., 2011), may influence whether a child will turn to others to cope with sadness and dysphoria. In fact, the attachment behavioral system, which emerges in infancy, is believed to be the foundation for affect regulation (e.g., Mikulincer et al., 2003; Zimmer-Gembeck et al., 2017). According to proponents, children's early experiences with parents give rise to a mental prototype of the benefits (or costs) of key relationships, which sets the stage for (or against) turning to others to regulate emotion in later years (e.g., Collins & Read, 1990; Hofer, 1994; Mikulincer et al., 2003). When caregivers are repeatedly ineffective at lessening a child's distress, the child learns that she *cannot* rely on people to help modulate dysphoria, which can lead to avoidance of emotional closeness and physical intimacy (Mikulincer et al., 2003). Indeed, as early as their second year, infants who were not securely attached were found to be less likely than their peers to positively engage their parent to regulate distress (Crugnola et al., 2011).

A longitudinal study of 2-year-olds found several paths from early attachment style to later emotion regulation: For example, secure early relationships were directly related to good self-regulation in the face of frustration as early as ages 3–5 (Boldt et al., 2020). Another longitudinal study of 9- to 17-year-olds confirmed that attachment security has positive effects on emotion regulation strategy use (Iwanski et al., 2021). Overall, reviewers have concluded that children who are not securely attached have problems in regulating their emotions and that avoidantly attached children are particularly less likely than well-attached peers to use social support to respond to stress (Cooke et al., 2019; Zimmer-Gembeck et al., 2017).

Key Mood Repair Response Mechanisms

As summarized in the previous sections, children (as well as adults) have at their potential disposal a large variety of adaptive responses when dysphoric affect needs to be repaired. One may therefore wonder how all the responses achieve the common goal of attenuating dysphoria. Although it is quite likely that some regulatory responses are underpinned by specific processes (the mechanism of affective touch was one example), given that regulatory responses number in the double (or possibly triple) digits, it is unlikely that each repairs mood via a unique mechanism or pathway. Instead, there probably are a limited number of processes that account for much of successful mood repair via some common processes. Knowing the mechanisms through which many mood repair responses accomplish their goals has practical implications, as I discuss in Chapter 10 on coping skills training.

There has been very limited research on emotion regulation mechanisms in childhood. However, I propose that at least three mechanisms or pathways account for many successful mood repair responses: a cognitive pathway that involves attention refocusing; a hedonic pathway that involves the activation of positive affect; and another cognitive pathway that involves the reprocessing of affect-related information.

Attention Refocusing

Up to this point, I discussed *attention refocusing* (often called *distraction*) as a specific cognitive regulatory response to dysphoria. However, refocusing of attention away from the experience of dysphoria and sadness also functions as a mechanism that underpins a large array of adaptive regulatory responses. Responses as diverse as organizing one's room, reading a book, fixing a broken toy, doing chores, or recruiting parents or peers for some type of help are likely to be effective in reducing dysphoria, at least in part, because they make it possible for the depressed youth to focus their attention on an affectively neutral goal or task and away from the experience of distress. It has been shown, for example, that attempts to recover from feeling sad and dysphoric through making art are beneficial only if the art is used to refocus attention, but not if it serves as the vehicle for venting (e.g., Drake & Winner, 2013). Bebko and colleagues (2011) have likewise proposed that attention deployment contributes to the success of various emotion regulatory responses.

Attention refocusing likely helps to repair mood via its association with working memory. *Working memory* refers to the ability to keep some information in short-term memory storage, while, at the same time, continuing to process some other information (e.g., Garrison & Schmeichel, 2022). Erber and Tesser (1992) have suggested that focusing attention on a highly involving task engages working memory and thereby constrains ongoing processing of negative mood–related information. This proposition has been verified by van Dillen and Koole (2007); they demonstrated in a series of experiments that more complex and difficult tasks, which make greater demands on working memory, are associated with the most improvement in experimentally induced dysphoria. Thus, many mood repair responses are successful, in part, because they use brain processing resources that cannot then be allocated to negative emotion circuits. The very same proposition has been voiced by Erber and Erber (2000): They note that the easiest way to attenuate sad mood is to get involved in tasks that are "cognitively taxing" or engaging, regardless of whether the engagement involves "doing crossword puzzles or yard work" or "watching hours of sidesplitting comedy" (p. 144).

The importance of working memory capacity in attention refocusing, and thereby in emotion regulation, has received empirical support. Adults with higher working memory capacity demonstrated more effective use of distraction for emotion regulation in the laboratory than did peers with lower working memory capacity (Kobayashi et al., 2021). Working memory capacity also plays a role in emotion regulation in daily life (Garrison & Schmeichel, 2022), and there is some evidence that attention control training can promote successful emotion regulation (e.g., Xiu et al., 2018). Attention refocusing allows the distressed child to stop processing and attending to his sadness and related information, which appears to facilitate a return to the prior emotional and physiological homeostasis. In turn, this process then frees up emotional and cognitive resources to respond to the problem at hand.

Activation of Positive Affect

There are responses in each of the three regulatory domains that appear to rely on the *activation of positive affect* as the mechanism of mood change. In the cognitive regulatory domain, examples include refocusing one's thoughts on positive topics (Garnefski & Kraaij, 2006), recalling happy personal memories (Werner-Seidler et al., 2017), responding to humor (e.g., Samson & Gross, 2012), and possibly some forms of positive reappraisal. Behavioral mood repair responses that have a positive affective core include engaging in play activity, listening to uplifting music, some forms of dancing, or spending time in an amusement park. Helping others is a mood repair response in the interpersonal domain, which has strong positive affective features. It can be argued that each of these responses involves attention refocusing, which therefore could be the mechanism. However, neuroimaging work has shown that experiencing positive affect recruits brain reward circuits that are distinct from prefrontal cortical brain regions that enable abstract thinking and forms of attention and thus behavioral control (Nestler & Carlezon, 2006). Therefore, while leveraging positive affect appears to be the hallmark of the regulatory responses enumerated just above, attention processes may also play contributory roles.

The importance of positive affect for well-being is widely acknowledged (Alexander et al., 2021), and seeking to experience positive affect to recover from dysphoria may occur automatically as a form of counter-regulation (Quirin et al., 2011; Schwager & Rothermund, 2013). However, it is worthy of note that cultural differences in how positive affect is valued can constrain its pursuit (Ma et al., 2018).

There is scant research on the relations of positive affect and mood repair in young school-age children. According to a study of emotionally well girls, assessed when they were 9 and 10 years old, the ability to draw on and display positive emotions in response to conflict situations protected them from depression symptoms 1 year later (Feng et al., 2009). Laboratory studies of adolescents and adults have confirmed that hedonic capacity can be harnessed for mood repair by conjuring up happy personal memories (Cooney et al., 2007; Joormann et al., 2007; Kovacs et al., 2015) or reading jokes and puns (Strick et al., 2009). Among college students, ready access to positive emotions (via memories) was one of the automatic regulatory responses to experimentally induced distress (DeWall et al., 2011).

The means whereby positive affect impacts mood, cognition, and behavior has been of considerable interest (for a review, see Vanlessen et al., 2016). Positive affect as a mechanism of change may help to repair dysphoric mood via its beneficial effect on attention and cognitive flexibility, but the results (e.g., broadening vs. narrowing of attention) are constrained by the motivational quality of the affect (for reviews, see Lacey et al., 2021; Paul et al., 2021). Possibly, positive affect also may enable mood repair by boosting working memory capacity (Figueira et al., 2018), a process that was described earlier in connection with attention refocusing as a mechanism of change.

Cognitive Reprocessing

Cognitive reprocessing of information is the mechanism of change when a person lessens the negative affective impact of a depressogenic event by altering how she thinks about it. As an example, let us consider a youngster whose peers left her out of a play activity, which can be a depressogenic trigger. Adaptive cognitive reappraisal on her part could take several forms: She may think that the omission was accidental because her friends thought she had been invited a while back, conclude that the event was of no consequence ("I wasn't sure that I wanted to go anyway"), or reframe the event in beneficial terms ("This will work out OK—I now have extra time for my school project"). The first two responses exemplify neutral reappraisal, while the last response is an example of positive reappraisal.

Cognitive reappraisal differs from other cognitive mood repair strategies because the emotion or mood that is being regulated and its context remain in the forefront of thinking. Although the neural basis of cognitive emotion regulation in general and reappraisal in particular have been researched mostly in adults (for a review, see Buhle et al., 2014), by late childhood adultlike brain activation patterns during reappraisal have been reported. Specifically, a developmental study of children, adolescents, and young adults (ages 10–22) during reappraisal found linear age-related increases in activation of the left ventrolateral prefrontal cortex, which is known to underpin reappraisal among adults (McRae et al., 2012). Belden et al. (2014) likewise reported that positive reappraisal of sad photos by 8- to 12-year-olds involved the same neural activation patterns (e.g., areas of the prefrontal cortex) as those identified during such tasks among older youth and adults.

How does the cognitive reprocessing of affect-related information achieve mood repair? Contemporary approaches have used mostly neuroimaging to answer this question. The findings suggest that reappraisal attenuates or reduces the responses of the amygdala to affective stimuli (for an overview, see Silvers, 2020). Given that the amygdala is a key brain structure that is involved in generating affective responses, its reduced activity is believed to signal decreased intensity of affective experience. Because reappraisal involves working memory (Silvers, 2020), it has been questioned whether working memory capacity may best explain reappraisal success (Lee & Xue, 2018). However, working memory has been separable from and negatively correlated with neural activation of prefrontal brain regions during reappraisal (Zaehringer et al., 2018), suggesting that a person with high working memory capacity needs less neural resources to reappraise. Thus, cognitive reprocessing of dysphoria-related information via reappraisal may help a youth to feel better because it both reduces amygdala activation and engages working memory.

Mood Repair among Depressed Children

Empirical research on how depressed children regulate sadness and dysphoria has been somewhat constrained because most studies have defined depression by self-rated symptom questionnaires rather than by psychiatric diagnosis and focused only on adolescents. For example, a comprehensive review, which found a robust association between dysfunctional emotion regulation and depression, covered studies of mostly 11- to 17-year-olds (Young et al., 2019). Likewise, a meta-analysis, which reported that depressive symptoms go hand in hand with lower use of adaptive affect regulation strategies and higher use of maladaptive ones, included only 13- to 18-year-olds (Schafer et al., 2017). Thus, while the research findings support clinical experience that depressed youngsters have emotion regulation (mood repair) problems, this relationship needs further empirical confirmation in younger school-age children with diagnosed depression.

The emotion regulation skills of depressed children have been assessed via their responses to affective stories, by parents' or youngsters' reports of youngsters' habitual regulatory strategies, or by children implementing regulatory responses in the laboratory. When asked to respond to vignettes of distressing scenarios, symptomatically depressed students in grades K–8 were less likely than nondepressed peers to endorse mood repair responses that alleviate negative affect, more likely to favor responses that worsen or intensify it, or not even attempt to regulate it (e.g., Garber et al., 1995; Reijntjes et al., 2007). A meta-analysis found similar trends among 13- to 18-year-olds: Depressive symptoms were associated with less frequent use of adaptive regulatory responses (cognitive reappraisal, problem solving, acceptance) and more frequent use of maladaptive strategies (avoidance, suppression, rumination) (Schafer et al., 2017). Another meta-analysis confirmed that depression in youngsters is closely tied to ruminative responses to negative mood and a disinclination to engage in distracting responses (Rood et al., 2009), although the associations were far stronger among adolescents than among children. Based on samples that bridged ages 8–16, it has been repeatedly confirmed that symptomatically depressed children frequently rely on maladaptive cognitive responses to distress, such as self-blame, other blame, catastrophizing, and rumination (Andrés et al., 2016; Garnefski & Kraaij, 2018; Garnefski et al., 2007; Uhl et al., 2019), and are less likely to use problem solving or positive reframing (Siener & Kerns, 2012). Testifying to the robustness of the association of depression symptoms and maladaptive mood repair, the findings have been replicated in very large community-based samples of 7- to 11-year-olds (Kudinova et al., 2018) and 12- to 16- year-olds (Betts et al., 2009), and in national and school-based samples of 8- to 12-year-olds in Norway and Spain (Loevaas et al., 2018; Melero et al., 2021), and among 7- to 16-year-old school children in Belgium (Van Beveren et al., 2018).

Studies that ascertained depression by psychiatric diagnosis are particularly relevant to CERT. In a sample of 11- to 17-year-olds, youth with major depressive disorder reported co-ruminating more and problem solving less with peers in daily life than emotionally normative peers (Waller et al., 2014). In a study of 697 psychiatrically diagnosed depressed children and 1,394 nondepressed control peers who were 7–14 years old (Kovacs et al., 2019), my research group characterized mood repair repertoires via the Feelings and Me Questionnaire, completed by children about themselves, and the Feelings and My Child Questionnaire, completed by parents about their offspring (these questionnaires as well as the adult self-report questionnaire and a scoring template are described later in Chapter 5 and included as reproducible Forms 1–4 in Appendix A). Depressed children reported an abundance of maladaptive responses to sadness (rather than a poverty of adaptive responses): Their maladaptive response repertoires were significantly larger than the repertoires of controls and grew increasingly larger with age.

Unexpectedly, up to about age 11, depressed children reported larger adaptive mood repair repertoires than their emotionally healthy peers: Possibly, younger depressed children attempt a variety of adaptive regulatory responses one after another because the previously executed response has failed to reduce dysphoria (Kovacs et al., 2019). Of particular clinical relevance, we also found that parents of depressed children described their offspring in far less favorable mood repair terms than the children described themselves and, regardless of offspring's age, reported significantly larger maladaptive response repertoires (but only slightly smaller adaptive repertoires) for their children than did the parents of controls.

We reexamined subgroups of these youngsters when they were 11–19 years old (Bylsma et al., 2016), by which time most of them had recovered from their depression episodes: But even in remission from depression, these youth reported higher rates of maladaptive mood repair responses and lower rates of adaptive responses in the face of sadness than controls. We also assessed the ability of these youth to repair sad mood in the laboratory. After watching a very sad film clip, the youngsters implemented either an attention refocusing task or were asked to recall positive autobiographical events. Regardless of the regulatory response that was implemented, youth with either past or current depression were less successful than controls at repairing their sadness (Kovacs et al., 2015): Thus, even a highly controlled laboratory environment that was designed to facilitate mood repair could not compensate for the mood repair problems conferred by having a history of depression episodes.

Finally, the reported difficulties of depressed youth to reduce negative affect via cognitive reappraisal has provided opportunities to probe the neural basis of impaired mood repair in such populations: The results have been equivocal. For example, in one study of 9- to 15-year-olds, neural activation during instructed emotion regulation (vs. baseline) was unrelated to levels of depression symptoms (Bettis et al., 2021). However, in a sample of 13- to 17-year-olds, those with major depression engaged less efficiently various prefrontal brain cortical regions during mood repair than controls (LeWinn et al., 2018). Examining the neural correlates of cognitive regulatory responses among children and youth remains a research priority but also a challenge because the cortical regions of interest continue to undergo development until (and even beyond) emerging adulthood.

Practical Implications of the Research Literature

Research on mood repair and its developmental unfolding has translational value and thereby can inform clinical practice. For example, the findings provide useful information about the normative mood repair responses that characterize different ages and developmental stages. Are there further critical takeaways from the huge, multidimensional developmental literature on emotion regulation? How well do research findings support CERT's approach to problematic mood repair responses?

One critical takeaway from the literature is that affect regulatory competence has a long and complex developmental history. There is no question that emotion regulation, including mood repair responses, and the skills that underpin them, begin to emerge in late infancy. Importantly, they are then subject to multiple interactive forces that shape regulatory competence. For example, having a negative temperament is associated with problems in emotion regulation in infancy, which then can adversely affect the subsequent unfolding of regulatory responses. But such an adverse trajectory can be prevented by parenting that is consistently responsive to the infant's affect regulatory needs. I suspect that the presence of siblings, and their temperaments as well as their own regulatory styles, also will influence a given child's affect regulatory trajectory. Indeed, the developing infant and child are exposed to a variety of inputs from caregivers, family, and the wider social milieu, which interact with the child's characteristics and jointly contribute to the unfolding of culture-specific (and family-specific) ways of responding to sadness and dysphoria. It is highly unlikely that the therapist can elucidate fully this developmental process or identify all the historical contributors to a given child's mood repair problems. Given the myriad of inputs to mood repair development and their variable timing, the most pragmatic approach is to focus on proximal events and processes related to sadness self-regulation. Furthermore, it is important to keep in mind that, for example, when the therapist seeks to change some feature of a 10-year-old depressed child's mood repair repertoire, the therapist is facing the child's nearly 10-year history of having learned how sadness ought to be managed. Therefore, even the smallest positive change in the young patient's mood repair approach should be regarded as a major achievement.

Another important takeaway from the literature is that while depressed children do have somewhat fewer adaptive mood repair responses than normative peers and appear to apply the responses less efficiently, they are primarily distinguished by the excess of maladaptive strategies in their emotion regulation repertoires. This is important because research has documented that it is the presence of maladaptive and dysfunctional emotion regulation responses (rather than the shortage of adaptive regulatory responses) that are associated with psychopathology (Aldao et al., 2010). Thus, the research evidence supports CERT's emphasis on replacing maladaptive regulatory strategies that support depression by reinforcing children's adaptive mood repair responses.

As the literature review suggests, we know a great deal about how regulatory responses unfold up to about ages 4 and 5, know far less about the process during the subsequent years of childhood, but the information base then expands dramatically around the years of adolescence. Relatedly, it is not clear whether the developmental trajectories of emotion regulation are positively linear and, if so, up to what age. Some researchers have argued that regulatory skills continue to develop linearly across childhood and adolescence and then level off; others have argued that during mid-adolescence, emotion regulatory development takes a temporarily maladaptive direction; while still others have noted that the picture of mood repair development will differ as a function of the specific regulatory response. There also is a lack of consensus on how best to define emotion regulatory development: Should the definition focus on the number of responses or the size of the regulatory repertoire, the types of regulatory responses, response effectiveness, some mechanistic feature of regulation, or a combination of the foregoing?

Regardless of the definition, the age-group targeted by CERT is still in the process of emotion regulatory development. To help the therapist recognize whether a given depressed young patient is "off" developmental course vis-à-vis mood repair, or if a particular style of regulatory responding is not age-appropriate, I included in the literature review available information about typical regulatory responses in each domain at various ages, and about the development of underlying skills. For example, given an 8-year-old patient with normative language development, the therapist can tentatively conclude that the patient is delayed in the age-appropriate use of interpersonal mood repair if he consistently fails to use language to summon a parent (a regulator) but instead relies on posturing, such as physically holding onto the parent. As a potential remedy, the therapist may model for the child age-appropriate versions of recruiting the adult regulator. As another example, by the age of about 10, all children should be able to implement strategies that entail attention refocusing. If a 10-year-old patient cannot deploy attention refocusing for mood repair, the therapist can target another cognitive regulatory response or a noncognitive response; a neuropsychological assessment would also be warranted to identify the source of the child's attention difficulties.

Another important takeaway from the research literature is that the developmental trajectories of the three regulatory domains and the skills that undergird them will differ within and across children. Mood repair via the intervention of others is developmentally the earliest to emerge (late infancy) but is followed closely by infant-initiated behavioral (self-soothing) and cognitive (gaze aversion/attention refocusing) regulatory responses. All other things being equal, by the age of 7 (the lower age target of our treatment program), all three regulatory domains should be "up and running." But levels of response sophistication and ease of response implementation will differ across the domains, and the unfolding of some responses may pose more challenges than other responses. For example, summoning a parent for help to provide distress relief is probably easier for younger children than cognitive reappraisal. Furthermore, whereas attention refocusing for mood repair can be implemented even by toddlers and essential components of this response remain the same as children age, elemental self-soothing (e.g., sucking, self-pleasuring), a critical mood repair response during infancy, goes mostly "underground" by preschool and may have to find a different form of somatosensory expression in later years. Overall, developmental patterns and challenges become evident as individual differences in mood repair repertoires and competence even among children of the same age.

Another takeaway from the literature is that only a few age-specific transition points in emotion regulation have been identified. For example, we know that children in Western society start to self-initiate emotion regulation when they are about 3 or 4 years old. However, we don't know at what age talking to a parent (or other trusted adult) about one's sadness becomes normative and effective, or the age at which a child can deploy cognitive reappraisal to repair sadness in everyday life. This lack of information can be partly overcome by recourse to the developmental literature on the various skills that support emotion regulation; earlier in this chapter, I provided examples of such an approach.

I acknowledge throughout this book that young patients have mood repair response preferences, which are to be accommodated. In Chapter 7, I nonetheless suggest that all patients be exposed to a discussion of mood repair via the social–interpersonal domain and that the response of giving or getting a hug from the parent be reviewed with all patients. These recommendations are based on the crucial importance of caregivers in children's emotion regulation, the very early developmental origins and functional importance of affective touch and interpersonal regulation, and the availability of other people across the life span as agents of positive mood change. The reader also will discover that, compared to some other interventions, CERT gives limited consideration to regulatory responses that involve cognitive *reappraisal*. The research on cognitive development that I reviewed supports this decision, particularly for patients in their earlier childhood years.

As can be seen in Chapter 7, CERT has a conservative approach: It focuses on reinforcing a limited number (rather than a broad set) of adaptive regulatory responses for any given child and mostly in his preferred functional domains. This approach is consistent with research findings that, in any actual depressogenic situation, children (and adults) typically deploy just a few regulatory responses and findings that most emotion regulation strategies are traitlike.

The research literature also reveals that, when it comes to emotion regulation and mood repair responses, what young patients say about themselves, what their parents say about them, and what young patients actually do when subjected to a depressogenic trigger do not necessarily correspond. That is not to say that patients or parents tell untruths; instead, the lack of concordance across these informants reflects the very different perspectives children and adults have on children's affect-related thinking and behavior. However, the lack of concordance can become a source of conflict. As shown in the remainder of this book's chapters, the team approach advocated by CERT can help in this regard: Children and parents have different and clearly defined roles and therefore are expected to produce different types of information, and the therapeutic emphasis is on a common goal rather than who is right or wrong.

The developmental literature buttresses other key elements of CERT. Findings on the early sequential unfolding of different types of regulatory responses support CERT's grouping them into multiple functional domains. The extensively documented social context of emotion regulatory development overwhelmingly supports CERT's emphasis that parents must play active and key roles in their offspring's treatment. Within the context of a team approach, engaging the parents as assistant coaches to reach treatment goals acknowledges and reinforces their historical roles as emotion regulatory agents in their children's lives. CERT's team approach also conveys a meta-cognitive message of distancing because the "I" that is the center of most evidence-based interventions is replaced by "we." This shift away from the use of personal pronouns is supported by the literature on the use of language to serve emotion goals.

Although I focus in this book on children who live and are treated in the

United States, basic elements of emotion regulation development and issues of coping with depressogenic triggers should be applicable within contexts other than North America. As part of the socialization of children, all cultures acknowledge the need for emotion regulation and, in particular, for the control of negative emotions. The reliance of infants and young children on caregivers to meet affect regulatory goals is not constrained by geography. The developmental unfolding of basic skills and the processes of biological maturation are also universal.

However, culture plays a role regarding which mood repair responses and styles are preferred or accepted, and the extent to which affective experience and expression are valued. For example, several Asian cultures put a greater emphasis on communal values than individualized and personal goals. Thus, during development, regulation via the social–interpersonal domain can be expected to be more reinforced in those cultures than regulation via cognition or behavior that focuses on the self. Relatedly, affective (nonsexual) touching of nonfamilial same-sex peers is a part of some Asian cultures, while it is often frowned on in North American settings, which has obvious implications for interpersonal strategies for mood repair. As a further example, suppressing facial expression of affect during certain social interactions is normative in some cultures but generally considered to be maladaptive in North American contexts. Therefore, if the cultural background of the parent–child pair and the therapist notably diverges, I suggest that the therapist seek information about how the young patient's culture views emotions and their optimal management. The information then can serve to modify CERT to meet the given child's and family's needs.

In closing, it is important to note that mood repair development, including the interactions of various sources of influence across the years, and issues of coping with stress both become more complicated in the presence of depression in the family. In the chapters that follow, it will be evident that CERT *distills* the most critical elements of affect regulatory development and coping and presents them to families in the simplest possible ways. By defining key concepts in plain words and asking the parent–child pair to engage in tasks that are doable and relatable, CERT seeks to bring about changes in affect and behavior without overwhelming a family already stressed by the young patient's depression. In the next chapter, I describe key aspects of CERT.

Chapter 3

Introduction to CERT for Children

Contextual emotion regulation therapy (CERT) emphasizes the adaptive self-regulation of dysphoria as the primary road to recovery for children with clinical depression. Informed by the empirical literature on typical development, CERT is directive- and skill-focused. But it is also a flexible intervention that accommodates individual differences among young patients with respect to their mood repair response repertoires, related basic skills, and social contexts. This chapter provides an overview of CERT's distinguishing features, its central goals and intervention strategies, and guidelines for treatment duration.

Three Distinguishing Features of CERT

Three features of CERT distinguish it from other interventions for pediatric depression: (1) its *explanatory framework*, which identifies poorly regulated dysphoria (usually in the context of stress) as the central problem in depression and therefore accords a key role to adaptive mood repair in recovery; (2) the *active engagement of parent(s) in the depressed child's treatment by using a "coaching" model;* and (3) a *developmentally informed and individually tailored approach* to young patients.

The Explanatory Framework

An explanatory framework in psychotherapy is a way of explaining why the patient is suffering from the disorder and what ought to be done to help the patient recover from it. CERT's explanatory framework integrates information about the relationship between stress, coping, and depression with developmental research on emotion regulation and mood repair. It posits that recovery from depression and the ability to stay depression-free depend on the young patient's ability to keep sad and dysphoric affect at bay so that those affects do not take over, a process called *adaptive mood repair* throughout this book.

The Mood Repair Formulation of Depression

CERT identifies *mood repair failure* (or *maladaptive mood repair*) as the mechanism responsible for the child's depression. Mood repair failure contributes to clinical depression in two ways. First, it accounts for how dysphoric emotion leads to a depressive disorder. Second, maladaptive mood repair then maintains the depressive episode by contributing to persistent sadness, distress, or irritability that are central to clinical depression.

According to CERT's explanatory framework, the child's depression has come about because she has been unable to modulate the initial sadness and dysphoria that had been triggered by a negative event or process (stressor). Once the dysphoric emotion becomes persistent and segues into dysphoric mood, it is followed by a cascade of other depressive symptoms, some of which (e.g., sleep problems, concentration difficulties) further exacerbate dysphoria and distress. The end result is an episode of a depressive disorder. The depressive disorder is maintained by the child's maladaptive mood repair responses to everyday perturbations in emotions, which are brought on by the inevitable hassles of life.

While clearly acknowledging the full range of a child's depressive symptoms, this formulation focuses the therapist's attention on the young patient's affective complaints and the regulatory responses that maintain them. Because adaptive mood repair responding unfolds as a part of normative development (as reviewed in Chapter 2), persistent mood repair failure can implicate atypical development that should be identified and remediated, whenever possible. But, persistent mood repair failure also can reflect the malignant effects of more recent contextual stress processes.

The mood repair formulation of depression has several practical implications for the delivery of CERT. One implication is that right from the start, the therapist has to share this particular view of depression with the young patient and parent. Being able to think about depression as a problem in mood repair provides them with a new perspective on their difficulties and points to new directions for recovery.

Another implication is that the therapist has to frame the presenting problem (the concern that prompted the family to seek help), and the specific issues brought into each session, as *reflections of the child's mood repair problems.* Such a framing is easy if mood symptoms are the main problems. It is more of a challenge if the parents identify behavioral issues as most pressing, such as noncompliant and disrespectful behavior, declining school performance, or sibling rivalry. In these instances, the therapist has to explain that it is the dysregulated mood that gives rise to and fuels such maladaptive behaviors and most other depressive complaints.

As soon as possible the therapist has to take rapid corrective action to replace the maladaptive mood repair response(s) that maintain or exacerbate the child's despondent, dysphoric affect and introduce the parent–child pair to alternative and adaptive ways to respond to dysphoria. Keep in mind, however, that much of mood repair is *automatic* (see Chapter 2). Thus, in the beginning of treatment, neither parent nor child may be fully cognizant of how the child's own responses to dysphoria or distress maintain it.

Viewing mood symptoms and problem behaviors as mirroring the child's mood repair difficulties, and then identifying how best to replace maladaptive responses that perpetuate the child's distress, are the initial steps for arriving at a *mood repair–based case formulation.* The case formulation goes beyond the observed mood repair problems and ways of correcting them and seeks to identify the contextual or developmental features of the child's life that may have contributed to the child's mood repair problems. It generally takes several sessions before the therapist has sufficient information to attempt an initial case formulation, which is likely to be revised as new data emerge.

Stress, Coping, and Dysphoria

The contexts of children's lives play important roles in the onset, course, and outcome of depression. Contextual elements that have been implicated in depression include acute or chronic stressors that impinge directly on children themselves (e.g., loss of a friend) or affect the entire family (e.g., parental unemployment), dysfunctional parental characteristics or family environment (e.g., mental illness, poor parenting style), limited availability of social and material resources, and stress-generating aspects of the community (e.g., Hammen et al., 1999; LeMoult et al., 2020). Recent research has also established early life maltreatment as a risk factor for depression and has started to identify some mechanisms (Hammen, 2015; Heim & Binder, 2012; LeMoult, 2020; Park et al., 2019). Notably, physical abuse is more strongly related to pediatric depression than sexual abuse (LeMoult et al., 2020).

CERT focuses on stressful life events as triggers in pediatric depression (see Chapter 1 for the supporting literature). It has long been established that stressful events that signify important real or symbolic losses appear to be specific provoking agents for depression (Beck, 1967; Brown et al., 1994), and this applies to youngsters as well (LeMoult et al., 2020). And, as already noted, there is evidence that psychosocial stressors may play a greater role in triggering the first episode of affective disorder than later episodes, possibly suggesting that the first episode sensitizes individuals to stress.

How does stress in a youngster's life lead to depression? The psychological construct of *coping* points to one pathway through which stressful events and depression are linked. Stress leads to depression only if the child has not been able to cope. According to a classical and enduring definition of coping, the word reflects the ongoing "cognitive and behavioral efforts to manage [those] specific external and/or internal demands that are appraised as taxing or exceeding the resources of the person" (Lazarus & Folkman, 1984, p. 141; 1991). *Emotion-focused coping* refers to efforts directed at managing the emotions and distress provoked by (or secondary to) the problem, whereas *problem-focused coping* refers to efforts directed at managing or altering the problem that caused the distress (Lazarus & Folkman, 1984, 1991). Emotion-focused and problem-solving coping are evident among children and adolescents as well (e.g., Compas, 1987; Compas et al., 1993). Although a third response type has also been proposed (Endler & Parker, 1990a, 1990b), the first two coping styles have received the most attention and researchers have consistently emphasized active problem solving as the best way to cope with stress.

Coping and emotion regulation clearly are overlapping constructs (e.g., Bonanno & Burton, 2013). This has been confirmed by an extensive meta-analysis of coping and emotion regulation in childhood and adolescence (Compas et al., 2017). And, as noted in Chapter 2, the study of coping has been one important antecedent of contemporary research on emotions (see also Gross, 1998, 1999; Tugade & Fredrickson, 2004). Having established the importance of coping with stress, research has segued into new directions, including the role of coping flexibility in depression (Bonanno & Burton, 2013; Kato, 2015).

In CERT, coping is regarded as the *broad area of stress management;* specifically, the responses to and management of adverse events and their impact on one's daily functioning and well-being. CERT's explanatory paradigm of depression, however, highlights the affective consequences of stress and underscores that coping requires the adaptive regulation of dysphoria provoked by stress. Furthermore, because many (if not most) stressful events in children's lives are outside their control and not amenable to problem solving (as would be recommended by traditional coping paradigms), children's ability to manage their emotional reactions to stressors is a crucial component of coping. Therefore, in CERT, the construct of emotion regulation, which includes mood repair, is super-ordinate to the construct of coping. Good affect regulation skills are essential for many areas of functioning and need to be deployed in the service of coping with stressful events.

Pathways from Dysphoria to Depressed Mood to Depressive Disorder

John Teasdale (1988) has noted that people who tend to get clinically depressed and those who are able to recover from an episode of sadness do not differ in the trigger events or the initial experience of dysphoria. Instead, they differ in how they respond to that affect: Depression-prone people are likely to respond in ways that impede "natural recovery." In other words, once a dysphoric emotion has been provoked, the normative and typically automatic response is to somehow lessen, diminish, or attenuate the dysphoria. But children who are prone to depression often fail to accomplish this goal. This opens the gateway to further depressive symptoms and undermines coping efforts.

Depressed mood may lead to clinical disorder via various pathways (e.g., Lyubomirsky et al., 2003; Lyubomirsky & Nolen-Hoeksema, 1993; Pomerantz &

Rudolph, 2003). For example, depressed mood elicits negative social responses, which range from being ignored to outright rejection (e.g., Joiner & Metalsky, 1995). Negative social responses, in turn, can have adverse effects on self-esteem, trigger ruminations, and thereby contribute to the downward spiral of clinical depression (e.g., Duggal et al., 2001; Feinstein et al., 2013; Joiner & Metalsky, 1995; Morrow & Nolen-Hoeksema, 1990). Protracted dysphoria also may adversely affect neurovegetative functions, most particularly, sleep. Sleep disturbance (e.g., Franzen & Buysse, 2008) can then contribute to fatigue (another symptom of clinical depression) and undermine the ability to concentrate (a further symptom), all of which then exacerbate negative mood and enable further depressive symptoms (e.g., Dahl, 1996). Self-regulatory responses, which may temporarily relieve dysphoria but engender other problems (e.g., the use of alcohol or other substances), also can pave the way to clinical depression (e.g., Cooper et al., 1995; Stapinski et al., 2016).

In general, pathways from dysregulated, dysphoric emotion to dysphoric mood and then to a depressive disorder probably are influenced by the affected individual's age and context. For example, negative family environment and parents who are emotionally unavailable or unsupportive are likely to contribute to the unfolding of depression in childhood (e.g., Cicchetti & Toth, 1998; Duggal et al., 2001), while contextual constraints, external pressures, or lack of material resources may be more decisive from adolescence onward. Regardless of the pathways whereby a depressed youngster's sad mood segued into a depressive disorder, CERT focuses on the youngster's mood repair response repertoire.

Engaging the Parent by Using a "Coaching" Model

According to a meta-analysis of clinical trials, the inclusion of parents in their children's treatment led to better outcomes than did treatments that only involved the young patients (Dowell & Ogles, 2010). However, most of the early (typically CBT) trials of depressed children and adolescents (usually conducted in school settings) did not include the parents, or only involved them in separate "parent groups" (for an overview, see Kovacs & Sherrill, 2001). In contrast, parental participation, which is consistent and active, is a critical component of CERT.

The Basis for Involving Parents in CERT

CERT's requirement of parental participation reflects practical as well as conceptual considerations. When parents are active participants in their child's treatment, they are more likely to feel involved in the therapeutic process and more likely to cooperate with the treatment regimen. Active parental participation also reinforces the important social and educational roles parents play in their children's lives.

But parents are involved in CERT primarily because of developmental considerations. As described in Chapter 2, emotion regulatory responding is learned in a social context and children's acquisition of mood repair responses is initially facilitated primarily by parents. Across infancy and childhood, parents act as regulatory models, as "teachers" who selectively reinforce some responses (but not others), and as key interpersonal regulatory agents for the child. Parents remain the most important interpersonal regulators of a child's distress, at least up to the years of mid-adolescence, which further underscores the need for their active involvement in their offspring's treatment.

Another important reason for active parental involvement in CERT concerns the importance of reestablishing reasonable parent–child interactions. As any parent can testify, part of the glue of the parent–child relationship is the ability of the child to respond positively to caregiving and nurturing parental behavior. However, a depressed child often is unaffectionate and unresponsive (Kovacs & Bastiaens, 1995), denies parents the satisfactions for which they strive (Coyne et al., 1992), and prompts negative parental responses. Such interactions can become recursive, disrupt the parent–child relationship, and undermine the attachment bond. Indeed, depressed children have troubled relationships with their parents, and even subclinical depression can adversely affect interactions with parents and siblings (e.g., Dietz et al., 2008; Messer & Gross, 1995; Puig-Antich et al., 1985a, 1985b). Indeed, it is not unusual that, by the time a family presents for help, the original psychosocial stress that instigated the child's depression is no longer salient. Rather, the child's depressive symptoms and behaviors, which triggered negative parent–child interactions, has become the major source of stress and the stimulus for seeking help. The active involvement of the parent affords the therapist the opportunity to fulfill one important (although implicit) goal of CERT, the *normalization of parent–child interactions,* particularly around affect-related topics.

The "Coaching" Model

In CERT, the therapist views the parent as an active partner, not as a "co-patient." The parent becomes involved in the child's treatment in several ways. The parent: (1) actively works with the therapist as the therapist selects treatment targets, (2) acts as information gatherer, facilitator, and observer by carrying out the agreed on plan or strategy with the child and reporting on its success or failure, and (3) provides both feedback and reinforcement to the child. To facilitate their involvement, parents are given a parent manual at the start of treatment that explains depression and the parent's role within the context of CERT, and also provides other key information. A reproducible copy is included in Appendix D.

The parental role as a helpful agent or collaborator establishes a particular bond between therapist and parent. A sports analogy then provides a framework for how the parent is expected to help and how the child is expected to contribute: The therapist is the "coach," the parent is the "assistant coach," while the child takes on the role of the special "player." The coach and assistant coach roles make it explicit that these two adults share the common goal of helping the child *and* that the focus of their interactions is the **child.** One consequence of this formulation is that, as assistant coach, the parent is expected to make objective observations of the child's behavior and thus becomes an information source for the therapist.

By defining the roles of the assistant coach and player and their implications in the presence of the young patient, the sports analogy also serves as a vehicle for **transparency:** The child now knows that the parent will have to report observations (and thus information is not being conveyed behind the child's back). Furthermore, the parental role as an assistant coach underscores that the young patient (not the parent) is the treatment focus. It is important to note, however, that while the parent plays a key role in CERT, the therapist has the final responsibility for the conduct, content, and format of treatment.

During each CERT session, the therapist takes every opportunity to get the parent involved as assistant coach in verbal exchanges: This can be introduced to the parent along the lines of "Can you now put on your coaching hat?" Furthermore, it is by identifying *coaching opportunities* for the parent that CERT provides the parent–child pair with the framework for new ways of interacting. Coaching opportunities can be structured as specific homework assignments or can be linked to the child's displays of adaptive (or maladaptive) mood repair responding.

Coaching interactions between parent and child (as well as between the therapist and the parent–child pair) *are guided by rules.* There are six rules for coaches and six rules for the child player. These are introduced in the first CERT session and are prominently displayed as posters in the treatment room. (See Posters 1 and 2 in Appendix B.) The rules are also included in the parent manual for CERT. (See Appendix D.)

Viewing the parent as a helping agent may not always be easy. For example, the parent could evidence behaviors or symptoms that may seem to be causally related to or reinforce the child's depression. The parent may appear to sabotage aspects of the child's treatment and/or divert the treatment focus from the child. However, focusing on the negative aspects of parental behavior is not likely to help the child. Instead (according to The Rules of Coaching), the therapist needs to focus on the strengths and assets of the parent to harvest them in the service of the child's treatment.

A Developmentally Informed and Individually Tailored Approach

The fact that CERT is developmentally informed is evident in several ways. As I discuss in Chapter 4, there is considerable emphasis on the therapist's use of age-appropriate language and oral communication. Furthermore, key elements of CERT are concretized for young patients by displaying illustrated posters in the treatment room. Foremost among these is the poster The House of Emotion Regulation. (See Appendix B, Poster 3.) This poster depicts the three functional domains of regulatory responding as "rooms" that contain corresponding "tools" (mood repair responses).

On a conceptual level, CERT acknowledges that there are developmentally mediated differences in the extent to which the various mood repair responses can be used effectively even among children of similar ages. For example, one depressed 11-year-old may successfully use cognitive reappraisal to minimize the effects of a depressogenic trigger, whereas another 11-year-old's cognitive mood repair repertoire may only extend to the use of attention refocusing. Furthermore, responses also can be deployed in a developmentally inappropriate manner. Consider, for instance, a 10-year-old girl whose mood repair responses rely on interpersonal regulators. If, under circumstances of distress, this child starts crying and typically waits for the parent to initiate mood repair, her method of trying to recruit the parent is characteristic of a much younger child.

CERT also takes into account that, independent of psychopathology, children's developmental stage (which encompasses both psychosocial and physiological maturation) constrains the range and sophistication of mood repair responses. While there are no standardized or formal ways to assess a child's developmental level vis-à-vis mood repair, the key developmental trends were discussed in Chapter 2. The therapist should be fully cognizant of these trends (as well as the developmental trajectories of the skills that underpin them). This means that the therapist's expectations should reflect patients' developmental levels. For example, it would therefore be unlikely to have the same mood repair expectations of a 12-year-old and a 7-year-old.

Intrinsic to a developmental approach is the recognition of individual differences. Indeed, an individually tailored approach to depressed youngsters lies at the heart of CERT. This means that, while CERT sets the same **overall** goals for all depressed children (symptom elimination and mood repair competence), the ways in which those goals are achieved will differ across patients even of the *same age and same developmental level.* For example, CERT does *not* assume that one mood regulatory domain is better or more desirable than another; instead, it focuses on the functional domain that is "the best fit" for or preferred by the particular child. Thus, CERT easily accommodates the fact that for one child, tender hugs from the parent along with reassuring words may be a guaranteed path to feeling better; for another distressed child, the promise of some rewarding activity may work magic; yet another child may need to be engaged in some absorbing task to attenuate distress. Furthermore, for one child, the therapist might need to focus on modifying key contextual features in the home (e.g., parental affect-related behavior), while for another child, the challenge may be to assist the parent in securing material resources relevant to mood repair (e.g., access to a basketball court).

The individually tailored approach of CERT also accommodates the fact that contextual and cultural differences affect the availability and utilization of mood repair responses. For example, it may be perfectly acceptable in one culture for teenage boys to hug each other as a way to alleviate emotional distress, whereas in another culture, such responses may cause boys unanticipated problems. Finally, an individually tailored treatment approach takes into consideration the fact that mood repair success is affected by children's temperament and existing parent–child interactions around affect displays. Thus, the CERT therapist works with the child within the framework of the child's developmental tendencies, functional strengths, and contextual reality. The flexibility inherent in CERT is captured in the following tenets:

- Youth vary in their inclinations and abilities to deploy responses from the behavioral, cognitive, and interpersonal response domains.
- Mood repair responses that "work" for some youth may not work for other youth.
- Youth vary in the extent to which their mood repair repertoires consist of adaptive versus maladaptive (and automatic vs. conscious) responses.
- Youth vary in the skills that underlie effective mood repair.
- The stage of psychosocial development (and likely neurocognitive maturation) mediates the type of mood repair responses on which a child can draw.

Goals, Pacing, and Duration of Treatment

CERT aims to reduce depressive symptoms and prevent relapse. These goals are achieved by focusing on the affective symptoms of depression, along with attending to other key symptoms as needed. A further (albeit implicit) goal is to normalize parent–child interactions particularly around topics that concern dysphoric emotions, moods, and their regulation.

CERT can be delivered across varying time periods, depending on individual need. Ideally, the duration of treatment should accommodate the temporal features of the child's depressive disorder. One possible rule of thumb is that the intervention should be about one-third (or more) of the length of the average episode of depressive disorder being targeted. That means, for example, that for psychiatrically referred (but medically well) children with major depression, CERT should be provided for *at least* 3 months, while for youngsters with dysthymic disorder, a treatment duration of about a year should be considered (see Chapter 1 for related information). However, in clinical practice, treatment duration may be constrained by financial issues, including the health insurance coverage of a family. In any case, it is highly advisable to have a *predefined treatment duration,* even if it is presented to the family as a goal that can be renegotiated at some later point in time.

Irrespective of its total duration, the intervention should include at least three phases that are distinguished in part by the "dosing" of sessions and in part by the goals of treatment. In Phases I and II, the major goals are reducing symptoms and reaching favorable emotional homeostasis. In Phase III, the goal turns to maintenance of treatment gains and prevention of depression recurrence through mood repair–related coping skills training. Thus, treatment should be delivered in a graduated fashion, with a decreasing "dosage" as follows:

Phase I: Intense intervention involving two sessions per week across an overall period of no longer than 2–4 weeks

Phase II: Regularly paced treatment, delivered on a once-a-week basis across a specified number of months

Phase III: Tapering and/or maintenance sessions separated by increasingly longer intervals, starting with 2 weeks and up to 4 or more weeks in between sessions across a specified number of months

The high frequency of contacts in the beginning helps to address the acute distress that usually accompanies initial presentation of pediatric depression. It also helps to actively engage the parent and lays the foundation for a therapeutic relationship. It was established quite a while ago that a substantial part of symptomatic improvement in adults occurs by the eighth session of psychotherapy (Howard et al., 1986); one would similarly expect an early response phase in child psychotherapy. Thereafter, weekly or less frequent sessions may be sufficient (and preferable) to achieve further symptom remission.

The therapeutic goal of Phase III in CERT is recurrence prevention, with an emphasis on the adaptive regulation of distress and a proactive approach to coping. As already noted, this phase focuses on affect-related coping skills training. The transition to Phase III takes place only after the child has few, if any, depressive symptoms. Coping skills training is most likely to be fruitful if implemented over an extended period of time with sufficiently long intervals between sessions to allow practice and consolidation of the learned information.

For example, given a child with major depression, a plan can include a 22-session intervention across a 6-month period, with 4 sessions in weeks 1 and 2, followed by weekly sessions until the end of month 4, and then tapering to 1 session every 2 weeks for months 5 and 6. In a treatment study of children with dysthymic disorder (a more protected form of depression; see Chapter 1), CERT was delivered as a 30-session intervention across a 10-month period (Kovacs et al., 2006). Month 1 included 2 sessions per week, and months 2–4 included weekly sessions (up to a total of 13 sessions). Tapering was delivered in two phases: 1 session every 2 weeks in months 5–6 and then monthly sessions across months 7–10.

To accommodate individual differences in the speed of therapeutic response, a young patient may be advanced across the various phases based on symptom criteria. For example, a predefined percent drop in initial depression severity (by self-rating or clinical evaluation) could be required to progress from Phase I to Phase II. Maintenance of gains may be required for several weeks before moving from Phase II to Phase III. In general, some combination of the just noted criteria (time, or number of sessions, along with symptom severity) may be the most useful guide to progress a patient across Phases I to III.

How CERT Accomplishes Its Goals

Overall Approach

CERT is directive. In practice, this means that the therapist explicitly sets the focus of the session and, as "head coach," makes sure that the session's actual content remains true to the goal. To accomplish this, each session starts with "setting an agenda," which is basically a session plan. Likewise, the CERT therapist is directive when she guides the family to focus on a particular symptom or complaint. The symptom-oriented chapters provide numerous examples of the directive nature of CERT.

CERT is skill-focused. This means that teaching, demonstration, and practice are important elements of each session. CERT's skill focus is one reason why homework assignments, and practicing mood repair responses and related skills, are key treatment components. The didactic aspects of CERT can take the form of psychoeducation, such as when the therapist explains to the parent–child pair CERT's approach to depression. However, CERT typically promotes an approach involving the therapist posing questions in ways that help the parent and child to connect the dots themselves.

CERT's skill focus also means that the therapist takes every opportunity to demonstrate (rather than just talk about) how mood repair works. For example, if a child experiences an upsurge in distress *within the session,* the therapist can demonstrate how to attenuate it by having the parent and child engage together in physical activity for a few minutes (like jumping jacks or vigorously throw a ball back and forth; see Chapter 6). The fact that physical activity can reduce the child's distress *in vivo* then is fodder for a discussion of "what just happened," including which aspect of the intervention (e.g., mood repair response domain) made it effective.

CERT is also a practical intervention: It recognizes that the needs of a given young patient at a given point in time may override directives in the treatment protocol. For example, although there are guidelines for topics to be covered in the first CERT session (see Chapter 6), the therapist can elect to address only some of them if the situation warrants it. Likewise, during coping skills training, practical considerations may limit the range of topics that are addressed. All in all, the empirical and practical approaches imbedded in CERT mean that the road to recovery is not straight, but is likely to include some trial and error on the part of the therapist and the parent–child pair.

Symptom Reduction

Young patients can manifest a variety of depressive and nondepressive symptoms; parents may also identify behavioral issues, including the child not listening, having tantrums, or being disrespectful of elders. The CERT therapist prioritizes the reduction of affective symptoms of depression (see Chapter 7) but can readily intervene with nonaffective symptoms as well (see Chapter 8). However, the nature of some acute symptoms may not be clear, while other symptoms may persist or change across contexts or interactions. The template for working with target symptoms offered in the next section can help the CERT therapist decide how to approach a symptom and what to do about it.

A Template for Working with Target Symptoms

The template identifies five steps for working with a target symptom. For some symptoms, the sequence listed here may be followed exactly. However, interventions with some other symptoms may emphasize only some of the five problem-solving features of the template. In addition to the two brief examples given, the symptom-focused chapters (principally Chapters 7 and 8) contain further illustrations of how parts of this template can be applied.

The five steps for working with a target symptom are: symptom verification, contextual mapping of the symptom, symptom (re)formulation (if warranted), selecting an intervention point and strategy, and assessing the outcome of the intervention. See also Table 3.1.

1. ***Symptom verification:*** The therapist, parent, and child need to agree on what the target symptom is, that it has been present recently, and that it has been a problem. As amply illustrated in this book, it is very important to clarify what the symptom is. For example, what parents may perceive as intentional meanness on

TABLE 3.1. Steps for Working with a Target Symptom

Symptom verification
Contextual mapping of the symptom
Symptom (re)formulation (if warranted)
Selecting an intervention point and strategy
Assessing the outcome of the intervention

the part of their child often turns out to be extreme irritability. It is also important to identify and isolate the most recent example of the symptom. If agreement cannot be reached on these three points, work should not proceed on the symptom in question and an alternative target should be selected.

2. ***Contextual mapping of the symptom:*** Symptoms are embedded in particular contexts, which can have ramifications for how the therapist elects to intervene. For any symptom, it is helpful to identify at least three contextual elements: the interpersonal interactions within which the symptom became manifest, the behavioral and environmental antecedents or concomitants of the symptom, and the interpretations attached to the symptom by key actors. More specifically, a symptom is mapped by asking, "what, how, when, who, and where" it occurred. The resulting information helps the therapist to select an intervention point. For example, the therapist may focus on the parent–child interactions that typically precede a symptom for a given child in order to reduce the likelihood of its occurrence. Or, the intervention focus may be to reduce the child's tantrum that occurs concomitant with his display of acute dysphoria.

3. ***Symptom (re)formulation (if warranted):*** With some families, it may be necessary or useful at times to formulate (or reformulate) what a symptom signifies in order to place it within the explanatory framework of CERT, provide parent and child with a new way of looking at that difficulty, and lessen the sense of personal blame for the patient's and family's dysfunction. One formulation of a symptom is that it is a sign of depression. For example, if the parents regard a depressed child's lack of interest in joining family functions as being oppositional, the behavior can be reformulated as mirroring the anhedonic aspect of depression. The symptom also can be reformulated as resulting from the child's problems in mood repair, rather than as evidence of willful disobedience.

4. ***Selecting an intervention point and strategy:*** Should the therapist focus on the symptom itself, its precursors, or its consequences? That is a clinical decision, which is influenced by the nature of the symptom. As noted in a prior example, if the target depressive symptom arises amid a parent–child dispute (symptom antecedent), then the therapist may wish to focus on and resolve the interpersonal interactions between parent and child and thereby reduce the child's exposure to that particular depressogenic process. Such stress reduction can be especially helpful early in treatment when the patient–therapist alliance is still being formed. But if the symptom is known to have multiple adverse effects (e.g., marked sleep disturbance), then it needs to be the treatment target. Later in this chapter, various intervention strategies are listed that the CERT therapist may use to alleviate depression symptoms.

5. ***Assessing the outcome of the intervention:*** After an intervention has been applied, the next step is to assess its outcome: Did it achieve its goal? If not, why not? Exactly when this step is implemented depends on whether the intervention

is applied in the treatment session (in which case, its effects can be immediately recognized), or if it is to be carried out by the child and parent as part of a homework assignment (in which case, the outcome can be reviewed only at the next session).

Intervention Strategies

An intervention strategy may be deployed in-session or assigned as part of homework for the parent and child to implement between sessions. The therapist can draw from a broad array of focused and goal-directed techniques that have been documented in the professional literature as feasible and effective with pediatric samples, as follows:

- **Behavioral techniques:** These techniques require the child or parent to engage in a specific action or overt behavior. It can involve assignments that the parent and child complete together, such as keeping a log of a target behavior, monitoring of symptom frequency and/or severity, "behavioral experiments," or keeping "temperature charts" of moods. It may entail the parent setting up differential reinforcement schedules for the child. Other examples include implementing various behavioral regulatory responses to dysphoria, such as assigning physical exercise to be performed by the child at preset occasions or intervals, having the parent and child engage in affect-related interpersonal interactions like long hugs twice each evening, implementing a sleep hygiene protocol, role playing within or outside the session, social skills training, or improving communication skills.

- **Cognitive techniques:** Cognitive techniques are used in CERT differently than they are in traditional cognitive therapy. In cognitive therapy, cognitive techniques are used to correct the patient's negative and biased information processing about the self and related issues; in contrast, in CERT, cognitive techniques are used to reinforce adaptive cognitive regulatory responses and deter the deployment of maladaptive cognitive responses to sadness and dysphoria.

The following cognitive techniques can help the child to interrupt sadness and/or thoughts that maintain or worsen it: visual and/or auditory imagery (e.g., a magic sign or phrase, "Pretend in your head . . . ," "Make believe you see a picture of . . . ," "Sing a song in your head"); thought interference (e.g., "Think of an opposing idea"); refocusing attention on a nonaffective problem-solving task (e.g., picture puzzle, word puzzle); thought substitution using nonaffective content ("Think about the room layout of your house," "Think about a favorite object"); or using positive affective content (recalling a fun-filled or happy event). With older youth, the therapist may try to counter cognitions that exacerbate distress with cognitions that entail alternate and neutral interpretations of the source and implications of the distress.

• **Contextual–environmental manipulation:** Changes in a child's physical environment can bring about surprising improvement in various depressive symptoms. Here are several examples: reducing negative stimulation by changing physical features of the home environment, such as where the child sleeps (see the discussion of sleep disturbance in Chapter 8) or does his homework; altering aspects of the school environment, such as changing the child's sitting arrangement in a classroom to facilitate attention; and working with community resources to provide safe exercise space to be used for behavioral mood regulatory responses.

Relapse and Recurrence Prevention

As the child achieves symptom relief, the focus of CERT turns to the maintenance of treatment gains, and the prevention of depressive relapse and recurrence. This part of CERT is called *coping skills training*, which includes emotion regulation coping goals and problem-solving coping goals. The concepts and strategies that were articulated to the child and parent in the symptom-reduction phase of the treatment become the basis of a preventative and hence a proactive (as opposed to a palliative and reactive) perspective. This shift in framework prepares the child and parent for the fact that recovery from the current episode by itself is unlikely to alter future risk of depression. However, continuous efforts at adaptive mood repair responding and willingness to strengthen one's existing mood repair response repertoire should lower the likelihood of depression recurrence.

Coping skills training focuses on the child's mood repair strengths (while remaining mindful of vulnerabilities) and builds in great measure on what the child and parent have learned and achieved throughout the symptom-reduction phase of CERT. It also introduces problem-solving coping as either a proactive or reactive response to impending or existing stressors, as one way to minimize their depressogenic effects. Coping skills training focuses on the following issues:

- Ongoing reinforcement of adaptive mood repair responses that have "worked" for the young patient to reduce dysphoria
- Ways to strengthen further the young patient's existing adaptive mood repair response repertoire
- Awareness of personally significant depressogenic stressors
- Use of proactive and reactive problem solving to eliminate stressors or mitigate their depressogenic effects

By the time this phase of CERT is reached, the therapist will have considerable information about the child's and parent's achievements in CERT and the child's depression history, including depressogenic stressful events (or processes). Based on such information, the therapist formulates a tentative "training plan" with specific goals for the child and how to best achieve them, which is then implemented by the parent–child pair.

Coping skills training differs from the symptom-reduction phase of CERT in several ways. One difference is that coping skills training involves substantially more teaching (didactics) or psychoeducation. The purpose of didactics is to help the child–parent pair identify and integrate what they have learned in treatment, distill essential lessons that may be of help in the future, and provide conceptual schemata that will serve to anchor information about a preventative approach to depression. Additionally, coping skills training is future-oriented, while the symptom-reduction phase is present-oriented. Finally, because coping skills training is implemented while the frequency of patient–therapist contact is reduced (as noted earlier), this third phase of CERT also involves considerable demands for self-motivation and self-reinforcement on the part of the child and parent.

Homework: Why, How, and What

Homework assignments are an essential part of CERT and present the greatest demand for parent–child treatment adherence. In CERT, *homework* refers to a task that is assigned to the parent–child pair to complete before the next therapy session. Because homework usually involves gathering evidence or information, and changing behavior or aspects of the child's environment, it typically requires the use of one or more of the techniques noted in the prior section "Intervention Strategies." With few exceptions (usually involving adolescents), homework assignments are implemented by the parent serving as the coach to the child.

The Why of Homework

One reason for homework assignments is that the results provide the therapist with factually more accurate information than the family's narrative recall of events. The importance of getting parents and children to monitor and report on tasks in real time cannot be overemphasized because research has shown that memory is reconstructive and both negative and positive mood act to bias (to filter) the way in which memories are recalled. Consequently, the narrative information the therapist obtains in the session from child or parent is likely to be somewhat distorted as compared to the actual flow of events. For example, a frustrated mother may recall a day when her daughter was "always cranky." But a homework assignment involving the mother and child completing a mood log each morning and evening may show, for example, that the child was cranky in the evening but not during the day (see Appendix A, Forms 5–7, for examples you can photocopy and/or download). The therapist can use this information to explore the context of the irritable mood and factors that feed into it. The results of homework assignments also provide the therapist with information on whether the therapeutic decisions were appropriate and suitable to the young patient's needs.

Another important reason for homework assignments is that many of them provide the parent–child pair with the opportunity to implement approaches, behaviors, and mood repair skills that have been addressed in the therapy sessions. Recall that CERT seeks to reduce the child's depressive symptoms and teach the parent and child to be more effective in managing the child's dysphoric affect in everyday life. These goals can only be accomplished by an iterative process that involves the parent–child pair repeatedly implementing specific symptom-reduction and mood repair tasks outside the treatment setting. Learning new skills or improving existing ones requires practice, which can be facilitated by the structured nature of homework assignments.

And finally, homework assignments in CERT provide the parent–child pair with a new paradigm for interacting with one another in daily life. This is important because, as already noted, by the time they seek treatment, the interactions between parents and their depressed children tend to be conflictual and dysfunctional. However, homework assignments involve specific roles and rules as well as a commonly agreed on goal. The parent serves as coach, the child is the team player, and the rules of coaching and of being a good player have to be followed: These features maximize the likelihood of positive outcomes. Additionally, a well-designed homework assignment gives the parent–child pair the opportunity to engage in role-appropriate interactions and thereby serves as implicit proof that the parent–child relationship can be mended.

The How: Rules for Assigning Homework

There are three rules for assigning homework:

Rule 1: The therapist must have a clear rationale for the homework, which is integrated with the goal of treatment at that point in time. A task assigned just to give the parent–child pair something to do is unlikely to be completed and unlikely to contribute to therapeutic progress.

Rule 2: The young patient and the parent both have to understand the reasons for the assignment; the reasons have to "make sense" to them.

Rule 3: The assignment has to be doable. In other words, the parent–child pair must have the internal and external resources to implement the assignment. Even if the results are negative, or not as expected, completion of homework assignments greatly furthers therapeutic progress.

To implement these rules, the homework has to be discussed and rehearsed in detail, with the following questions in mind:

Does it make sense to parent and child?

Do parent and child understand how it can help to deal with the symptom or target problem?

Do parent and child believe that they will be able to implement the assignment?

Homework assignments should be graded across CERT sessions. This means that the CERT therapist must start with relatively simple tasks, even if the child presents as unusually precocious and the parent as very eager. The first one or two homework assignments should involve monitoring no more than two important parameters, for example, the occurrence of irritable mood (yes/no) using an hourly log and the patient's location at logging. Tasks can gradually be increased in complexity by adding further parameters: For example, while monitoring irritable mood, each occurrence can be rated on a severity scale as well.

With all homework assignments, the therapist presents the strategy, explains its rationale, obtains parent–child agreement on its implementation, and reviews in detail with the family how to do it. It is especially important for the therapist to ask the parent and the child to explain, in their own words, their understanding of the homework assignment. The therapist must listen carefully for signs of any misunderstanding of the nature of the assignment, which needs to be corrected.

For example, after a therapist asks a parent about her understanding of a mood-monitoring homework, it is not unusual early in the treatment for the parent to respond along the lines of "You want me to write down for you each time [the child] is cranky and upset." The therapist needs to correct such a statement by saying, "I don't think I explained this homework well" and then adding, "It is not that I want this, but that it is a good idea because it will help us to see if there is a pattern to [the child's] distress, so then we can talk about what we could do about it." The corrective statement emphasizes that the homework is a collaborative task, one which will yield information that can be used on the path to help the child feel better. The symptom-focused chapters provide examples of how homework assignments are introduced and used in CERT.

The What: Types of Homework

There are two general categories of homework assignment: tasks that involve monitoring and recording, and behavioral experiments that involve some action with the goal of changing some variable. However, the range and content of homework assignments are limited only by the imagination of the therapist and the topic.

Monitoring and Recording. Monitoring or recording of symptoms, mood, and behavior is the strategy of choice in the beginning of therapy; it is the simplest and easiest to do. This type of homework provides the therapist with real-time data regarding the ebb and flow of the young patient's emotions, symptoms, and behaviors and the effects of context on them. The therapist also can use the successful completion of this assignment as proof of the ability of the parent and child to effectively work together to help the child get well. Thus, completed monitoring homework can provide parent and child with a sense of accomplishment early in treatment.

The easiest monitoring and recording procedure is completion of a daily log of any given behavior, activity, mood state, or context. A log can focus on how *frequently* a particular behavior or symptom occurs on a typical day (e.g., recorded as a "yes" or "no"). The recording window can be the entire day until the child goes to bed or only selected segments, such as after school or after dinner. See Appendix A, Forms 5 and 6, for reproducible daily feelings logs to track dysphoric mood.

After the child and parent have mastered simple monitoring, they can be asked to provide information about additional dimensions, such as how severe or disruptive a given symptom or complaint was (rated on a Likert-type scale). A further rating dimension can be the context at the time that the mood is logged (e.g., at school, at home) or the child's reaction to her affect (e.g., "Write down what you did or thought when you had this bad feeling"). Form 7 in Appendix A is a blank reproducible version of a daily log of affect, including severity ratings and context.

When monitoring affect intensity with younger children, line drawings of faces can be used to indicate the strength or severity of the target experience. Alternatively, colors can be used, with dark blue signifying great sadness or upset and increasingly paler blue colors signifying less and less sadness or upset. If a numeric scale is used with younger children, it should be simple, ranging, for example, from 1 (little; not strong) to 4 (a lot; very strong). Older children should be able to rate affect intensity on a more differentiated numeric scale (e.g., from 0 = not at all to 9 = very strong). To lessen response bias, try to avoid a metric with a natural midpoint. A more difficult assignment, generally suitable only for older children (and their parents), is monitoring both the affect and the young patient's response to it. An equally challenging monitoring task is to record target cognitions or thoughts that emerge in association with particular mood states. These types of assignments require trial runs in the session so that the therapist can determine whether the assignment is understood and if the child can complete it on her own.

Behavioral Experiments. Some homework assignments are defined as experiments because: (1) They involve attempts to change or explore something and (2) neither the therapist nor the parent–child pair know the outcome beforehand. The results will be learned only after the assignment has been attempted. Most behavioral experiments entail overt behavior change, including the implementation of new mood repair responses. Note that, by definition, in an experiment, both negative and positive results are equally important and informative! Chapters 7 and 8 contain examples of homework assignments focused on adaptive mood repair responses that were presented by the therapist as behavioral experiments.

Homework Compliance and Noncompliance

Because most families may not be familiar with the concept and practice of therapeutic homework assignments, do not expect perfect compliance. It is not uncommon in the beginning of CERT for many parent–child pairs to return to the next session with partially completed homework assignments or assignments that were executed incorrectly. However, families should always be praised for any effort that has been exerted on behalf of homework, even if the task was not completed or was executed incorrectly (e.g., "I am really happy to see that you gave [the task] a try! This is very important—and you can now tell me about it!"). The fact that the parent and child had tried to implement an assignment signals that both are engaged in the treatment.

If there is full noncompliance, the therapist should make every effort to determine the reasons for it. During such questioning, be sure to be supportive, which can be conveyed by statements like the following:

> *Yes, homework can be a real pain and hard to do, so why do you think you had trouble getting it done?*
>
> *I was wondering if I explained it to you correctly. Was the explanation too complicated?*

It is particularly important to find out whether noncompliance reflects solvable issues such as the parent–child pair having failed to understand or agree with the homework's rationale and/or not having the needed resources, or the homework being too taxing or cumbersome.

If task complexity was the reason for noncompliance, simplifying a homework assignment by breaking it into subcomponents (if possible) can facilitate its completion. Further explaining the homework's rationale may motivate young patients and parents, who otherwise may have failed to see any beneficial consequences of the homework. And proposing an alternate homework may be the solution if noncompliance reflects insufficient parental resources. Parents and young patients also can be asked to propose modifications to some homework. Regardless, always be willing to negotiate the scope of any homework.

In closing this chapter, I wish to reemphasize the importance of homework in CERT. In the earlier phases of treatment, homework assignments generate very important information for the therapist and provide the parent–child pair with learning experiences. And depending on the issues at hand, homework assignments can comprise significant portions of a child's coping skills training.

Chapter 4

Getting Ready to Deliver CERT

To deliver contextual emotion regulation therapy (CERT), the therapist must be prepared to meet the general demands of a therapeutic relationship with children and the specific demands of this emotion regulation–focused intervention. Namely, the therapist is mindful of nonspecific factors that facilitate the psychotherapeutic process (e.g., empathy) and developmental issues (e.g., extent of language skills) that constrain psychotherapy with children. The therapist is ready to enter into the CERT mindset (see Chapter 3), engage the parent–child pair, and focus on the young patient's dysphoric affect and its regulation. The therapist also recognizes that the generic treatment plan provided here has to be customized for the given young patient and delivered via a standardized session structure.

Finally, because CERT makes extensive use of props and didactic aids, the therapist prepares the treatment room. CERT-related posters (see Appendix B) should be affixed at eye level on the treatment room's walls or displayed in other appropriate ways. Additional aids to be provided include toys and objects that can serve to engage young patients; small bins labeled with key emotions into which the children can place marbles or other small objects to indicate severity or strength of a given affect; as well as a jump rope, a ball, and mats that can help to implement *in vivo* behavioral responses to dysphoria.

Prepare the Treatment Room

The chairs for the therapist, parent, and child should be arranged as a triangle to allow full visual communication among all parties. To facilitate the treatment process and because some youngsters may be unable to use oral communication to express themselves, CERT utilizes various visual and behavioral aids. Some visual aids, such as posters, also help the child and family to remember key constructs.

The liberal use of props, graphical aids, and other illustrative materials is encouraged.

Posters

Posters that display key CERT concepts and rules should be affixed to the wall of the therapy room at heights that make them easy to see and read. They are frequently referred to during the course of treatment to teach and reinforce basic concepts. The therapist can point to a poster while discussing its content and young patients may be asked to read text aloud from a poster.

The posters used in CERT are next described; Appendix B provides facsimiles that can be copied and enlarged for use in the therapy room. The text of these posters also appears in the Manual for Parents (Appendix D), which is provided to parents prior to the first session. Posters also can be homemade by therapists to provide more details or to meet specific needs of young patients and their families.

The Rules of Coaching

The six rules listed on Poster 1 are meant for the *parent-coach,* but children also can take advantage of them. For example, one of our young patients noted in a treatment session that during a specific homework assignment, his mother did not quite follow one of the rules of coaching; she criticized rather than positively reinforced the child.

A Good Coach

1. **Focuses** on the player's abilities and strengths.
2. **Works** with the player on new ways to do things.
3. **Helps** the player to use different abilities to reach goals.
4. **Praises and encourages** the player to keep going!
5. **Hangs in there** and works with the player even if the coach had a bad day!
6. **Learns and practices** because coaches are made, not born.

The Rules of Being a Good Team Player

Poster 2 shows a set of rules intended for the child-patient. If warranted, a copy can be provided to children for their own use.

A Good Team Player

1. **Will try new ways** to do things.
2. **Works with the coaches** on game plans and goals.

3. **Uses words** to tell the coaches how he or she feels.
4. **Asks for help** when things get tough or confusing.
5. **Does *not* give up** even if a game plan doesn't work right away.
6. **Practices, practices, practices** because that's what it takes to reach a goal.

The House of Emotion Regulation

Poster 3 in Appendix B, The House of Emotion Regulation, is a child-friendly graphic that represents the three mood repair response domains as discussed in Chapter 2 (and also calls attention to their physiological infrastructure). Each domain is depicted as a room in the house that contains specific mood repair "tools" or responses. The number of tools listed on the sample poster in Appendix B is constrained by size. On a larger poster created by the therapist, additional tools could be listed in the various rooms. For example:

The Thinking (Cognitive) Room

Imagine a magic picture, word, or phrase.

Count backward from a specific number.

Think of a funny idea or scenario.

Sing a special song in your head.

Read something interesting.

Imagine yourself in a different or favorite place.

Think about a favorite thing.

Imagine the stores in the shopping mall you usually visit.

Plan your next birthday party in your head.

Think differently about something that is upsetting.

The People (Social–Interpersonal) Room

Ask your mom, dad, or grandparent for a hug.

Talk to your mom or dad about the feelings you are having.

Talk to your friends about what is going on.

Spend time and do fun things with your friends.

Ask your family or friends for help to feel better.

Help someone who needs help (a grandparent or friend with a disability).

Ask your favorite teacher for help.

Talk to a counselor or minister.

The Things to Do (Action or Behavioral) Room

Choose an exercise or sport (do some push-ups, swim, jump rope, walk, shoot baskets, etc.).

Work on a project or hobby (rearrange your closet, update your baseball card collection, knit, build toy trains).

Pick up an old hobby or start a new one.

Fix things that are broken or otherwise need care.

Play with toys or a game.

Do a personal chore, like clean your room.

Help with a family chore, like washing the car.

Sing, dance, listen to happy (high tempo) music.

Take a bath.

Paint, draw, do other forms of art.

Make brownies, help with dinner, go grocery shopping with Dad.

Go to the movies with your mom, dad, or siblings.

Learn a relaxation exercise such as yoga.

In addition to the rooms of emotion regulation, the House of ER poster includes an acknowledgment that regulatory efforts have biological or physiological foundations. In practical terms, what that means is that young patients' physiological functioning and well-being influence their emotion regulatory efforts. For example, as discussed in Chapter 2, attention is one of the basic skills that support regulatory processes. Experimental and neuroimaging work have shown that attention is supported by the interactions of various brain cortical and subcortical circuits (Knudsen, 2018; Miller & Buschman, 2013). Therefore, events that may impair cortical functioning (e.g., a fever, poorly controlled diabetes) are also likely to have a negative effect on a child's attempts at mood repair. The therapist has to decide whether a discussion of the physiological foundations of emotion regulation is likely to be helpful to a given child and family, which will partly be a function of the young patient's age as well as the nature of the potentially impairing events.

WWW.Solve: Solving a Problem

Poster 4 (Appendix B) displays problem-solving steps that can be applied in some stressful situations. Chapter 10 contains examples of its application.

W **What** is the problem?
W **Who** can help to solve this problem?
W **Ways** to solve this problem.

Children's Facial Expression of Emotions

A large poster of facial emotion expressions can help young patients to identify their emotions and moods. There are various *commercially* available posters that show children's facial displays. Because these products frequently undergo changes, I have no recommendations. However, experience suggests that portraits of actual faces may be more appropriate than line drawings of them. Please make certain that the displayed faces are diverse.

An alternative is to create a poster using a wide array of emojis to represent emotional expressions. It may be particularly useful to locate "stick-on" emojis that the young patient can use to indicate the severity of a target emotion when engaged in affect monitoring.

Behavioral Aids

Various tools and objects can serve as behavioral aids for children. These should be placed next to the young patient's chair, or on a table in a basket or similar display unit, so that they are readily available. Include a collection of different-colored marbles (or glass pebbles) that can be sorted into bins labeled with the names of specific emotions (sadness, anger, unhappiness, upset, fear, happiness). The youngster then can indicate "how big" each emotion is at a given point in time by the relative number of marbles he places in the designated emotion bins. To show changes in those emotions after some event or intervention has taken place, the child can sort marbles into a second set of bins labeled with the same emotions.

To convey how "big" a given emotion (or behavioral tendency) is at a particular moment, plain LEGO or Jenga blocks can be assembled to different heights. Such a representation can then be compared to the same emotion (or behavioral tendency) as displayed, or not, after some response was deployed in the treatment session. Pencils, highlighters, and crayons, along with drawing paper, should also be made available to help the young patient keep her hands busy and to depict (draw a picture of) the emotion she is experiencing. A whiteboard (along with colored markers) is additionally very useful and can make it easier for young patients to illustrate certain concepts.

Jump rope, various-sized balls, and an exercise mat should also be available to facilitate the *in vivo* deployment of behavioral mood repair strategies. Finally, if young patients become restless or impatient, access to objects such as a wiggle ball, Etch A Sketch, and Slinky can help them to settle down. Such objects are familiar and provide a form of physical/manual engagement.

The Therapeutic Framework

The CERT therapist's mental template regarding the cause of depression and its optimal treatment (described in Chapter 3) will largely frame interactions with patients, along with the treatment's highly collaborative nature and its emphasis on the use of evidence from daily life to resolve issues. The use of evidence in therapy has been labeled collaborative empiricism (Beck et al., 1979), although *guided collaborative empiricism* is a more accurate description. In practice, guided collaborative empiricism is a process that is directive, skill-focused, and practical within the framework of a supportive therapeutic relationship.

Guided Collaborative Empiricism

Working in a collaborative manner requires the active participation of the therapist, parent, and child. Consequently, therapy is not something being done to the patient and family, but a process in which change is achieved in large measure through the efforts of the child and parent. However, the collaboration that occurs in therapy differs from other forms of collaboration.

Iconic therapists long ago sought to identify unique features of the psychotherapeutic process. For example, Sullivan (1954) specified that the therapeutic collaboration involves a trained mental health professional who guides the patient in resolving specific difficulties. A parent may generate four possible approaches to a particular problem, but the therapist might believe that one of these approaches will exacerbate the problem. Therefore, the job of the therapist is to steer the parent toward the more helpful possibilities and avoid the potentially harmful alternative. Or, a family may generate a list of several problem behaviors to be addressed. Based on clinical experience, the therapist might decide that several problems are too deeply entrenched to be readily workable. The job of the therapist is to guide the family toward working with the more easily remedied problem and thus provide the family with an initial successful experience.

The CERT therapist facilitates collaboration in the session through a variety of means, such as routinely asking the parent–child pair for feedback regarding the therapist's statements and about treatment targets and intervention strategies. Here are some examples of questions the therapist may use to encourage participation of the parent–child pair during the treatment session:

I want to be sure that what I said about [the child's] depression makes sense. So, can you tell me your understanding of what we just talked about?

Let me go over the homework again. Do these [summarize the key features] make sense to you? Do you see any problems in doing this homework?

What I think you are telling me is [summarize the parent's or child's response] do I have it right?

Let me summarize what we just discussed [review the content or theme of the conversation] is that how you see it?

Empiricism refers to making decisions based on objective information that has been gathered through observations, behavioral experiments, and other practical approaches. Homework assignments (discussed in Chapter 3) are key vehicles for empirical data gathering. Empiricism also means that the therapist does not dictate decisions or present potential solutions as right or wrong. Rather, the therapist encourages the parent–child pair to gather the needed information, which will be used for further decisions, and to experiment with alternative ways of resolving difficulties.

Taking an empirical stance also helps the therapist to disentangle facts from emotional reactions to, or personal interpretations of, facts. For example, one parent was upset that her child was "always sad and never wants to do anything." Instead of disagreeing or agreeing with this conclusion, the therapist sought more information. The parent and child agreed to keep a log in which the child's mood was recorded multiple times each day. The log revealed that the child was sad at home and mostly in late evening, but not at school. Faced with this empirical information, the emphasis shifted to uncovering depressogenic triggers in the home, along with the young patient's regulatory responses that could be perpetuating the dysphoric mood.

Empiricism also helps to maintain a nonjudgmental attitude toward symptoms. In the just noted example, the conclusion that the child was sad more often at home was not introduced with the question "What's wrong at home?" Instead, it was discussed as one source of data about the youngster, something that could be understood better in the context of further information. Therefore, the parent continued to use a mood log to monitor contextual variables that might affect the child's moods at home. The resulting log revealed that it was mostly during times when the parent had to attend to another offspring in the evenings that the child tended to become physically inactive and sad. The empirical method therefore helped the parent and child to better identify the nature of the problem at hand.

A Directive, Skill-Focused, and Practical Approach

As noted in Chapter 3, CERT is directive, skill-focused, and practical. The directive nature of CERT is at play when the therapist explicitly sets the goals of each session and, as head coach, ensures that the session's content runs true to the planned goals as much as possible. Thus, each session starts with *setting the agenda,* which is basically a session plan (for an example, see the section titled "Opening Statement: Setting the Stage" below). Likewise, the CERT therapist is directive when she guides the family to focus on a particular symptom or complaint. The symptom-oriented chapters provide numerous examples of the directive nature of CERT.

CERT's skill focus means that teaching, demonstration, role playing, and practice are important therapeutic elements. It is one reason why homework assignments, and practicing mood repair responses and related skills, are key treatment components.

CERT is also practical; it recognizes that the needs of a given young patient at a given point in time may override directives in the treatment protocol presented here. For instance, although there are guidelines for topics to be covered in the first CERT session (see Chapter 6), the therapist can elect to address only some of them if the situation so warrants. Likewise, during coping skills training, practical considerations may limit the range of topics that can be addressed. All in all, the empirical and practical approaches embedded in CERT mean that the road to recovery is not straight, but likely to include some trial and error on the part of the therapist and the parent–child pair.

Supportive Therapeutic Relationship

Getting ready to deliver CERT means that the therapist is prepared to establish a supportive therapeutic relationship. Although this is believed to be necessary when working with young patients (McDermott & Char, 1984), most of the related theoretical literature has concerned adults and empirical research has remained scarce (for an overview, see DiGiuseppe et al., 1996). One of the giants of psychotherapy, Carl Rogers (1961, 1980), whose influence continues to shape the field, posited that empathic understanding, genuineness, and unconditional positive regard are key elements of a therapeutic relationship. Beck et al. (1979) likewise proposed that warmth, accurate empathy, and genuineness on the part of the therapist are important treatment factors. In general, there is agreement that empathy, genuineness, and trust are the building blocks of a supportive therapeutic relationship.

One feature of a therapeutic relationship, *empathy*, has been described as the therapist entering into the patient's feelings and inner reality and experiencing them almost as if they were his own (Rogers, 1961) The therapist's empathy can be communicated as "unconditional positive regard" (Rogers, 1961) or as congruence between therapist and patient on emotional and intellectual levels (Beck et al., 1979), which can be conveyed through empathic verbal responses, body language and eye contact, and accurate summaries of the child's and parent's statements. *Genuineness*, another feature of a therapeutic relationship, means that the therapist experiences himself as an integrated person, can express appropriate emotional reactions, and can admit to being fallible. Genuineness does **not** mean being inappropriately personal or blunt. Finally, *trust* has long been regarded as an essential component of therapist–patient exchanges (e.g., Sullivan, 1954). In general, trust is a process that builds gradually in psychotherapy. It is facilitated by the confidentiality inherent in therapy and by the therapist behaving in a consistent, reliable, and predictable manner, maintaining a consistently noncritical stance, and not making promises that cannot be kept.

However, it is questionable that children and young adolescents experience therapeutic trust in the same way as adults do partly because trust is a cognitively based and developmentally mediated phenomenon (Hermes et al., 2018). Although empirical data are scant and much of what is known derives from studies of economic decision making (e.g., Evans et al., 2013; Sutter & Kocher, 2007) or social perspective taking (van den Bos et al., 2010), it appears that trust increases in a typically linear fashion, that developmental gains can be detected even when 9-year-olds are compared to 12-year-olds (Sutter & Kocher, 2007; van den Bos et al., 2010), and that aspects of trust continue to develop through adolescence (e.g., Wray-Lake & Flanagan, 2012). More psychologically oriented research suggests that between the ages of 7 and 11, trust involves reciprocity, namely, "You'll do something for him, and he'll do something for you" (Selman et al., 1977). It may not be until age 12 or later that children experience trust as involving the sharing of interpersonal concerns (Kovacs, 1986). Therefore, it may be appropriate for the CERT therapist to engage with the young patient in some form of reciprocal exchange to facilitate trust, such as to accept and display in the treatment room a drawing made by the young patient.

The therapeutic relationship in child psychotherapy has become a topic of research interest. According to a meta-analysis of child and adolescent psychotherapy studies, there is a modest but consistent positive association between treatment outcome and the therapeutic relationship across both behavioral and nonbehavioral interventions (Shirk & Karver, 2003). Furthermore, in one study of depressed, suicidal adolescents, the quality of the therapeutic alliance was more contributory to outcome in a cognitive-behavioral than in a nondirective, supportive intervention (Karver et al., 2008). Thus, the therapeutic relationship is an important component of manualized, directive interventions, including CERT.

Effective Use of Language

As with most forms of psychotherapy, CERT relies on spoken language as its primary means of communication. While supervising child psychotherapists over several decades, I frequently observed the failure of many trainees to monitor their own verbalizations, which often included college-level words and phrases. Thus, getting ready to deliver CERT also means that the therapist becomes mindful of the way she communicates and uses language. Effective use of language is important not only with regard to oral communication, but also when it comes to written materials that serve as props during CERT. To optimize accurate communication, an attempt should be made to adhere to the following guidelines.

Use Simple Words, Be Explicit, Be Clear

Several lines of evidence underscore that the therapist has to be mindful of his language. Language skills, including comprehension and expression, are developmentally mediated and substantially shaped by education. Thus, children of any age can vary widely in their language skills and even a 14-year-old may not comprehend text that mirrors a third-grade reading level. Additionally, the parents may have limited communication skills. For example, a national literacy survey found that up to 23% of the adult population functions at the lowest level of literacy (involving very simple skills such as following instructions on a questionnaire) and that an additional 25–28% have somewhat better but still limited literacy skills (Kirsch et al., 2002). Importantly, this survey also determined that performance and self-perception do not correspond; many people at the lowest literacy levels rated themselves as having good English-language skills.

Given both child developmental and adult verbal competency considerations, it is therefore critical for CERT therapists to use the plainest possible vocabulary and avoid complicated sentences. This is important not only because the patient is a child, but also because the more sophisticated and complex the words and sentences, the more likely that a miscommunication may occur. It can be helpful for the therapist to videotape or audiotape several treatment sessions and then review them with a focus on the vocabulary level used. In general, the best approach is to use language at lower-grade reading levels. Here are a few examples of desirable and undesirable utterances:

Say . . .	*Rather than . . .*
"We will try . . . "	"We shall attempt . . . "
"Things you did show . . . "	"Your behavior mirrors . . . "
"We'll work together . . . "	"We will collaborate . . . "
"I would like to know about . . . "	"I need feedback regarding . . . "
"You did a great job of . . . "	"It was commendable that . . . "
"One important thing in CERT . . . "	"A salient feature of CERT . . . "
"Why did you . . . ?"	"What motivated you to . . . ?"
"I will call you . . . "	"I will reach out to you . . . "

Clear and explicit communication also means that the therapist answers direct questions and avoids language that is tangential or vague. For example, if the parent or child asks a question to which the therapist does **not** know the answer, it is better to say, "I don't know, let me think about this," rather than to beat around the bush or answer with another question. But being explicit and clear does *not* mean being rude or inappropriate. For example, if a mother is not paying attention in the session, the therapist could say: "You seem to have something on your mind, is it something we should talk about?", which is an explicit but appropriate statement. If a parent or child starts complaining about something tangential, such as having had to wait for the bus, a direct comment such as "Yes, it can be a real hassle having to wait!" is preferable to an obscure statement such as "I hear you," or ignoring the comment altogether.

Explain and Illustrate Keywords and Concepts

The therapist has to be as certain as possible that key (even simple) words or phrases are clearly defined. A good operational rule is this: *Do not assume that the family knows what you mean and, conversely, do not assume that you understand exactly what the parent or child has in mind.* Chapters 6–8 contain examples of dialogues that address the definition of a keyword or concept.

It is particularly important that the therapist ask for specific examples of behaviors that have given rise to global judgments or assertions about the child. For example, the parent of a depressed youngster may complain that the child is mean or has an attitude. These words imply not only that the child has exhibited socially undesirable behaviors but also that the behaviors in question were willful and purposeful. However, it would be a mistake for the therapist to interpret such complaints as reflective of the child's intentional cruelty or insensitivity if the parent has not provided specific examples of the behaviors in question.

If a girl complains, "My mom hates me," do not assume that the mother is rejecting and not affectionate. Ask for examples of what that mother does that suggest hatred. It may be that the mother won't allow the child to associate with certain children (possibly for good reasons) or won't buy the child a desired object (possibly because she cannot afford it). Such examples would indicate that the statement "My mom hates me" has become a shorthand way for the child to communicate her dysphoric affect if she cannot have her way.

Be mindful of verbally precocious young children. Such children frequently use sophisticated phrases and expressions in generally appropriate contexts, but without really knowing the meaning of the words. For example, a 7-year-old girl reported that she and her mom get into arguments because "I am not responsible enough for my behavior" but was unable to define the words or even provide examples when asked.

Be mindful of verbal labels that the family may have learned in the past. For example, a mother consistently described her 9-year-old boy as having "an anger problem." This label apparently was coined by the mother's own therapist, who never met the child and had only the maternal account to go by. When questioned by the child's CERT therapist, it turned out that the mother was referring to the boy's displays of distress whenever she ignored his evident sadness and unhappiness.

In addition to offering straightforward definitions, the use of analogies from everyday life is an excellent way to explain or illustrate some principles. As already noted, CERT uses a sports analogy to define the child's role, the parent's role, and the therapist's responsibilities (see Chapter 3). Additionally, CERT's emphasis on the importance of practice in skill acquisition readily lends itself to analogies. For example, the need to practice mood repair responses can be conveyed by comparing it to riding a bike, break dancing, or some other appropriate activity involving skill acquisition. How is the need to practice some mood repair response similar to learning how to ride a bike? Well, learning to ride a bike is hard in the beginning, but if you keep at it, riding will become easy and *automatic*. Learning to ride a bike also involves multiple attempts at getting it right, falling down, and even bruising your knees a few times. But with repeated practice and riding, you can ride the bike without having to think about it. The same is true when learning to become better at mood repair.

Engage Both the Parent and the Child

Getting ready to deliver CERT means being prepared to translate into practice CERT's key strategic components; the involvement of the parent–child pair requires special attention. As emphasized in Chapter 3, CERT requires that the parent and young patient both attend treatment sessions together and also be active participants throughout and in-between the sessions.

How does the CERT therapist get the parent–child pair to become actively involved in each session? Indeed, engaging concurrently both the parent and the young patient can be challenging. As revealed during training sessions, trainees appeared to be most comfortable focusing either on the young patient, or the parent, consecutively one after another, rather than getting both of them involved simultaneously. Unfortunately, such an approach means that, much of the time, one or the other of the parent–child pair is not an active participant and may feel or be effectively ignored.

Without question, the young patient is the primary focus of attention during the sessions. However, concurrent parental engagement is made easy by the fact that the parent has been identified from the start as assistant coach. Thus, the therapist should take every opportunity to involve the parent in his coaching role, which can range from active listening to actual coaching interactions with the child. Starting with Chapter 6, there are numerous examples of how the therapist can accomplish this goal.

Here are some prompts to the parent that should be helpful:

Mom [Dad/both], can you now put on your coaching hat? Listen with your coaching ear?

Can you think about what would be a good coaching response to [the child or the item under discussion]?

Mom [Dad/both], I'd like you to put aside your role as [Mom/Dad/both] and take on the coaching role.

The parent also can be engaged by asking her to assist the child who is reporting on a homework assignment, or by monitoring the child's performance during *in vivo* attempts to regulate dysphoria (see Chapter 6). Addressing a question to both parent and child also will engage both of them. After a verbal exchange with either the parent or the child, immediately asking for feedback from the other participant can facilitate that person's engagement (e.g., "What do you think about what your mom just said?"). Another strategy for concurrent engagement of both parties is to encourage the young patient to pose a direct question to the parent about the issue being discussed (or vice versa). For example, the therapist may say to the young patient:

> *Hmm, you believe that Mom did not notice what a nice job you did in keeping track of your feelings for this homework.*
>
> *So, why don't you just ask her? Turn to mom and ask her to look at your log sheet and tell you what she thinks of how you did.*

At times, however, it may be necessary for the therapist to pay undivided attention to the parent. Under such a circumstance, the therapist should explain what is to come and engage the young patient as an active listener, or in some other way. For example, the therapist may say to the young patient:

> *OK—for the next few minutes, let's hear your mom tell the story of what happened that made you guys so late today. Can you [the child] listen along with me—maybe you can add to it?*

Or

> *I would like to hear from Mom about what happened at work to make you guys late. This should take a few minutes—can you help out by keeping time? Watch this clock and tell us when this hand has gone around three times?*

Identify the Affect and Regulatory Response in All Complaints

Remember that according to CERT, the key problem in depression is the dysphoric, despondent mood that the patient has failed to decrease or terminate owing to his mood repair deficiencies. It is mood that initially triggered the cascade of other depressive symptoms and now maintains the depressive syndrome or disorder. Thus, the patient's dysphoric mood is the initial target symptom in CERT; it is ameliorated by strengthening the child's adaptive mood repair response repertoire (see Chapter 7).

In every presenting complaint and problem scenario, the therapist searches for and hones in on the young patient's sad, dysphoric affect and associated regulatory response. When children and adolescents suffer from depression, their affective dysfunction (e.g., sad, dysphoric mood and associated behaviors) usually is in the forefront of parental accounts of the offspring's difficulties.

Follow a Session Structure

Getting ready to deliver CERT means that the therapist is aware of the need to introduce and maintain a consistent structure in each treatment session. The structure helps to achieve the session's goals, maintains its focus, and enables the therapist to redirect the parent–child pair if they go off on a tangent. Structuring means that the therapist defines the framework and content of the session and reiterates this information as needed. Session structure involves the following elements during the typical session length of 50 minutes:

1. Opening statement: setting the stage
2. Review the child's depressive symptoms
3. Set a working agenda
4. Follow the agenda
5. Set intersession goals and assign homework
6. Closing statement

Opening Statement: Setting the Stage

At the start of each session, the therapist provides a brief overview of what is to come by outlining the goals and content of that particular session. The goals of a given session will vary as a function of the phase of treatment, the extent and severity of the child's symptoms, the level of the child's functioning, and the need to attend to crises or problems, should they arise. Except for the first session (covered in Chapter 6), opening statements should sound something like the following:

> *I'd like to review what we will be doing today. Let's start by spending a few minutes going over how [child] has been doing since we last met—also, I'd like to know if there have been any new problems.*
>
> *Then, we will decide on our plan for the rest of the session: If something new has come up, we will talk about it, and we also will go through [the assignment/monitoring/experiment the family agreed to at the last session]. Depending on the results, we will see where we go from there.*
>
> *At the end, we'll do a wrap-up and decide on things to do before the next session.*
>
> *Does that sound OK to you? So—is there anything important—and new—that has come up which we should talk about today?*

Structuring should be carried out even if the circumstances appear to be unfavorable. For example, the parent–child pair may arrive for the session in the middle of a heated argument or crisis, which may preclude the usual opening statement. In such a case, the initial structuring should focus on setting some constraint on how the family's presentation will be handled. For example, the therapist might say:

> *Well, we usually start out by going over how things went since the last time we met and then by planning our session. But I can see that we have a problem* right now. *So, let's spend the next 5–10 minutes on figuring out what this [argument, etc.] is about and what happened. And then we will move on to our usual steps—we review what we will be doing, and make sure that you [parent and child] give me a progress report. OK?*

Review the Child's Depressive Symptoms

Every session must include a brief review of the child's recent mood and other depressive symptoms and general functioning. One way to facilitate this is to have the parent and child complete the relevant questionnaires before the session (e.g., the parent version of the CDI-2; see Chapter 5). The therapist can quickly examine the completed questionnaires and inquire about any new or troubling symptoms (e.g., suicidal ideation, sleep difficulties). For example, in moving to establish the agenda, the therapist might say:

> *Let's start with how [the child] has been feeling.*
>
> *It looks from this form that his mood has been OK, but he has been having sleep problems—that is new, is that right? So, let's put this on our agenda, our list of things to talk about.*

Otherwise, a general inquiry, such as the following, may suffice:

> *To start with, can you [mother] give me a quick idea about how [child] has been doing since [last meeting]. How has [he or she] been feeling?*
>
> *[If appropriate] Last time, we were concerned about [him or her not eating, crying a lot, etc.]. Has that continued?*
>
> (To child) *How have you have been [doing/feeling/etc.] in the past few days?*

Set a Working Agenda

Establishing a working agenda helps to focus the session and assure progress in symptom reduction or relapse prevention (depending on the phase of treatment). Introduce the agenda setting along the following lines:

OK. I have some idea how [the child] and you have been doing.

Now, let's make some plans for what we will do today—OK?

[If appropriate] First, I want to hear about this new symptom that you noticed this week and then also . . .

I would like to hear about what happened with [whatever the assignment was last time] and how it went.

Also, we want to be sure to spend some time on [if any further issues were identified]. Anything else you want to add for today?

At the end, we will decide on new things to do before the next session. OK?

The easiest way for the therapist to redirect the parent and child (if they are about to go off on a tangent) is to refer back to the agreed on structure. This is an important consideration because some therapists may feel that if they do not attend to every matter unexpectedly brought up by the parent or child, they may offend the family or undermine the therapeutic relationship. However, by having previously structured the session, the therapist can refer to the agreed on framework and content, without giving offense. For example, if the parent suddenly introduces some family issue, the therapist can say:

Oh—I see that [reframe the issue] is important to you—if we have time [or I'll make sure that] at the end of the session—let's talk about that then. But, we agreed to deal with [review the agreed on contents or items], can you tell me about that now?

Follow the Agenda

Implementing the agenda should take the bulk of the CERT session. Remember that if the child or parent brings up an issue that was not part of the agenda, the therapist has to refocus their attention. One way to do this is to acknowledge the importance of the distraction but then remind parent and child of the agenda that was previously set. If relevant, the issue can be put on the agenda as its last item. For example, if the child starts a fight with his mother about something she promised but did not deliver, the therapist can say to the young patient:

OK, I see that you are upset with Mom because she promised . . . but she didn't. . . . I can see that is upsetting—right?

Why don't we do this—let's try to find time at the end of our session to talk about what happened. But now, if you remember, we agreed to go over the [monitoring homework that was assigned]. I see that you brought it with you—that is great that you remembered!

So, how about going through this with me?

Set Intersession Goals and Assign Homework

After working through the issues that were targeted for the session, it is important to set goals that the parent–child pair can work toward prior to the next session. These goals typically involve a homework assignment, the importance of which in CERT cannot be overemphasized. Throughout this book, there are multiple examples of various types of homework and how they can be assigned.

Closing Statement

End each CERT session with a brief summary of what was accomplished and what has been planned for the time interval prior to the next session. Parent and child should be asked for their own summaries to be sure that there is consensus about any plans that were made. It is particularly important that the therapist clarify any misunderstandings about the assignments to be completed between sessions. The closing statement could be along the following lines:

> *Well, let's finish by going through what we did today. [Review progress.]*
>
> *We also agreed on [review the specific homework] which you [parent] and [child] will work on together before the next session. Is this about right? Good!*
>
> *Now, I want to be sure that I explained everything clearly. So, can you [parent and then the child] tell me in your own words what this new [homework/exercise/experiment] will be, and what you think the purpose is?*

If the parent's and child's responses accurately reflect the homework assignment, the therapist should say so. But misunderstandings need to be corrected before the session can be ended.

Chapter 5

Assessment, Case Formulation, and Treatment Planning

Contextual emotion regulation therapy (CERT) includes two types of assessments. The goal of the initial broad-based assessment is to determine the child's suitability for CERT. The second type of assessment typically has a narrow symptom focus and is conducted at any time during the course of treatment.

The initial broad-based clinical assessment should include a full psychiatric and psychosocial evaluation of the young patient, along with queries about the family situation. Psychometric testing of key functions also may be conducted. Consideration should be given to administering self-rated questionnaires to the young patient and parent(s) about a range of issues and functions because they are efficient and cost-effective ways to obtain information.

By the end of the initial assessment, the clinician will have sufficient information to decide if CERT is suitable for the young patient, which then can be communicated to the parent–child pair. If the decision is made to offer CERT, the parent(s) should be provided with the Manual for Parents (Appendix D; see Chapter 6 for further discussion). At this point, the therapist is also likely to have developed a tentative case formulation and potential treatment plan: The details of both will undergo changes as the treatment progresses and as the therapist becomes increasingly familiar with the parent–child pair and the child's mood repair response repertoire. As the case formulation becomes confirmed, it also provides leads about the areas to be emphasized in coping skills training.

Assessments throughout the course of treatment are conducted within a given session or assigned as homework: They typically involve gathering information about the young patient's symptoms and behaviors, with the parent often serving either as a primary informant or coach.

The Initial Clinical Evaluation

During the initial clinical evaluation, it is best to first interview the parent alone about the presenting problem, the child's symptoms, the family situation, and the parents' well-being, while the child may complete self-rated questionnaires or undergo psychometric evaluation. Then the clinician can proceed to conduct a shorter interview with the young patient about current/recent symptoms and difficulties.

The Presenting Problem

Ask the parent why she is bringing the child for treatment, in what context the problems are most obvious (at home, with peers, in school), and what has made these problems pressing *now*. Ask for specific recent examples of problems and difficulties. The child also should be asked why he thinks he has been brought to see the clinician. Keep in mind that the presenting problem may not mirror the child's diagnosis.

Demographics and Background Information

Information about demographic and background characteristics helps the clinician to understand the context of the child's difficulties and become aware of the family's resources (or lack of them). Ask about the child's living arrangement; the employment, educational, and mental health status of his primary caregivers; and ease of access to the clinic or treatment venue. Ask about the child's developmental, educational, and medical history and the date of his last pediatric examination and its results. Inquire about recent (within the past 6 months) major life events or overall stresses for the child and family.

Differential Diagnosis

In research settings, diagnostic evaluations are conducted via standardized, semi-structured, psychiatric interviews, such as the Kiddie Schedule for Affective Disorders and Schizophrenia—Present and Lifetime Version (K-SADS-PL; Kaufman et al., 1997) or the Interview Schedule for Children and Adolescents—Diagnostic Version (ISCA-D; Kiss et al., 2007; Kovacs et al., 2019). These interviews yield systematic information from parents (or other adult informants) about young patients, and from young patients about themselves, and cover the most frequent major psychiatric diagnoses (e.g., mood disorders, anxiety disorders, eating disorders, and externalizing disorders).

While semi-structured diagnostic interviews may be too unwieldy in the usual clinical practice, the evaluator can implement the underlying rule; namely, systematically checking for the presence of major psychiatric disorders by first asking about gating symptoms. Gating symptoms (and their features) *must* be present for a disorder. For example, depressed, irritable, or anhedonic mood for at least 2 weeks, and most of the time, is a gating symptom for various types of depression. If the gating symptom is *not* present, then there usually is no need to ask about the remaining symptoms of the disorder under consideration.

I strongly recommend that the evaluator ask about gating symptoms for all major disorders because depressed youngsters are likely to have comorbid anxiety disorder, oppositional defiant disorder (ODD), and/or conduct disorders (discussed in Chapter 1). Also keep in mind that symptoms of depression can mirror an undiagnosed medical condition. Therefore, it is a good idea to require a pediatric examination of the young patient, especially if the patient's symptoms have had an acute onset, there is a lack of meaningful explanation, and no prior history of emotional or behavioral difficulties exists.

Differential diagnosis is important to decide if CERT is the appropriate treatment for a given child. CERT is *not* recommended for youngsters who are severely mentally disabled or psychotic and those whose primary problem lies within the externalizing disorders domain (attention-deficit/hyperactivity disorder, ODD, and conduct disorder). If the young patient has a depressive disorder superimposed on an externalizing disorder, he is likely to benefit from CERT with respect to the former condition (but probably not the latter). CERT is appropriate for depressed children with comorbid overanxious disorder or separation anxiety disorder. But comorbid posttraumatic stress disorder or disabling phobia is a *contraindication* for CERT because these conditions have been shown to respond to other specific evidence-based behavioral interventions. Furthermore, the conceptual paradigms and treatment strategies of some interventions (e.g., exposure therapy) for disabling phobias and stress-related disorders are the direct opposite of CERT's approach to mood regulation.

Suicidal Behavior

The clinical assessment of suicidal behavior, one of the symptoms of an episode of depression, warrants a separate section because of the potential threat to life. The DSM system specifies that suicidal behavior can manifest as recurrent thoughts of death, recurrent suicidal ideation, specific suicide plans, and having made a suicide attempt (see Chapter 1). The presence of some form of suicidal behavior is not a contraindication for CERT. But suicidal symptoms require careful assessment to determine if the child can receive CERT as an outpatient or needs inpatient hospitalization. (The use of CERT to treat some suicidal symptoms is discussed in Chapter 8.)

Queries about the child's suicidal behavior should establish its *timing* (e.g., "When was the last time you thought about killing yourself and/or made plans to do so?"), *frequency* (e.g., "Did you have ideas of wanting to kill yourself a few times, more than just a few times, many times?"), *persistence* (e.g., "Do these ideas come and go? Or, stay on your mind?"), and *controllability* (e.g., "Can you make the ideas go away? If your favorite game show was coming on—could you pay attention to it?"). It may be useful to ask about the source of the suicidal ideas (e.g., "Can you tell me—where did these ideas come from? Did they just pop into your head? Did you hear about them from somebody? Do you know someone who has talked about suicidal ideas?").

Be sure to ask if the young patient has a suicide plan and if he considered ways to implement it (e.g., "Did you think about how you were going to kill yourself? How were you going to do it? And when?"). Determine the accessibility of the methods the child has considered, such as firearms or medication (e.g., "Where will you get the gun from? How will you get it? Whose medicine are you planning to take? Where is it kept?").

The following signify that the child needs immediate clinical attention and most likely within an inpatient setting: persistent suicidal thoughts and related actions, ideation not within the young patient's control, specific and highly lethal plans for suicide (e.g., strangulation, firearms), accessibility of the considered method, and having started to implement the plans (see Spirito & Esposito-Smythers, 2006).

If the decision is to treat the child with CERT as an outpatient, be sure that the family meets minimal standards for the management of suicidal youngsters, which includes close and continuous monitoring and supervision of the child by adults (American Academy of Child and Adolescent Psychiatry [AACAP], 2001). If supervision and risk-reduction provisions (e.g., removal of firearms from the home, keeping potentially lethal medications away from the child) cannot be met, treatment options other than outpatient CERT should be considered.

The clinical assessment of suicidal behavior can be repeated as warranted during the course of CERT.

Emotion Regulation (Mood Repair) Characteristics and History

As part of the clinical evaluation, the clinician should gather information about how the child deals with emotions in general, particularly with sadness and dysphoria. Given that there are no accepted guidelines for how to assess a child's emotion regulation characteristics and history and what factors the assessment should cover, the best approach is to gather narrative information about how the child has recently responded to sadness and dysphoria. Ask about what triggered the uptick in negative affect, how the child responded, and whether the distress got worse or better. Time permitting, also inquire how the young patient managed sadness and distress at earlier ages, what may have helped him (and what did not) to feel better, and whether any family member is able to get the child to settle down when distressed.

In the "Quantitative Assessment of Symptoms and Functional Domains" section later in this chapter, I discuss two questionnaires that can be used to obtain information about the child's emotion regulation response repertoire: the Feelings and Me Questionnaire—Child Version and the Feelings and My Child Questionnaire—Parent Report. These questionnaires yield information about the range (and type) of adaptive and maladaptive responses the child typically deploys when feeling sad and dysphoric. Not surprisingly, young patients' answers on the child version will reveal that they usually react to distress in ways that make the emotion worse. The adaptive mood repair responses that characterize a given child (and mirror her regulatory domain preference) should be noted because these responses have failed to attenuate the child's sad mood, as evidenced by the presence of a depressive disorder.

Characteristics of the Young Patient's Sadness and Dysphoria

To determine whether the young patient meets diagnostic criteria for a depressive disorder, the initial clinical evaluation will have included the assessment of all the criterion symptoms, including sadness and dysphoria. However, sadness and dysphoria also are key treatment targets. Thus, they need to be monitored during CERT and characterized on several dimensions—namely, severity/intensity; persistence; type of onset (sudden vs. gradual, presence vs. absence of a trigger); and context—which then inform the therapist's choice of intervention or the regulatory responses to be pursued (this is discussed further in Chapters 6 and 7).

Sadness intensity is important given evidence that very intense affect is best regulated by refocusing the person's attention away from the distress (one type of cognitive strategy), rather than by having her reevaluate or try to understand it (other types of cognitive strategies). Sadness duration is important because if the child suffers from chronic periods of sadness, for example, then mood repair success may depend on implementing "portable" regulatory responses that are mostly within her control. The context and type of onset of an acute episode of sadness may indicate the feasibility of proactive intervention: For example, if a dysphoric episode occurs within a specific interpersonal framework (e.g., with the young patient's father) or environment (e.g., a particular school class), it may be possible to reduce the child's exposure to the context-specific depressogenic stimulus (see later discussion in this chapter).

There are two ways the therapist can obtain timely and detailed information about the young patient's sadness and dysphoria: via direct questioning during the CERT session and by assigning sadness monitoring as homework.

Information Gathering during the Session

As discussed in Chapter 4, each CERT session should start with a review of how the child has been doing and feeling. As relevant, direct questioning can establish the characteristics of the young patient's sadness and dysphoria currently (in the session) and recently (over past 24 hours).

The information gathering can be introduced by saying, "And now, I would like to know more about [the child's] sadness" and then proceeding with specific questions. The inquiries about severity, persistence, type of onset, and context should first be addressed to the parent and then confirmed (if appropriate) by asking the child selected questions.

In the first treatment session only, it may be useful to ask the parent(s) whether the characteristics of the young patient's sadness and dysphoria have recently differed from those across the past several months. In later sessions, the inquiry need only address the current (most recent) and interim (since last contact) time frames.

Ask about the following symptom features:

- **Severity:** How sad, despondent, or dysphoric has the child recently been (use a numeric severity rating scale ranging from 0 = not sad at all to 10 = extremely sad)? Has anything helped to lessen it?
- **Persistence:** How long has the child been feeling this sad/despondent? Has the dysphoria been continuous or episodic? Has it gotten worse recently?
- **Onset:** How did the current dysphoric episode *or* increase in sadness severity start? Did it come out of the clear blue sky? Did anything trigger it?
- **Context:** Is the child's affect/mood different depending on context (home vs. school, with family vs. with friends)? What was going on when the current mood grew worse?

Information Gathering via Homework Assignment

Homework assignments involving sadness monitoring are used after the first CERT session; they can provide more accurate and timely information about the child's affective dysfunction than retrospective recall because recall is likely to involve distortions. Furthermore, recall is influenced by many factors including one's current and past mood, the importance of the event being recalled and its context, or innate attention to detail.

Gathering information about the young patient's despondent affect in daily life via homework can involve hourly (or less frequent) monitoring for one or more days, portions of days (e.g., in the evenings), or some combination of frequency and time of day (e.g., four times a day after school). The type of monitoring depends on the nature of the information the therapist seeks, the young patient's maturity, and the quality of the parent–child coaching relationship. Thus, sadness monitoring can range from a simple exercise (e.g., confirming at predetermined times whether the young patient is sad/dysphoric) to an increasingly complex assignment that includes further dimensions to be rated (e.g., intensity, context).

When such a homework assignment is discussed with the parent–child pair, it is important to emphasize that the task needs to be done at the agreed on times and not from memory at the end of the day (see Chapters 6 and 7 for examples).

Common sense and practical considerations should be at the forefront when assigning real-life mood monitoring for a given patient. For example, the desired frequency of monitoring may not be feasible in some school settings without the child calling attention to herself (which is to be avoided). As another example, mood monitoring in the morning is likely to be contraindicated for families with two working parents, who need to get several children to school each day. In general, the goal should be for the child to complete the log with the parent as coach. But, under some circumstances, a mood log may be completed by the parent alone about the child or the young patient alone about herself. Chapter 6 includes a partially completed simple affect monitoring form. Chapter 7 includes a completed custom-made log for monitoring completion of homework. Blank reproducible versions of these monitoring logs can be found in Appendix A, Forms 5–8.

Quantitative Assessment of Symptoms and Functional Domains

The completion of self-rated questionnaires by parents about themselves, the young patient, and the family, as well as by the young patient about himself, is an efficient way to obtain information, can provide the clinician with quantified indices of various areas of functioning, and round out the clinical picture. The so-called Buros Mental Measurements Yearbook (Carolson et al., 2021) is one reliable source of information about a wide range of questionnaires. The list given here includes several recommended questionnaires that can be helpful as pre- and posttreatment measures, or to track changes in symptoms across time.

Depression and Overall Psychopathology

The Children's Depression Inventory—Second Edition (CDI-2; Kovacs & Multi-Health Systems Staff, 2011) has been a frequently used self-rated depression scale for youngsters ages 7–17. The *child self-rated version* contains 28 items that cover a wide range of depressive symptoms. A 12-item short self-report version may be particularly useful to track changes in overall depression severity across time. The *parent-rated version* contains 17 items that focus on observable manifestations of depression in the child. All versions are rated for the past 2 weeks. In clinical trials of CERT, both the child and parent usually complete the CDI before the first session and once every 2–3 weeks thereafter. In addition to yielding raw total scores, which mirror the extent of depressive symptoms, each CDI tool also yields a standardized score, allowing the therapist to compare the child's ratings with those of similar-age and same-sex peers in the normative sample.

The Child Behavior Checklist (CBCL; Achenbach, 2001) provides an index of the young patient's overall psychopathology as well as its various domains. The CBCL is one of the most widely used tools of its kind: It has parent-rated, teacher-rated, and youth self-rated versions and is typically completed to reflect behavior over the past 6 months. The CBCL yields standardized scores that indicate a given child's ranking (compared to typically developing peers of a similar age and the same sex) on global dimensions (i.e., externalizing and internalizing problems) and specific syndrome scales (e.g., "anxious/depressed," "aggressive behavior"). It also yields six dimensions that tend to reflect various DSM categories. If the therapist can administer, score, and review the parent-rated CBCL before the first assessment session, the results may help to focus the diagnostic interview on troublesome domains. Use of the CBCL before and at the end of treatment may provide the therapist with information about the overall impact of the intervention.

It is also helpful to ask the parents to complete questionnaires about themselves. One of the most widely used depression self-rating scales for adults is the Beck Depression Inventory—Second Edition (BDI-II; Beck et al., 1996). This is a 21-item questionnaire that surveys a range of depressive symptoms over the prior 2 weeks. The item scores yield a total raw score, for which clinically meaningful cut-offs have been established. The higher the score, the more depressed is the respondent; a total score of 11 or above traditionally has been considered as the lower end of clinical depression.

As an index of overall psychopathology, parents may be asked to complete about themselves the Symptom Checklist-90—Revised (SCL-90-R), which queries about a wide range of symptoms associated with major mental disorders (Derogatis & Unger, 2010). The questionnaire yields several indices of global severity, along with scores on nine primary symptom dimensions (e.g., "anxiety," "paranoid ideation"). In addition to the SCL-90-R scores, it may be informative to examine which particular items have been endorsed by a given parent.

Negative Life Events or Stress

Standardized questionnaires that quantify life stress for adults typically consist of a list of events, each of which is rated by the respondent for its presence or absence in a given time frame (e.g., past year) and possibly for its subjective impact. The Social Readjustment Rating Scale (SRRS) of Holmes and Rahe (1967) is one of the most widely used tools to assess life stress in adults (reviewed by Scully et al., 2000): Its completion by parents would be most informative at the initial assessment. A revision and update (Hobson et al., 1998) outlines 51 major life events and includes an impact rating (from 0 to 100) for each event. By asking parents to check which events have happened in their lives during a specified time frame (e.g., the past year), the clinician will have a framework within which to view the stress burden on the family, which undoubtedly has an impact on the young patient.

The standardized measurement of stressful life events for children and adolescents has been problematic, partly owing to developmental reasons (for a review, see Grant et al., 2004). The Coddington life event scales are the only ones suitable for younger children (Coddington, 1972): Although developed quite a while ago, these forms continue to be used (reviewed by Shaw et al., 2008). There are three separate Coddington questionnaires to accommodate youngsters in elementary school, middle school, and high school; they usually are completed by a clinician based on an interview with the parents. Although there are no normative data against which the summed scores can be interpreted, the higher the score, the more stress the child has experienced. The clinician also benefits from knowing which stressful events have occurred.

Emotion Regulation or Mood Repair

The development of CERT included the construction of self-rated questionnaires that survey a young patient's (and adult's) mood repair response repertoire. As already noted, the Feelings and Me Questionnaire for Children is completed by youngsters about themselves and the Feelings and My Child Questionnaire quantifies the parents' observations of their child's mood repair responses. Asking the parents to complete the Feelings and Me Questionnaire for Adults can provide the therapist with information about how the parents themselves regulate sadness, These three questionnaires (collectively called the Feelings and Me [FAM] scales and available as reproducible Forms 1–3 in Appendix A) should be administered prior to the first CERT session, at midpoint, and toward the end of treatment to assess changes in the young patient's mood repair repertoire.

The respondent indicates on the FAM questionnaire the degree to which a variety of behavioral, cognitive, social–interpersonal, and body-focused mood repair responses are typically deployed when feeling sad or dysphoric. The three versions contain the same number and type of items. Each version yields three main scores. The Adaptive Regulatory Response score and Maladaptive Regulatory Response score mirror the extent (size) of an individual's adaptive and maladaptive response repertoires, respectively, and are derived by simply adding the item endorsements in the given functional domain. A review of the child's item-by-item answers can help the clinician to identify maladaptive responses that the youngster typically deploys, which need to be eliminated, and adaptive responses that reflect the child's preferred regulatory domains and should be reinforced. The Adaptive/Maladaptive Balance score, or ratio score, mirrors the extent to which a person's mood repair repertoire is dominated by adaptive responses: It is derived by dividing the total number of (adaptive plus maladaptive) responses that were endorsed by the total number of adaptive responses endorsed (see Appendix A; Kovacs et al., 2009; Tamás et al., 2007). The FAM ratio score is informative because for emotionally well individuals that score is typically .75 or above, while it is about .50 or less for those with depression histories (Kovacs et al., 2009). In other words, although the mood repair response repertoires of emotionally well individuals are dominated by responses that attenuate sadness and distress, this is not the case for depression-prone youth.

The Cognitive Emotion Regulation questionnaire is another self-rated scale suitable for youngsters (Garnefski et al., 2007). That questionnaire (for 9- to 11-year-olds) focuses solely on cognitions and queries children about their thoughts after a stressful event has happened. However, the items are framed as responses to "something unpleasant" with which the child was confronted, rather than as responses to the child's own emotions. Thus, it provides a picture of the cognitive strategies a child may use to cope with stressful events but yields limited information about the child's response repertoire to manage dysphoria.

What to Do When Parental Psychopathology Exists

Depression is the most likely psychiatric disorder among parents of depressed children and is of concern because it compromises the parent's ability to manage the demands of CERT. Up to about 70% of the mothers of clinic-referred depressed youngsters were found in one study to have had *histories* of depressive disorder and about 30% were in a depressive episode *concurrently* with their child's depression (Hammen et al., 1999). Using a different ascertainment method, another study reported that about 31% of mothers seeking help for their depressed children had a psychiatric disorder; depression and anxiety disorders were the most common (Ferro et al., 2000). The strong concurrent (and reciprocal) relationship between depressive symptoms in clinically treated adults and their young offspring has been confirmed longitudinally (Garber et al., 2011).

While successful treatment of parents' depression can have a positive impact on the mental health of their children (e.g., Weissman et al., 2015), it is a considerable challenge to engage in their own treatment the depressed parent of a depressed child (Verdeli et al., 2004). In our pilot study of CERT, maternal depression was associated with failure to complete the child's treatment (Kovacs et al., 2006). Indeed, according to a review, it is current rather than past parental depression that undermines the depressed offspring's response to treatment (Gladstone et al., 2019).

Both the clinical evaluation and the adult self-rated questionnaires will yield information about parental depression. The therapist also may observe expressions of maternal depression during the treatment session. Presumptive depression (and other serious emotional and mental problems) should prompt a referral for an independent clinical assessment. The mother (or father) should be advised openly as to the purpose of the referral, along with a discussion of why diagnosis and treatment of parental psychopathology are critical for the child's progress.

If the parent is unwilling to follow up on an assessment or treatment recommendation, one approach is to get the parent to agree to a short period of monitoring (i.e., 2–3 weeks) while continuing with CERT. The goal of such a contract is to be able to determine the parent's ability to optimally help the child. If parental (maternal) psychopathology is so impairing that the parent cannot sustain the level of motivation, energy, or attention needed for her role as an assistant coach, a temporary solution is to have the other parent or other responsible adult (who resides with the child) serve as a substitute in the CERT sessions. While this solution is not optimal, it is better than terminating the child's treatment.

Case Formulation and Treatment Planning

Case formulation generally involves an explanation of the nature or origin of a patient's difficulties and what maintains them, along with potential strengths that can offset them. Case formulation can be theoretically or conceptually based. The treatment plan identifies the therapeutic goals for the given patient and ways to achieve them. The case formulation and treatment plan have overlapping components and are partly intertwined.

Components of Case Formulation

A CERT case formulation is a hypothesis about what factors may account for the given child's mood repair difficulties and how best to mitigate them to prevent future depression. Toward that aim, the case formulation needs to identify how the young patient's mood repair problems are manifest, the responses that are involved, the response repertoire at the child's disposal, key developmental and historical information and familial variables (including the ability of parents to serve as coaches) that bear on the young patient's mood repair problems and strengths, and relevant contextual issues.

To construct a picture of a young patient's regulatory repertoire, focus on response domains. And then be attentive to the responses that the child appears to favor. The goal is to identify the child's domain preference(s), the adaptive responses that need to be strengthened, the relevant skills to be reinforced, and the maladaptive responses that need to be discouraged.

Keep in mind that the three regulatory response domains (social–interpersonal, cognitive, and behavioral) can overlap. The rule is to classify responses according to the primary route, or essential area of functioning, through which affect change seems to be eventuated. In other words, identify in a given response the component or domain that appears to be *most critical* for affect change. Here are some examples:

> An adolescent girl always goes for a run when feeling distressed and prefers to run with friends. However, even on rainy days when her friends will not join her, she will run when feeling down. For her, running exemplifies a behavioral

(rather than a social–interpersonal) mood repair response because the crucial reparative ingredient appears to be the physical experience of running, rather than the company of friends.

A depressed boy usually seeks out his mother when he is distressed, which inevitably brings him emotional relief. The mother's approach is to discuss what is happening and help the child to view matters in a less negative way. Is this a social–interpersonal response (seeking the mother's help) or a cognitive response (reevaluation)? The answer is the former, if it turns out that this child also obtains relief if he seeks out his father (who plays softball with him to alleviate distress) or his grandmother (who bakes him cookies when he is dysphoric).

Identifying a young patient's domain preference helps to pinpoint future regulatory response options and calls attention to relevant skills. For example, if a young depressed boy is responsive to physical comforting by his parents (social–interpersonal domain), the therapist may eventually consider more symbolic forms of interpersonal nurturance as mood repair responses. Social skills are highly relevant to the competent deployment of social–interpersonal mood repair responses, begging the question: How effective is this boy when he needs to summon social regulators? Is that an area to be considered for modification?

Case formulation should take into consideration atypical developmental and familial variables that may have compromised the child's mood repair competence. For example, having an attention-deficit disorder may make it challenging for a young patient to master regulatory responses that build on attention refocusing. Or, as discussed in Chapter 10, a developmental history of parental abandonment is likely to engender mistrust of people, with negative implications for the social–interpersonal regulation of distress.

Familial variables that may affect case formulation include how the parents respond to and regulate distress emotions. For example, if a mother responds to her child's distress repeatedly by yelling or berating the offspring, which upregulates the child's distress, that the mother is a stable "up-regulator" of her child's dysphoria. Therefore, options for dealing with this problematic issue need to be identified. As another example, if a mother's prototypical response to her own distress is crying and complaining that nobody loves her (unlikely to be an adaptive response), there is a chance the daughter will learn and adopt that response via social modeling. In such a case, the therapist may need to identify other adults in the family who can serve as alternate regulatory models, or the therapist herself can model in the treatment session different ways to react to distress.

Case formulation also should note depressogenic stressful events or contexts in the young patient's life. If various past depressogenic situations have aspects in common, then such common features can help to identify sensitivity to certain triggers. In some cases, problem-solving coping approaches may be the best way to manage depressogenic triggers, as illustrated in Chapter 10.

Components of a Treatment Plan

CERT's major goals are depression symptom reduction and relapse prevention (see Chapter 3), to be achieved primarily by strengthening affect-related regulatory skills and responses and thereby correcting the young patient's mood repair deficits. However, the treatment plan for a given patient has to be more detailed and customized and reflect the presenting complaint and clinical picture. It should answer this question: "What exactly do I want to achieve for this given patient and how am I going to go about it?" Thus, the treatment plan guides the therapist's behavior and the choices he makes in the interest of the young patient and the parent–child pair.

Treatment planning in CERT is made easier by the fact that its explanatory framework (detailed in Chapter 3) points to the child's sad, dysphoric, or anhedonic affect as the *initial symptom target,* which reflects his problems in mood repair. The therapist's plans to strengthen the child's adaptive mood repair response repertoire should include the intervention strategies that are likely to be used.

The treatment plan should also enumerate the nonaffective depressive symptoms that comprise the patient's clinical picture and how they are to be prioritized for intervention. Suicidal thoughts and behaviors are always prioritized for intervention because they may have fatal consequences (see Chapter 8). Otherwise, two considerations can help guide the process of prioritizing for treatment among the *nonaffective* symptoms of depression: the patient's distress or functional impairment due to the symptom, and the availability of an effective intervention for the symptom. Thus, the therapist may prioritize for intervention sleep disturbance over fatigue, in light of the former's wide-ranging functional consequences and the beneficial effects of sleep hygiene training (see Chapter 8). Or, reduced motivation may be prioritized over reduced appetite since the use of graded task assignments is known to help with the former symptom. However, once the young patient has recovered from affective symptoms, the severity and problematic nature of most nonaffective symptoms often decrease as well. Thus, the initial symptom priority list is likely to undergo major changes over the course of treatment.

A treatment plan may need to consider areas of development with potential bearing on the child's ability to participate in CERT. For example, immature social development may mitigate against the optimal deployment of strategies in the social–interpersonal regulatory domain. As another example, a child's history of having been overprotected may pose a challenge to the consistent self-initiation of mood repair responses.

The treatment plan should consider contextual issues, such as whether the parent(s) can serve as assistant coaches and the psychosocial and material resources available to the family. As already noted, parental inability to function as the assistant coach indicates the need to identify other responsible adults (e.g., a grandparent, another relative) to help implement CERT. If limited resources prevent attendance at every session, alternative plans may have to be considered, such as occasional online therapy meetings.

The CERT treatment plan has to address the child's coping skills training, which is the last phase of therapy. While Chapter 10 provides examples of how various coping skills training goals are implemented, the personalized plan of a given patient is built on that patient's mood repair strengths, trait characteristics that impact mood repair competence, and clinical history, some of which comprise the therapist's case formulation.

Finally, given the high rate of comorbid psychiatric conditions among depressed children (see Chapter 1), the therapist may be faced with symptoms of other disorders after the child has recovered from depression. It is recommended that the treatment of such further symptoms be discussed and negotiated with the parent, but its coverage is beyond the scope of the present manual.

Appendix C contains the case formulations and treatment plans, including coping skills training plans, for four young patients described in this book.

Chapter 6

The Initial CERT Sessions

In some clinical and treatment environments, the assessment and treatment of potential patients are conducted in separate sessions (and/or by different individuals). This chapter, which presents a general template for the initial *treatment* sessions, assumes that to be the case.

The initial contextual emotion regulation therapy (CERT) sessions should include the following: (1) an opening statement, including structuring or setting the agenda and information about the phases of treatment; (2) summary of the presenting problem, highlighting the importance of dysregulated emotions; (3) an explanation of how CERT will help the child overcome depression and the role of coaching in that process; (4) identification of depressed, dysphoric affect as an initial target symptom and showing how a response can change its subsequent course using *in vivo* demonstration or didactic explanations; and (5) a homework assignment that ensures continuity with the session to follow. If the assessment and the start of treatment are combined in one session, time constraints may prevent the therapist from covering the entire content reviewed in this chapter. In that case, a distilled version of the topics just enumerated should focus on identifying sad affect as the target symptom, the importance of coaching, the *in vivo* demonstration, and the homework. The *in vivo* demonstration is critical because the initial sessions *must* provide the patient with some symptom relief and the parent with hope.

Opening Statement

Just like all sessions (see the "Follow a Session Structure" section in Chapter 4), the initial meetings must start with structuring, or setting the agenda, which is basically an overview of what is to come in that session. In the first session, information about the phases of treatment or how long the therapy is expected to last should be provided.

The content of the opening statement will partly depend on the information the therapist already has available. If the therapist is familiar with the presenting problem, a brief summary may suffice. If not, then eliciting the presenting problem is part of the session. Assuming the former scenario, the opening statement may be along the following lines:

> *I'd like to tell you what we will be doing today. First, I want to summarize my understanding of [or discuss the child's] problem.*
>
> *Then I will explain to you how this therapy works and how we will work together to help [the child] get better. If there is anything specific you want to talk about, we will discuss that, too.*
>
> *At the end of our meeting today, we will review what we did and agree on a project you can do before we get together again.*
>
> *We'll have regular meetings—in the beginning twice a week and then once a week and then once every 2 weeks. Toward the end, we will meet about once a month or less often. Every time we meet, we will go over some basic problem or issue.*

Summarize and Reframe the Presenting Problem

After setting the agenda, the therapist should state her understanding of the presenting problem or key issue (or elicit it *de novo*). If the parent has brought the child for treatment because she suspects that the child is depressed, then the therapist's task is to confirm and summarize the presenting complaint. However, if the child is depressed but the parent views the main problem as some other behavior, it may need to be reframed within the conceptual framework of CERT. Basically, this means that major complaints of the parent about the child (and child about herself or others) are reconceptualized as the youngster suffering from a depressive disorder, with its key feature being problematic mood repair.

For example, lack of motivation as well as crying episodes can be identified as symptoms of depression, rather than evidence of laziness or attempts to manipulate family members, respectively. Irritable, noncompliant behavior and rejection of presumably friendly overtures from a sibling can be reframed as examples of difficulties in mood regulation, rather than intentional meanness or evidence of sibling rivalry. Thus, the reframing highlights the child's affective disturbance, which may be described by the parent–child pair as sadness, distress, dysphoria, or feeling miserable and cranky.

When there is *a need for reframing,* the presentation may follow a script something like this:

I see that there are several issues about [the child] that have been of great concern, like his attitude, his behavior at home with the family, and his school performance. So, he has been difficult to deal with and is moody and cries a lot, and you also noticed that he is more tired than usual and not eating that well. And you have been concerned that there is . . . [e.g., sibling rivalry or anger with other family members]. I can see how people may think that [child] has a bad attitude, and Dad has worried because [child] is disobedient and acts out.

It may not be that obvious on first sight, but everything you told me about [child] points to a clinical depression. That is more than feeling sad and bad—it means that sadness and being miserable have gotten out of hand—it is like those feelings control [the child], rather than [the child] having control over those feelings. And when sad or unhappy feelings get out of hand, they have a negative effect on other areas of functioning: You start having trouble getting along with people, with paying attention and getting things done, you may have trouble with sleep, and the like. This can explain many of [child's] symptoms you described.

So, I want to tell you about what this treatment is and how we work together to help [the child].

Explain CERT to the Child and Parent

Explaining CERT demystifies the treatment and provides the family with a framework of what to expect. By the end of the first meeting, the parent and young patient should have some understanding of CERT's approach to depression and its ground rules. It is most important that the parent–child pair recognize the emotion-focused emphasis of CERT, the key role of the parent in the treatment, and the importance of active participation by both parent and child in carrying out homework assignments, which is facilitated by the coaching model. The gist of the explanation will have to be repeated during several sessions.

CERT can be described in terms of the four features that are next addressed. Note that the proposed text on CERT's definition of depression has to be modified if the presenting problem was reframed because the reframing also addressed the nature of depression (see the prior discussion). The following sections provide scripts describing the essential features of CERT with which the parent and child need to become familiar.

Script Addressing Depression

The purpose of this treatment is to help kids who are depressed. What does it mean to be depressed? Well—when kids have a lot of stresses, they can feel sad and miserable and bad. And that is OK, but *when these feelings last for a while or become very strong, they take over!*

And when sad and unhappy feelings take over, other things also start to go wrong, like you have trouble paying attention, getting things done, sleeping, or eating. And soon, you are in a depression, which is more than just feeling sad.

So, being depressed means that feeling sad and bad has gotten out of hand, which then created other problems. That is why in this therapy, we pay a lot of attention to feelings.

Script Addressing Treatment Focus and Goals

This treatment is called contextual emotion regulation therapy or CERT for short.

We will use CERT to help [the child] recover from depression and be able to better manage sad and upset emotions in the future. In CERT, we do this in the context of your lives—all the things that have been going on.

So, when things don't go right, many kids (and adults) feel sad or upset or disappointed. Everybody feels this way sometimes. But these feelings become a problem if they take over.

In our treatment, we start with focusing on [child's] feelings and on what to do so that feelings like being sad, upset, and cranky do not *take over. This is called* emotion regulation, *and it means changing how strong a feeling is and how long it lasts.*

Some of these pictures (pointing to CERT posters) *show important parts of emotion regulation, like the different things than can help to feel* less *sad, miserable, upset, unhappy, or cranky.*

As we go along, we also will work on other things like sleep problems or problems with getting schoolwork done, but obviously only if those things present problems.

Script Describing the Team Approach and the Coaching Team

In CERT, I [the therapist], you [parent], and you [the child] form a team. I [the therapist] am the coach; you [the parent] are the assistant coach; and you [the child] are the player. Just like in a sport, the team has to work together to reach its goals. To make [the child's] depression better, both you [parent] and you [child] have to pitch in!

I will always explain what I am doing and why. That's my part of the deal. Your part of the deal is to work with me because I cannot make [the child] feel better by myself.

Script Describing the Roles of the Parent and Child

A very important part of helping [the child] is that you [parent] will be my assistant coach. I will be counting on you to help me figure out ways to improve things and to do what is necessary to help [the child] feel better. And you [the child] will have an important part, too.

Because this is a little unusual, there is a list of rules that make a good coach and a different list of rules that make a great team player. You can see these here (pointing to posters) *on the posters titled The Rules of Coaching and The Rules of Being a Good Team Player.*

The optimal approach to be taken by the therapist is to list each rule, provide an example (some examples are suggested in the next section), and ask the parent and child to contribute further examples. It also may be helpful to provide the parent–child pair with small index cards on which both sets of rules have been printed. The rules of coaching and of being a good team player have to be revisited throughout treatment because adherence to them is important to the success of homework assignments and experiments.

Script Describing the Rules of Coaching

Start with The Rules of Coaching. The explanations can be changed and shortened or lengthened as needed:

1. ***A good coach takes you [child] as you are and pays most attention to things you do well and your abilities (not your weaknesses).*** *For example, let's say [child] has trouble with schoolwork, but is very good about helping out at home. So, we could pay more attention to the things she does well at home and see if any of those abilities could work at school.*

2. ***A good coach works with you [child] on new ways to do things.*** *Let's use an example from sports: Let's suppose you have been practicing swimming for a while, but you can't speed up. So, your coach can show you a new way to do the strokes to increase your speed. But it will work only if you will actually try it! And do it bit by bit or step by step.*

   In the same way, to get [child] out of her depression, we'll have to try new ways of doing things and go step by step, and you [parent] will be the assistant therapy coach.

3. ***A good coach helps you [child] use your abilities to reach your goals.*** *So, let's say [child] knows how to swim, and she wants to enter a race. Now that means a lot of things. You would have to plan when she should practice, how long, which stroke, and what sort of exercise would make her stronger.*

   So, you [parent] and I together will help [child] to use the skills she already has so that she feels better.

4. ***A good coach praises you while trying to help you keep going.*** *Let's again use the swimming example. Now, if [child] wants to be part of a swimming race, she needs to practice. But she may worry that she cannot get better! So, you [parent] would make sure to tell her about how far she has come already and would stay with her and give her a little extra push.*

So, you [parent] and I will help [child] to practice feeling better and give a little extra push when needed. OK?

5. ***A good coach works with you [the child] even if the coach has a bad day or has gotten up on the wrong side of the bed.*** *Almost everybody has a bad day once in a while. Right? So, this rule means two things: first—it means that it is OK to have a bad day, and second—it means that even if you [parent] are in a bad mood, if it is a swim practice day for [child], you would hang in there with her and coach her.*

   It's the same thing in helping [child] to get better. Even if you [parent] or I have a bad day, we will hang in there as therapy coaches. Right?

6. ***A good coach also needs to learn and practice because a coach is made, not born!*** *OK—this is important. What this means is that for you [parent] or anybody to be a coach, you also have to learn some things about coaching.*

   For example, you may have to learn how to pay the most attention to what a player can *do (instead of what he or she cannot do). And just like with anything new or important, the coach has to practice.*

(To child) *Have you ever been on a sport team?*

[If "yes"] If you remember, the coach would work with you . . . [Briefly review key features of coaching previously noted.]

[If "no"] You must have seen kids being coached at school, on the playground, on TV. Yes? So . . . [Briefly review the points just made.]

But, having a coach is only one part of making things better. The other part is that you [child] also have to try! For example, if I'm going to teach you swimming, there is no way I can do it if you won't go to the swimming pool with me. I cannot teach you swimming in the kitchen. Right? So, one big part of what we will do depends on you. OK?

Script Describing the Rules of Being a Good Team Player

To make your part easier, we also have rules for kids—you can see them here. (Points to poster on the wall.) *These are things that make for a good team player. Let's go through them.*

1. ***A good team player will try new ways to do things.*** *This means that—even if you don't really feel like doing something—you'll* try *it. Otherwise, you'll never know if something will help or not.*

2. ***A good team player works with the coach on game plans and goals.*** *This is important—this means that you have a say in what we do. What do you think about that? [Probe as needed.]*

3. ***A good team player uses words to tell the coach how she or he feels.*** *OK—so, why do you think that is important? Why is it important to use words? [Probe as needed.]*

4. ***A good team player asks for help when things get tough or confusing.*** *This is important because we work as a team. So, if one team player needs help, the others pitch in.*

5. ***A good team player doesn't give up even if a plan doesn't work right away.*** *Things don't always work right in the beginning. So, sometimes it may look like a plan won't work, but it is important to not give up. Can you think of a game where things didn't go right at first, but then everything worked out?*

And finally, the last rule:

6. ***A good team player continues to practice, practice, and practice.*** *This is really important. If you play basketball, or football, or if you are on a swim team, you have to practice so that your muscles don't forget how to react. With practice, things become easy. But if you stop practicing, your muscles forget.*

   It's exactly the same thing with learning to feel better. Once we learn what helps you, it is important to keep practicing it!

It may be useful to emphasize that the coaching model will help the parent–child pair when it comes to homework assignments: The parent will have to serve as coach while the child participates as the player.

So, now that we talked about coaches and players, let me go back to what we'll do in our treatment. We will spend time on different ways to change feelings like sadness or feeling miserable or cranky so that those feelings do not get out of hand.

We will also deal with other problems.

And after things get better, we will work on making sure that both of you have an easier time when problems come up in the future—that you are prepared for them.

OK. I want to be sure that I explained all this stuff clearly. So, [parent] can you tell me in your own words what we'll be doing? And [to child], what do you think about what I said?

Identify Sad and Dysphoric Affect as the Initial Target Symptoms

Given CERT's emphasis on the inability to adaptively regulate sadness and dysphoria as being at the root of depression, the child's affective disturbance is the initial treatment target. That decision can be explained by the therapist in the following way:

I think I understand what the problem seems to be with [child]. It looks like there have been various issues [enumerate as necessary].

But what really stands out to me are [child's] mood problems! And that makes sense because [child] is suffering from a depression, and in fact, sad, miserable, unhappy emotions, which last and last, are part of being depressed.

Most of the time, that is the first thing parents tell us about, and having such feelings every day make things tough for the child and the parents, too. And once the sad feelings have taken over, then other things also become problems, like sleep and paying attention.

I think it's clear that we have a bunch of things to work on here. But we have to pick one problem to start with.

I would like us to start working on [child's] feelings of being sad and miserable. *That is where we will start, but as we go along, we will get to all the issues. So, how can we get [child] to feel better, to feel less sad and cranky?*

At this point, the therapist can obtain information about the current severity of the child's dysphoria (discussed in Chapter 5). And then the therapist can proceed to the next issue, which is the need for the parent–child pair to understand the concept of mood repair.

Look for the Child's Dysphoric Affect/Mood

Identifying dysphoria as the target symptom initially or later in treatment may pose a challenge if the parents think of affect in a global way, and when parents' or young patients' framing of their complaints deemphasizes, or even obscures, the dysphoric component of the child's problems. Therefore, keep in mind the directive to "look for the dysphoric affect/mood" underlying the family's complaints.

The parent may complain about the child's affective dysfunction, but the account may still leave unclear what the child was feeling. If so, then be sure to elicit behavioral descriptions from the young patient, including an account of his nonverbal communication. For example, if the parent complains, "My child is always upset" or "My child is just too moody," inquiries along the following line may be useful:

Can you think back to the last time [the child] felt like that—as if you are watching a film—can you see [the child's] face just before [the scenario/event in question]? How did he look?

If you could have videotaped [the child] at that time, and we could play that now, what would I see in that video?

Did [the child] look at you or look away? What was [the child's] facial expression? What did [the child] say and do? Did he answer your questions?

Did [the child] cry? Or, yell? Did [the child] look upset or angry?

At other times, the challenge is that the parent's perspective on the child's problem may obscure the child's affective dysfunction or downplay its importance. If so, then the therapist needs to redirect attention to the child's dysphoria.

For example, while one mother focused on her child's depressed mood, the father emphasized that the family was seeking psychological help primarily because of the child's disobedient and uncooperative behavior. To illustrate the problem, he related the following incident. The child was scheduled for a pediatric checkup that took months to set up, for which he was to be picked up by the father from school, close to the father's workplace. On the morning of the appointment, the child didn't want to get out of bed, ducked under the covers, cried, and said that he did not want to go to school (although he did not appear to be ill). The parents then got into a fight over this, with the father opining that the young patient didn't want to go to school because it was raining and he just wanted to be oppositional.

In the telling of this story, the father emphasized the child's disobedient behavior because the father perceived the child as willful and oppositional. However, questioning revealed that the child's reluctance to go to school had happened before, occurred only on a specific weekday, and seemed to be associated with a school activity that the child had trouble managing. At that point, the therapist asked the father to think back to the problem scenario and focus on the child's facial expression and affect display: He then was able to report signs of dysphoria, crying, and emotional discomfort. Further questioning revealed that the child typically responded to academic challenges with a despondent mood.

Thus, by being on the lookout for the child's dysphoria, the therapist was able to ascertain that going to school on the day in question served as a depressogenic trigger, and that the resultant distress the child experienced was a central feature of the problem scenario for the family: The data then were used to probe for further examples of sadness and dysphoria, which then served as the target symptoms.

Look for the Child's Regulatory Response

In the beginning stage of CERT, do not expect parents and young patients to be able to differentiate a given affect experience from attempts to regulate it; even researchers do not always agree on the dividing line. And reporting on one's own mood repair responses may be challenging (even for many older children or adults) because this process often is *automatic.* Finally, individual differences in the ability to self-monitor and introspect will clearly influence young patients' reports of how they deal with dysphoria.

How does the CERT therapist identify the child's regulatory response? Recall that, by definition, a regulatory response occurs after an affect has been activated. Usually, the therapist can identify the young patient's regulatory attempts by obtaining a detailed chronological account of an affect-laden incident and the behaviors that became evident right away or closely following it. In the scenario previously described, the child's response to feeling dysphoric was to duck under the covers and withdraw from interacting with his parents, which probably exacerbated his distress. Chapter 7 includes several examples of how the therapist can elicit information about the young patient's regulatory response subsequent to an affective incident.

As just discussed in connection with identifying dysphoria as the target emotion, if the parents downplay the importance of the child's dysphoric affect, their accounts of regulatory responses also will be affected. Here is one example. A mother was concerned that her daughter's experiences in school were causing her depression and undermining her educational functioning. She related that her daughter had recently come home from school looking downcast and weepy and locked herself in her bedroom. This behavior occurred several times, and the mother determined that the child had been excluded from a particular social circle by a group of girls. During the most recent incident, the child ran away from the other girls in the schoolyard and hid in a stairwell. She then cut her next class and went home. The mother believed that the action of the other girls reflected their jealousy of her daughter's outstanding scholastic record. And the mother was particularly upset because she had several times asked school personnel to intervene, but to no avail.

In the mother's telling of this scenario, the emotional emphasis was on the dissocial, exclusionary behavior of the child's peers and the failure of the school to resolve the problem. While context does matter, CERT's emphasis is on the child's reaction to her own distress. In this case, the child's reaction was to hide and avoid contact with others, which is a maladaptive response because it maintained her distress. Therefore, the therapist's challenge in this case was to refocus the attention of the parent–child pair on the young patient's affective experience and to replace the maladaptive response with an adaptive one.

Here are examples of prototypical questions that can help to elicit information about a child's regulatory responses to sad and dysphoric affect. If the conversation is focused on a specific incident or interaction, the questions should be modified accordingly:

When something triggers [use specific examples] the child's sadness, dysphoria, or crankiness or makes the existing feelings worse, what is the child's usual reaction?

What does the child typically say or do after [triggering event]? How does the child look? How does the child act? Does the child ever talk about what is on her mind when she is dysphoric?

What (if anything) helps the child to feel better or calm down when sad or upset? Was that different in the past?

Has anything changed in the child's context or environment (at home, in school, in the

> *community) that may have made it harder for this child to overcome feeling sad and dysphoric?*
>
> *When the child feels sad, downcast, miserable, is there anything you [the parent] can do to make the child feel better?*
>
> *Is there anyone who can make the child feel better when he feels bad, sad, or cranky?*

It is likely that initial questioning about the child's mood repair responses will reveal mostly maladaptive responses, that is, ways of reacting to the affect that prolong or make it worse. Such responses include hiding or social withdrawal, yelling, throwing things, having a tantrum, arguing or picking a fight, and vocalizing depressive rumination or preoccupation with the trigger event, among other behaviors. If the questioning produces very few or no adaptive regulatory responses (ways of reacting to the affect that help to attenuate it), the therapist can probe by using examples from The House of Emotion Regulation (ER) poster (Poster 3 in Appendix B). This subject can be introduced along the following lines:

> *OK—it looks like [child] often reacts to being sad/dysphoric in ways that keep her feeling sad and bad. So, let's look at this poster—it has examples of ways to react that can stop sad feelings or make them not as strong. Thinking back, has there been a time when [child] would recover from sad feelings by getting involved in something that distracted her—like turning to play? How about . . .*

As treatment progresses and the parent and young patient become better informants about affect-related matters, information about aspects of mood repair development also can be sought, whenever it seems appropriate. One developmental feature of interest is the earliest age at which the young patient self-initiated seeking out caregivers when sad or distressed. Another milestone is the age at which the child consistently started to use words to convey that he was sad or distressed and needed help. A further milestone of interest is the earliest age at which the young patient seemed able to recover on his own from being sad, without parental intervention. The ages at which the just noted milestones were met provide clues as to whether the young patient experienced atypical mood repair development, which may make it more difficult for him to manage current dysphoria.

Demonstrate the Link between Regulatory Response and Subsequent Affect Experience

It is imperative that the child and parent understand a fundamental thesis at the heart of CERT: *How my child reacts to her own emotion and mood significantly alters the subsequent course of that emotion and mood and thereby her functioning.* Of course, this statement applies to every other person as well. Because initial affect regulatory responses typically are automatic, recognition of their impact on subsequent emotional experiences may mean *making explicit a process that has been mostly implicit.*

Several factors can make it difficult to render the affect regulation process more explicit. For example, it is difficult for many children and some adults to be aware of their own and other people's emotions. Some people are ill at ease having to discuss emotions, while others may believe that emotions are wild, unruly, or primitive, and best swept under the carpet. Relatedly, the concept of regulation may be misunderstood as either repression or rigid control of the affect. The therapist has to be mindful of such issues and explicate the affect–response relationship carefully. Make sure that the word *regulation* is not interpreted as blaming the young patient or the parent(s) for the child's affective difficulties and that it is regarded as a flexible process, rather than rigid and all or no control.

One would think that a didactic explanation of emotion regulation (mood repair), illustrated by The House of ER poster, anecdotes, or a discussion of imaginary affect-laden scenarios would be the way to go: Indeed, that may be the best explanatory approach for some young patients and their parents. Keep in mind, however, that, at the start of treatment, young patients and parents are likely to be upset and distressed, and that such affective states may not be conducive to listening to didactic explanations. The best way to initially convey to the parent–child pair how a response to an affect influences its subsequent course is for the therapist to intervene within the treatment session to decrease the young patient's evident negative affect.

As the therapist seeks to demonstrate, *in vivo,* the affect–response connection, the question arises as to which regulatory domain and which specific response to introduce. Having examined the child's and the parent's answers to self-rated questionnaires about how the child reacts to sadness, and based on the clinical interview, the therapist may have an initial picture of the adaptive responses (and corresponding domains) already in the child's repertoire and whether the child is most comfortable with cognitive, behavioral, or interpersonal regulation.

An intervention representing each domain is discussed in each of the sections that follow, to demonstrate the affect–response connection. In general, however, and particularly when in doubt about the child's domain preference(s), it is best to focus on the social–interpersonal regulatory domain. Linking affect and regulatory response within the session provides the parent–child pair with a real-life experience of a key CERT principle. This also can serve as the backdrop to a discussion of what responses to dysphoria have been historically helpful to the young patient.

Each of the following interventions showcases a relatively simple response in its respective domain in The House of ER: (1) Getting and giving a hug exemplifies The People (Social–Interpersonal) Room, (2) jumping jacks exemplify a response from The Things to Do (Action or Behavioral) Room, and (3) mental imagery exemplifies The Thinking (Cognitive) Room.

Reducing Dysphoria via a Social Regulatory Response

Getting and giving a hug exemplify social–interpersonal emotion regulation, which means that another person influences the intensity and duration of a given individual's sadness or dysphoria. While adaptive interpersonal regulation via touch or caress is relatively simple to execute, it is particularly important because it is one of the developmentally earliest and effective regulatory response to which a child is exposed (see Chapter 2). Getting a hug when distressed may not only activate sensory mechanism that can counter low mood but also signals being loved, comforted, and accepted. The use of "getting a hug" to demonstrate the affect–behavior connection is illustrated next in a session with Mary.

Mary, an 8-year-old, only child, was brought for treatment by her grandmother. Grandma, a still employed nurse's aide, in her sixties, has been Mary's primary caregiver since Mary's mother walked out when the child was about 3–4 years old and remained only in sporadic long-distance contact. The mother's difficulties appeared to have been exacerbated by substance abuse issues. About 9 months prior to seeking help, Mary's mother unexpectedly reentered the picture only to disappear again. Shortly thereafter, Mary started to show symptoms of depression, including moodiness, social withdrawal, unwillingness to help Grandma at home, and problems with getting schoolwork done. In the session, Grandma seemed a bit frustrated, but she was affectionate and invested in Mary's recovery. While it appeared that Grandma's material resources were limited, she had an ample amount of social support. Mary did not talk much and was clingy. She impressed the therapist as somewhat younger than her chronological age of 8 years.

Early in the first session after the basic features of CERT had been reviewed, the therapist determined that Mary's sadness and bad mood were problems and that she was consistently dysphoric (see Chapter 6). In the dialogue that follows, the therapist confirms with the child the nature of her emotion. Given that Mary is only 8 years old, the therapist uses a facial emotion expression poster to do this. In view of Mary's age and clinical history, the therapist then focuses on the social–interpersonal regulatory domain to illustrate how a response can alter the course of an emotion and tries to establish if a response from that domain can help this child to feel better. Note how the therapist (T) introduces the relevance of the rules of coaching and of being a good team player, identifies the relationship between affect and regulatory response, and repeatedly reinforces the importance of Grandma (G) as the parent-coach for the child (C).

T: (*To child*) So, Grandma feels that being sad is a problem for you. Mary, which picture (*pointing to the affect expression poster*) shows how you feel right now? (*Child points to a sad face.*) Yes, that girl *is* feeling sad and unhappy. Can you tell me about one thing that can make a girl like you sad? [Further confirming the affect]

C: Uhmm.

T: That's a tough question—so, what do you think?

C: When your Ma goes away?

T: Yes, that would make any kid really sad!

How sad do you feel right now?

Can you show me how big this feeling is? (*Therapist gestures various lengths with her hands.*) This big, this big, or this big?

C: Big sad!

T: Hmm—I guess it's hard to make sad feelings go away, especially when they are big.

OK (*to grandmother, child*), I have an idea we could try. Would it help if Grandma gave you [Mary] a *big* hug right now?

C: Dunno.

T: (*To grandmother*) In the past, when Mary got upset about something, did it help if you gave her a hug?

G: Well—let me think. Yeah, usually.

T: So, let's try this. Grandma, can you give Mary a *very big* and *long* hug right now?

At this point, the therapist encourages Grandma to leave her seat, approach Mary, and give the child several long hugs with brief pauses in between. The therapist then positively reinforces Grandma's behavior and proceeds to make explicit the link between feeling better and getting a hug from Grandma.

T: (*To Grandma*) I can see that you are a really good hugger! That is great—because hugging is very important for children.

T: OK, Mary, it looks like you are feeling a little better. I guess it's nice to get hugged by Grandma—isn't it?

C: Yeah.

T: (*To child*) That's good—

Are you feeling a little better, a lot better, or in between? (*Using hand gestures to illustrate size*)

C: (*Nods to the "small" gesture.*)

T: That's good. Can you show me on these emojis here, which shows how you feel? Hmm—that's good!

T: (*To Grandma*) Can you put on your "coaching hat"? Let's put this in words—let's put it together.

So, when Mary feels sad and unhappy, *one* way to make her feel less sad is to give her several *big* hugs. Right?

G: Sure.

T: So, that means that how we *react* to Mary's sadness can change that feeling—it can make it smaller, make it go away, or it can make it worse.

Can you think of one reaction to Mary's sadness that could make it *worse?*

G: Hmm. When it gets on my nerves and I yell at her.

T: *Right!* That is a very good answer. Yelling at a person who feels sad will make the sadness worse, although you do *not* mean it.

But hugging that person—like you just did with Mary—will make her feel better.

(*To child*) But Mary, sometimes Grandma may not know that you need a hug. So, *how* could you let her know? What do you think is the thing to do?

C: Tell her?

T: Yes. You could ask for a hug. Right? Can you do that now, show me how that would work? (*Mary reaches her arms out to Grandma.*)

That's great! And let's look at the Rules of Being a Good Team Player—which rule fits what you just did?

C: Dunno.

T: I can see that's not easy because there are six rules.

But you just showed how well you can follow the first two rules—you tried out the plan we had about hugging.

At this point, the therapist proceeds to ask for one more demonstration, while simultaneously verbalizing the lesson to be learned (as just illustrated), based on what is ongoing. Given Mary's chronic dysphoria, the therapist elects to bypass mood monitoring as homework for now; instead, she plans to use hugging as homework because it was so successful in the session and the grandparent–child pair was comfortable with it. Furthermore, given the apparent cause of Mary's depression (abandonment by and inconsistent presence of her biological mother, an important element of the emerging case formulation), the therapist feels that nurturing physical contact is particularly appropriate. At the end of the session, the therapist can introduce the homework as follows:

T: (*To Grandma and child*) If you remember, we talked about the fact that sometimes you will have homework in between sessions. That's a project that you do at home and then report back on how it went.

So, this homework is called "giving and getting a hug." That is the major part—like what you just did here.

It means having *huge hugging* sessions. Let's say four times a day. So, this would be before Mary goes to school, when she comes home from school, after dinner, and before going to bed. OK? Each session should have three long hugs. Three *big* and *long* hugs!

G: How long?

T: Very good question: about 10 seconds, each time. You can set the timer on your phone.

(*To child*) And *extra* hugs every time you feel sad. You can ask Grandma for a hug at any time. Does this make sense?

(*To Grandma*) And you have to be the coach. This means that you keep time and know when the two of you are due for a hug session and remind Mary.

Also, I would like you to write down on this paper here each time you practice the hug session. [To log the assignment, the therapist gives the pair a copy of Form 8, a blank reproducible version of which can be found in Appendix A.] You see. Here are the names of the days and the hours. So, before 8 A.M. is before she goes to school, after 3 P.M. is when she comes home—and the other two entries depend on when you have dinner and bedtime.

(*To Grandma and child*) And Mary, each time before the hug, you tell Grandma how strong your sad and bad feeling is—you pick between very strong, in-between strong, a little strong, and no sad feeling. So that Grandma can write it down. And then, the same thing *after* the hugs? OK?

(*To child*) Remember what you and Grandma did and how it worked out? We now know that *hugging* is one way to feel better when you feel sad.

Let's see if this homework can help you to feel a little better. That's why we are trying it.

(*To Grandma*) Looking at this poster [The Rules of Coaching], which rule will best apply to you when you are coaching this homework? (*Grandma points to Rule 2.*) Yes, you are right—it is Rule 2!

OK, I want to be sure that I explained everything correctly. So—can you tell me in your own words what you will be doing as coach?

(*To Grandma*) Finally, let's practice filling out this sheet—and remember to bring the sheet with you when you come next time.

As with all homework assignments, the therapist needs to be confident that this grandparent–child pair understands the assignment and the reason for it, and that both parties are capable of executing it. Practicing the assignment with the therapist in the session can help to identify potential misunderstandings. In the next session, feedback from the grandparent–child pair about the hugging homework will be a priority.

It is a safe bet that Mary and her grandmother are likely to carry out the homework, and that the exercise will bring about positive change by reducing her dysphoria. Thus, at this point, the therapist's treatment plan for the next few sessions is to continue to reinforce the social regulation of sadness, link the response to the appropriate room in The House of ER, and expand the range of people who can serve as regulatory agents for Mary (illustrated later in this chapter). However, if Grandma and Mary fail to carry out the homework, the therapist needs to find out the reasons and act accordingly. See the section "Homework Compliance and Noncompliance" in Chapter 3 for details about possible homework noncompliance and several ways to handle it.

Reducing Dysphoria via a Behavioral Regulatory Response

For some children, it may be more appropriate for the therapist to turn to the behavioral response domain to demonstrate the effects of regulatory attempts on mood. Physical activity and exercise are tools from The Things to Do (Action or Behavioral) Room of The House of ER. Physical activity and exercise involving effort are among the *most* effective ways to counter depression and its affective components. As a regulatory response, it is entirely within the control of the young patient. As homework, it can be deployed within a social–interpersonal context (e.g., a child may exercise with a sibling, or join a sports team). In the next example, jumping jacks demonstrate how a particular behavioral response can bring about a desirable change in the child's affect, *in vivo.* If the young patient dislikes jumping jacks, other related options in the behavioral domain include jumping rope, doing sit-ups, or modified triceps push-ups.

Nine-year-old Pete is the youngest of three children and gets along well with his older brother and sister who have expressed concerns about him. Pete was brought to the clinic by his mother because of mounting worries over the past 8–10 months. While Pete's mood started to change several years earlier, just after his parents' divorce, this year he developed additional symptoms of despondency and worthlessness: feeling unlovable, an inability to tolerate the slightest frustration, and more recently sleep loss. The mornings seem particularly difficult. Mother also notices fatigue. His school performance has suffered, and he has stopped playing with friends. Family context includes a positive history of mood disorder with several affected people both on the paternal and maternal sides, the recent remarriage of his mother, financial disagreements between the new couple, and the stresses and related arguments of joint custody. Additionally, Pete started attending a new school this year.

Earlier in the session, the therapist reviewed the basic features of CERT and the coaching model, and identified sadness as the target symptom. While Pete was cooperative and agreed that feeling sad and unhappy was a problem, he looked somewhat lethargic and uncomfortable, and his answers had a cynical tone. The therapist elected not to use getting and giving a hug to demonstrate the affect–response connection because he noticed friction between mother and child, the nature of which was unclear. Because Pete was visibly depressed, the therapist decided to focus on behavioral regulation and selected physical exercise as the response.

T: (*To mother and child*) Now, the important thing we want to do here is to help Pete feel a little better. We want Pete to feel less depressed. Right?

(*To child*) How strong is this feeling right now? (*Pointing to a container of glass beads*), let's say one bead equals not sad at all. Here is a container; put in some beads to show *how bad* this feeling is right now. So, one bead equals not sad, one or two beads equal a little sad—see what I mean? (*Child proceeds with task.*)

Oh, that's a lot of beads! That means being really sad. Yes, that is hard. Let's see if we can do something about it.

(*To Mom*) Can you put on your coaching hat? I would like you to help with something.

(*To child*) Can we do an experiment? Do you know how to do jumping jacks?

Note that at this point in the treatment, the therapist is not likely to get an enthusiastic response to any proposition. The goal therefore is to prompt the young patient *to just try* something new and *different.* The basic idea is that even if the task does not fully yield the expected results, the therapist has now witnessed the young patient actually engaging in a new initiative, for which he can be praised. Explaining the goal of the task being proposed is one way to attenuate resistance. The therapist may thus proceed as follows:

T: So, here is the experiment—let's see how many jumping jacks you can do in 1 minute.

I am asking because it turns out that some kids feel better if they exercise, like shooting hoops or riding a bike. It would be good to see if exercise works for you.

We can't shoot hoops here, but we can try something like jumping jacks and see if it helps.

(*To child*) So, how many jumping jacks do you *think* you can do?

C: Dunno. Some [after prodding], maybe 15.

T: (*To Mom*) Here is a stopwatch. We will set it to 1 minute. Can you hold it and also start counting *aloud* the number of jumping jacks while Pete is doing them?

This is one way to be a coach!

C: That's dumb. Don't want to do it.

T: Yeah, it could be dumb, but exercise *can* also help you feel differently. So, why don't we try?

Also, remember the rules of how to be a good team player? See here (*pointing to the appropriate poster*). Trying new things is one of the rules—right?

You know what—I'll do it with you! Let's start now.

Because the therapist is modeling the target behavior, the young patient is likely to do more than 15 jumping jacks, for which he can then be praised. And because jumping jacks can be fairly vigorous, there is a good chance that continuing to do them for a minute will bring about at least a mild decrease in dysphoric mood. Indeed, if the young patient has mastered the exercise, the therapist could propose an extra minute of it to increase its beneficial effects on mood.

Note that the therapist praises the child and also engages the parent (P). Then the therapist links the behavior to improved mood and helps the parent–child pair to locate this tool in the appropriate room of The House of ER.

T: That was really good.

(*To Mom*) Didn't you think he did great? And how many jumping jacks did he do?

P: He did 50!

T: (*To child*) Yeah! That was great. *And* you also followed the first rule of being a good team player.

Let's look at this container with the beads—this was how much you were feeling bad before. And how do you feel now? The same number of beads as before or less sad, which means not so many beads?

(*To Mom*) What *do you think?*

P: Well, he does look like he is in a better mood—he did really good with the jumping.

T: (*To child*) You can take out beads to show that you feel better. If you feel a little bit better, take out a few beads; if you feel a *lot* better, take out many beads. What is *left* shows me how sad you feel right now. (*Child takes out a few beads.*)

So, you feel a little better!

(*To Mom and child*) Can we put into words what just happened?

We started out with Pete feeling really bad, and then we did this experiment with jumping jacks, and what happened after that?

P: Well—he looks better.

T: Yes, I think he feels a little better. The idea is that when we feel sad, sometimes we can *do* something to make the feeling *less strong,* just like we did here. Feeling better makes it easier to do other things, like get schoolwork done.

(*To Mom and child*) You remember that we talked about The House of ER—that there are three rooms there and many tools in it that can help with feeling better.

OK, Pete (*pointing to The House of ER poster*), in which room do you think jumping jacks belong?

After an acceptable initial answer, mother and child can be asked to list other possible tools from The Things to Do Room that can help a person to feel less sad, and comment on which one would be most likely to work for Pete. The session ends with homework involving mood monitoring across specified hours during the day, along with jumping jacks for a certain number of minutes, several times a day, with Mom acting as coach; the purpose of the jumping jack homework (which also qualifies as an "experiment") is to see how it affects Pete's mood in daily life. As noted in the previous case, reporting on the homework becomes one of the first items on the next session's agenda. Depending on the outcome, the therapist may elect to continue to reinforce the use of jumping jacks or some other physical activity for mood repair. The therapist's treatment plan at this point includes both a continuous focus on reducing Pete's dysphoria via behavioral responses and the need to broaden his regulatory options most likely by introducing a nonphysical behavioral response.

Reducing Dysphoria via a Cognitive Regulatory Response

In CERT, cognitive regulatory responses are described to children as "things that go on in your head." The regulatory tools in The Thinking (Cognitive) Room include thoughts, ideas, interpretations, mental pictures or images, and internal sensory experiences (like hearing music in one's head). Deliberate refocusing of attention away from the source or experience of dysphoria is another important cognitive strategy that can serve mood repair.

The responses that exemplify the social or behavioral regulation of dysphoria are typically observable when they are being deployed. In contrast, the therapist must rely on the oral report of the young patient regarding the implementation of cognitive regulatory responses. In other words, the therapist has no direct proof of whether, and how well, a cognitive regulatory response is being implemented. Lack of information regarding a young patient's introspective and linguistic abilities, and younger age, both signal that the therapist needs to proceed with care when targeting the cognitive regulatory domain.

Generally, a cognitive regulatory response should not be the therapist's first choice with most children to demonstrate the principles of mood repair. Provided that the child or adolescent is reasonably articulate, a confluence of factors may warrant ignoring that guideline. For example, an initial focus on interpersonal regulation may be precluded when the parent–child relationship is very troubled, or if it appears that the parent will need training to be a good coach. The use of an activity tool from the behavioral domain may need to be modified or precluded if the young patient has some physical limitation.

In the following example, the therapist uses mental imagery (as attention refocusing) to demonstrate how a given response can alter affect experience. The aforementioned caveats notwithstanding, this intervention was selected because the young patient was verbally articulate and needed a regulatory tool that he could use on his own, and right away.

Davey, a bright and articulate 10-year-old boy, was brought for treatment by his father, who was concerned with Davey's ongoing sadness and the trouble they have had managing his asthma. Father revealed that Davey has been upset, dysphoric, crying, and has verbalized thoughts of death and suicidal ideation. He also has exhibited symptoms of anxiety, has been avoiding social interactions, and has been reluctant to go to school. Davey's previously outstanding school performance started to decline around a year earlier. That point in time corresponded to the onset of being bullied at school after he started dressing in all black, which appeared to be some sort of personal statement. Family context includes a younger sister who has been diagnosed with autism; Davey is responsible for caring for her a few hours on the days when his parents are busy meeting other obligations. There is a history of maternal mood disorder as well as a neurological disorder with a variable course. The parents, both of whom are professionals, also admitted to increased arguing in recent months but were unwavering in their support of Davey.

After being introduced to CERT, his father immediately voiced concerns about the child's dysphoric mood, which Davey acknowledged. It also appeared that Davey's recent dysphoria was related to the teasing and bullying in school, which contributed to his desire to avoid school. There was an urgent need to intervene because the parent's overtures to school personnel to stop the bullying had not been successful. The therapist therefore decided to target the child's affective reactions to the bullying and, given Davey's cognitive abilities, to focus on the cognitive regulatory domain, which is within the young patient's control. The therapist first confirms her understanding of the school situation and Davey's reactions via a short version of contextual mapping (see the section "A Template for Working with Target Symptoms" in Chapter 3). Note that while the therapist (T) focuses on helping Davey to implement an adaptive response to his distress, she also engages the parent (P) in his coaching role. C stands for child in the dialogues.

T: Let me put this together and see if I've got it correct. In school, during lunch, there are these three kids and sometimes they sit near you and keep saying nasty things, picking on you—sounds about right?

And many times, there are no teachers nearby to do something, and this situation happens several times a week?

And then what? What happens when these kids act like that? You sit and do what?

C: Nothing.

T: Well, I am guessing that you also feel really bad, really sad—and you are thinking: "Why are they picking on me?" Like "What's wrong with me? Is that how it goes?

C: Hmm.

T: So, you feel really miserable and upset, and you kind of think that it is your fault?

C: Hmm.

T: Is this one of the reasons that you don't want to go to school?

C: Yes, when they are doing it.

Davey's reactions to his own distress included blaming himself for being bullied, which is a maladaptive cognitive response that perpetuated and intensified his dysphoric mood. The therapist therefore proposed an alternate way to respond to the bullying:

T: So (*to child*) what if you did something, not just sit and blame yourself—something so that it did not matter what those three kids did—so that it didn't bother you?

C: Not go to school?

T: No, something else! Something in your head. Something using your imagination? Let me ask you this—can you see pictures in your mind? Like running a video show in your head?

C: Yeah like, sure.

T: Kind of *make-believe* in pictures! So, what would happen if you used your imagination when kids tease you in the lunchroom? Like, you sit in the lunchroom but *not* think about how mean they are and why.

Instead of thinking like that, maybe you can imagine a picture—seeing them doing things that are silly or funny, something like that.

(*To parent*) What do you think?

P: Sure, if he didn't pay attention to them, that would work.

T: (*To child*) Hmm. What would be a silly or stupid-looking picture? Can you think of something?

C: I got it. Their pants got loose and fell off and they are standing there in their underwear!!

T: That sounds great.

So, here is my question: Don't you think you would feel *much* better if you were thinking of those guys in their underwear and *not* thinking that everything is your fault?

C: Dunno, guess so.

T: Tell me more about this funny picture or video you are creating in your head. And (*to parent*) can you take some notes for your later use in coaching?

At this point, the therapist asks the child to describe his visual imagery and encourages him to provide as much detail as possible. More elaborate visual images are likely to be more potent in countering and replacing Davey's negative cognitive responses to being bullied. The therapist then engages Davey in role play to expose him to the actual experience of response implementation.

T: (*To child*) OK, so how about trying this now?

(*To parent*) Can you put on your coaching hat? Can you help Davey practice this exercise?

(*To both parent and child*) Let's pretend that you are at school. You are in the lunchroom, and some kids walk by and make some comment. Give me one example of what they might say.

Now . . . imagine hearing them say that stuff! But right away, have that video running in your head about these same boys walking around in their underwear.

(*To parent*) Let's start again with imagining the scene at school and then right away having the special video on his mind. Can you read off your notes about his video so that he can see it in his head?

(*To child and parent*) The reason why we are doing this is that if you have a negative idea in your head that upsets you and makes you miserable, one way to feel better is to replace it with a more helpful idea or an image that is funny.

C: Yeah, this is a funny picture.

Such a role play and technique rehearsal should be repeated several times until the child and parent appear to be fully comfortable with the task. The child and parent should also be asked to formulate in their own words the purpose of the strategy and its relationship to The House of ER. In Davey's case, it was apparent that the intervention might help him fend off distress; it was therefore assigned as a twofold homework: practicing the imagery twice in a row each weekday evening at home with Dad acting as coach and using it as a mood regulatory response when being subjected to bullying in school.

The therapist also made a mental note to assign mood-monitoring homework at the next session just to confirm whether (or not) Davey's dysphoria is entirely related to school. And as part of his emerging treatment plan, the therapist made a further note to be on the lookout for suicidal ideation because it was one of Davey's depression symptoms.

As noted in the previous case examples, reporting on homework becomes a focal point of the subsequent treatment session. If the homework was implemented with some success, the therapist can continue to focus on reinforcing the use of mental imagery as well as other cognitive strategies for mood repair. If the homework was implemented but failed to achieve its goals, the therapist can use contextual mapping to identify why the assignment failed. For example, the mother may have deviated from following the rules of coaching (e.g., got angry at the child) or others may have interrupted the sessions. Discussion of such problematic features needs to focus on how to correct them so that the parent–child pair can give the homework another try.

If the homework was not implemented, the best approach is to ask the parent–child pair what might have interfered with the assignment. For example, the mother's job may have required her to work extra hours, which left insufficient time for the homework or the family may have been too busy to set aside enough time for the homework: Such scenarios suggest that the frequency and timing of the assignment should be renegotiated. (See also the discussion about homework noncompliance in Chapter 3.)

End the Session with a Homework Assignment

Although homework is a crucial part of all phases of CERT, it is particularly important that the initial CERT sessions end with a homework assignment because the early sessions set expectations and serve as general templates for the sessions to follow. A homework assignment also assures continuity with the next session, underscores the key role of the coaching relationship, and gives the parent–child pair hope that new directions are possible. Chapter 7 includes several types of homework as integral treatment components.

Each of the initial sessions presented in the prior section concluded with homework that built on the mood regulatory response demonstrated in that session.

However, at this early stage in treatment, the therapist may decide that she needs further information about the characteristics of the young patient's dysphoria, rather than assigning for homework the practice of a mood repair response. Such a decision may reflect the therapist's concern about the severity of the child's sad affect and the most suitable mood repair response for it. As noted in Chapter 5, monitoring of sad, dysphoric affect is a logical and relatively easy homework, which can provide data about the persistence of the child's dysphoria as a function of time and setting and also can include severity ratings.

The case of Lisa illustrates the use of homework assigned in an initial session to gather further information about dysphoria. Lisa, a bright, 12-year-old only child, was brought for treatment by her mother due to increasing dysphoria, irritability, and social withdrawal over the prior 6 months. Her school performance in some areas had also declined, and recently she developed sleep disturbance and started to complain about not wanting to go to school. Lisa has a long history of learning disability, for which she had received continuous multifaceted interventions, including special education and behavioral support, until earlier in the year, at which time she was fully integrated into regular classes. Family context includes some financial stresses over the past 12–16 months and, relatedly, increased arguments between her parents. However, the clinician was impressed by the young patient's overall adjustment until recently, her school achievements in several areas, and the fact that both parents were clearly supportive of their child and appeared to be quite capable of functioning as coaches. The later factors were important in the therapist's emerging case formulation.

Much of the session focused on the presenting complaint and a discussion of CERT, including the role of the parents as coaches. But the therapist believed that she did not have a full picture of the persistence or severity of Lisa's dysphoria in daily life. So, toward the end of the session, she introduced the monitoring homework assignment and proposed to Lisa that she keep a log of her sad and dysphoric feelings. The therapist explained how the log would serve the treatment goals. Because Lisa is older and more articulate than many child patients, the therapist asked her to monitor not only her dysphoria (yes/no) but also its severity and context.

As described in the section "Homework: Why, How, and What" in Chapter 3, the therapist models the actions that will be required and checks that the parent–child pair understands and will be able to carry out the task. Note that the therapist integrates the homework and reinforcement for the coaching model (which had been introduced previously) to support this new pattern of parent–child interaction.

In introducing the task, the therapist emphasizes several issues, as follows:

T: Let's see how we can help Lisa so that she'll feel better. We'll try to get the sad feeling to be smaller. So, it is important to know more about it, like how often Lisa feels sad and what goes on when she feels that way.

One way to do this is to keep a record of sad feelings during the day. This is a type of homework.

We call this homework "keeping a log"—it is like a diary. It will show us if there are patterns to how you [child] feel. For example, some children feel sad in the morning, while other children only feel sad in the evenings. Some children feel bad every day, other children feel bad only on some days!

Here is the idea: I would like Lisa—with your [parent's] help—to make a note in the log about how sad she feels four times a day: in the morning before school, after Lisa comes home from school, after dinner, and before going to bed.

P: Like every day?

T: Hmm. How about doing this for 3 days before we meet again?

(*To Mom*) I am going to ask you to be the coach and work with Lisa on this. It is important that you do the log entries at the times we agreed. *Not* at the end of the day. Because it is hard to remember, thinking back, how we felt hours ago. If you had a tough or busy day, that can make it even harder to remember.

(*To Mom and child*) For this log, I will ask you to pay attention to two things: how strong Lisa's sad feeling is and what is going on at the time you rate that feeling.

And remember that this homework is part of the *coaching* we talked about (*pointing to the posters about being a good coach and a good team player*).

(*To child*) So, Mom will help you with this—like a coach and you will be the player—right?

Let me show you how this works.

(*To Mom*) Let's pretend that you had this log sheet to fill out this morning. You told me earlier about when Lisa was just sitting on her bed, and you couldn't get her moving, and she looked miserable.

(*Mother and child are handed a daily feelings/activity log.*) What time of day was it? [A blank version of the same log is provided as Form 6 in Appendix A.]

P: In the morning—I don't know—around 7 or 8?

T: OK, so here on the left side you can put down the hours. But now we will put down the four times you would do this. Next to the morning, 7 A.M. box, there we would ask Lisa to write in how she feels: "sad, miserable."

And (*to child*) how strong was that feeling? Let's use numbers: 1 equals very little to 10 equals very strong. So, a 5 would be middle to strong, for example.

C: Dunno, about 7?

T: (*To child*) And what was going on at that time?

C: Nothing, I was in bed.

T: OK, so now, in the space here, we write "in bed." Good? Let's make believe you are back from school. . . . [Figure 6.1 shows Lisa's partially completed form.]

The therapist should continue to work with the parent and child until it is clear that they understand the task. If further practice is indicated, the therapist, the parent, and the child can complete the mood log *in vivo* for the prior 3 hours or so. Then, the actual *homework* assignment has to be negotiated. For example:

T: (*To parent and child*) Like I mentioned before, could you do this four times a day? If you remember, we talked about this—homework is very

Daily Feelings Log by Location

Day/time	TODAY! Place (for example, home)	Feeling	How strong was the feeling? (pick a number between 1 = not strong and 10 = very strong)
7 a.m. morning	? in bed	sad misrable	7
Back from school			
After dinner			
Before going to bed			

FIGURE 6.1. Lisa's partially completed feelings log.

important because we want to get complete information about this sad feeling.

Do you think you can do this? Does this homework make sense?

Negotiating homework means that the therapist adjusts his initial expectations if the child or parent raises any concerns. For instance, if, in the prior dialogue, the parent interjects that she and the child won't be able to do the morning monitoring on the following day given an early event they must attend, the frequency can be decreased until a mutually agreed on goal is identified.

At the next CERT session, the outcome of such a homework assignment will be one of the first agenda items. If the assignment was attempted, both the child and parent should be generously praised (even if they did not complete it), particularly as a coaching team. Then the content of the mood log has to be examined to determine whether it provides leads that can be pursued. Look for patterns such as diurnal variation (e.g., sad affect is always worse in the morning and lessens as the day goes by, or the other way around), discontinuities (e.g., marked changes in severity ratings), and context specificity (e.g., mood is always worse at home after dinner). Any aspect of the log can become the focus of further inquiry.

At the next session, a review of Lisa's homework showed that she was consistently more despondent in the late afternoon and early evening after school: This may suggest that her dysphoric states are context-related. Thus, the next goal was to explore whether it is something at school or something about coming home that engenders Lisa's sadness and if any presumably causal features are amenable to intervention. A similar approach would be pursued if her dysphoric affect was typically present in the morning, not in the evening.

But let's assume that the mood log reveals no meaningful daily diurnal or context-related variation, which is also important information. If that is the case, the task completion and its meaning still have to be acknowledged by saying, for example:

T: You did a great job at completing this. Both of you! We now know much more about Lisa's feelings of sadness. It looks like Lisa is sad quite a lot. Also, it doesn't seem to matter if she is at home or at school.

The consistency of Lisa's dysphoria during the day may reflect that she ruminates, which is a maladaptive mood repair response. The therapist could therefore reassign the mood log homework but ask Lisa to monitor an additional dimension, the regulatory response being deployed ("Write down what you were doing or thinking each time you logged that you felt sad or bad"). Depending on the results, to be presented in the next session, the therapist may choose to explore the relations between dysphoria severity and Lisa's response, which may or may not be primarily cognitive, or focus on replacing a particular maladaptive regulatory response with an adaptive one.

Summary and Next Steps

In addition to forming the basis of the therapeutic relationship, the initial CERT sessions provide the young patient and parent with a general understanding of this intervention, its focus, and their own roles in the process of recovery. The psychoeducational information the therapist shares with the family further underscores why CERT emphasizes the role of dysphoric emotions and their regulation in depression and the process of recovering from it. *In vivo* demonstrations of how a given response to sadness and dysphoria can change the subsequent course of that affect experience further support the rationale of CERT; importantly, they also provide some symptom relief, which is critical to maintaining the engagement of the parent–child pair at this early point in treatment. The homework assignments contribute to patient engagement as well and establish continuity across the sessions.

The treatment plan of patients at this early stage reflects the explanatory paradigm of CERT, namely, that sad, dysphoric emotion and mood have to be the initial target symptoms. The subsequent sessions then continue to focus on alleviating dysphoria by strengthening the young patient's adaptive mood repair response repertoire and typically involve new regulatory directions. The emerging treatment plan is likely to specify nonaffective depression symptoms as well, which can be targeted (if they are still problematic) along with dysphoria or after that symptom has remitted.

The initial sessions provide the therapist with useful information about the emotion regulatory response (and domain) with which the young patient appears to feel comfortable. In later sessions, the therapist's emerging understanding of the young patient and the family (the case formulation) will influence whether the therapist continues to focus on the initially identified regulatory response and domain or pursues other mood repair responses and domains. Elements of this ongoing decision-making process in which the therapist engages are addressed further in Chapter 7, which also includes several illustrative case examples.

Chapter 7

Treatment of Sadness and Dysphoria

The treatment of sadness and dysphoria essentially involves achieving better mood repair. While the main treatment goal is to reduce the young patient's distress, contextual emotion regulation therapy (CERT) does not seek to eliminate sadness and dysphoria from the child's affective life: Adaptive mood repair responding does not mean the absence of distressing emotions. Instead, CERT seeks to change the power balance so that the young patient has control over her sad and dysphoric experiences, rather than those affects having control over the child.

This chapter provides guidance about how to proceed after the initial sessions (described in the prior chapter). It thus assumes that sadness and dysphoria have been identified as treatment targets, that the therapist has established at least some of their key features (e.g., severity), that the therapist has linked an *in vivo* regulatory response with reduced sadness, and so has tentatively identified a mood repair response that helps the child to feel better (as also described in Chapter 6).

CERT's main focus is on the alleviation of a young patient's affective distress by strengthening her adaptive mood repair response repertoire; the sections that follow illustrate various ways to approach that goal in each of the three regulatory domains. To help the therapist in decision making with his own patients, each section also enumerates the pros and cons of regulatory responses in the domain being addressed. In closing this chapter, two other approaches are also discussed that can lead to symptom relief: improving the process whereby a mood repair response is implemented and contextual manipulation to prevent the emergence or intensification of dysphoric symptoms.

The parent–child–therapist exchanges in the present chapter include multiple references to the posters displayed on the walls of the treatment room (described in Chapter 4), especially The House of Emotion Regulation (ER) that pictures its *rooms* (regulatory response domains) and some of the tools (adaptive regulatory responses) each room contains. The posters with the rules for coaching and being coached are also often referred to. This approach helps to reinforce the parent–child pair's understanding of basic CERT principles. Remember: Repetition facilitates learning. Eventually, emotion regulatory concepts can be integrated with problem-solving approaches (exemplified by the WWW.Solve poster; see Poster 4 in Appendix B) in the interest of better mood control.

As treatment progresses, the therapist develops an increasing understanding of how the given patient experiences dysphoria, the accompanying mood repair strategies (evident in the treatment sessions and the child's daily interactions), how the parents respond to the child's affect displays, and the presence of important thematic and contextual features. These variables form parts of the case formulation (see Chapter 5). In turn, the case formulation plays a role in which emotion regulatory responses the therapist reinforces for a given young patient (see the section to come, "Chantel, Age 9") and also sets the stage for the individually tailored coping skills training plan in the last phase of CERT (see Chapter 10).

Strengthening Adaptive Mood Repair Response Repertoires

The road to improved mood repair and associated remission of affective symptoms is unlikely to be a straight one. In fact, brief relapses (i.e., occasional increases in sadness and dysphoria) tend to be the rule rather than the exception. However, relapses should be framed for the parent–child pair as: (1) unsurprising given the child's history of depression that is likely to last several months or longer and (2) although unpleasant, as providing further opportunities to identify and practice the most useful mood repair responses for that given child. Relapses in mood repair competence can be explained as similar to learning how to ride a bike (or any complex skill acquisition): It takes a bit of time; you are likely to fall off several times; but with continued practice, you can master the art of bike riding.

After the initial CERT sessions during which the therapist identified a regulatory response that appeared to suit the young patient, the treatment segues into strengthening the response that was just identified, its domain, and eventually the entire repertoire. The continuing focus on adaptive mood repair is necessary to keep sadness and distress at bay. Strengthening an adaptive mood repair response repertoire can take various directions such as improving and expanding the scope of the identified response; introducing new responses in the same domain; introducing a response from another domain; and teaching more effective ways of response deployment. The direction the therapist will pursue is influenced by his emerging case formulation, which acknowledges the young patient's vulnerabilities and strengths, and the availability (or lack) of parental support.

The Social–Interpersonal Regulatory Domain

Recall that the social–interpersonal regulation of dysphoria constitutes one of the developmentally earliest regulatory mechanism to which children are exposed, and it should therefore be considered with all young patients. Chapter 2 listed various forms that social–interpersonal regulation may take, including gentle touch, caress, and embrace; receiving emotional support or other symbolic forms of nurturance; and talking to or being in the presence of others (which may entail conjoint activities).

Social–interpersonal mood repair responses build on the developmental significance of social relationships and the key role of primary caregivers in the unfolding of emotion regulation skills. This domain should definitely be explored with young patients who are imbedded in supportive families and/or have wide extrafamilial social networks. However, deployment of this regulatory domain is constrained by the fact that the young patient is not in full control. Its implementation requires the willingness and availability of another person to serve as a regulator, and that person also needs to have the requisite skills. Children who are constitutionally very shy or have poor social skills are likely to find the social regulation of sadness rather challenging.

Strengthening the child's interpersonal mood repair response repertoire may involve reinforcing or increasing the use of existing responses and improving the *process* of recruiting social regulators (i.e., what the child has to do for other people to recognize his need), engaging existing regulators in new or alternative ways (see the example that follows), and enlisting nonfamilial regulatory agents (e.g., peers, a religious figure, family friends). Engaging extra-familial adults as regulators requires mediation by the parent in her coaching role because children do not typically initiate such contacts.

The vignettes of Mary and Chantel next presented illustrate different ways of strengthening social–interpersonal mood repair response repertoires. Note that the focus on the interpersonal regulatory domain naturally followed from Mary's and Chantel's prior CERT sessions during which both patients displayed a favorable response to getting and giving a hug and were supported by evidence of strong caregiver support.

Mary, Age 8

Let us return to Mary and her grandmother from Chapter 6. They discovered in an earlier session that getting and giving a hug (a tool from The People [Social–Interpersonal] Room) were effective regulators of Mary's distress. During that session, the therapist also helped Mary to recognize that, at times, she herself may have to initiate such regulatory responses. Recall also that the therapist assigned homework involving multiple hugging sessions, to be logged on Form 8.

After structuring the current session, the therapist turns to the homework assignment completed for the past 3 days (see Figures 7.1, 7.2, and 7.3). She notices that the grandparent–child pair did not do the morning hug on 2 days and the evening hug on 1 day, and that Mary asked for an extra hug twice. Thus, the therapist makes a mental note that the missing hugs could signal the need to

Homework to Do Log

Tuesday Day/time	What to do? What is the task?	Was it done?	Initiator	Mary's ~~Child's~~ feelings after + severity (from 1 = little/none to 10 = a lot/very strong)
7 AM	before school HUGS (3 times)	yes	gm	😐
8				
9				
10				
11				
Noon				
1 PM				
2	home from school HUGS (× 3)	2 hugs	Mary	😐
3		yes	gm	🙂
4				
5				
6	after dinner HUGS (× 3)	yes		🙂
7				
8				
9	before bedtime HUGS (× 3)	yes	gm	🙂

FIGURE 7.1. Mary's Tuesday homework. All scheduled hugs completed plus two additional hugs requested by Mary.

Homework to Do Log

Wednesday Day/time	What to do? What is the task?	Was it done?	Initiator	Mary's ~~Child's~~ feelings after + severity (from 1 = little/none to 10 = a lot/very strong)
7 AM before	HUGS			
8 school	3 times			
9				
10				
11				
Noon				
1 PM				
2 home from	HUGS	yes	JM	☺
3 school	(x 3)			
4			Mary	☺
5				
6 after dinner	HUGS (x 3)	yes	JM	
7				
8				
9 before bed	HUGS (x 3)			

FIGURE 7.2. Mary's Wednesday homework. No morning or bedtime hugs.

Homework to Do Log

Thursday Day/time	What to do? What is the task?	Was it done?	Initiator	~~Child's~~ Mary's feelings after + severity (from 1 = little/none to 10 = a lot/very strong)
7 AM	before school HUGS			
8 ↓	(x 3)			
9				
10				
11				
Noon				
1 PM				
2 ↓	home from HUGS		Mary	☺
3	school (x 3)	yes	gm	☺
4				
5				
6	after dinner HUGS (x 3)	yes	gm	☺
7				
8				
9 ↓	before bedtime HUGS (x 3)	yes	gm	☺

FIGURE 7.3. Mary's Thursday homework. No morning hugs.

renegotiate "hug frequencies." After praising the child and parent, and emphasizing that they make a great coaching team, the therapist asks them about their experience in implementing the homework: Was it hard and, if so, what caused that? Did it help Mary to feel better? The therapist asks about the missing morning hugs and finds out that the family is in a big hurry some mornings, which makes a hugging session unfeasible.

At this point, the therapist is fairly confident that, for Mary, The People Room represents a favored regulatory domain. She is therefore planning to have the grandparent–child pair continue with the hugging sessions although she will suggest a reduction in the task's frequency across the mornings. She is concerned, however, that Mary's history of having been essentially abandoned by her mother may have undermined Mary's trust in people, which, in turn, could render her unwilling to recruit social regulators other than Grandma.

As one approach to expanding Mary's interpersonal regulatory domain, the therapist decides to try to have Mary enlist another adult as a regulator. Note that while the therapist (T) is now charting a new direction, she continues to reinforce the regulatory (coaching) relationship established with the grandmother (G), verbalizes lessons learned, and repeatedly refers (directly or indirectly) to how a response changes the course of a given affect. The dialogue may go something like this:

T: (*To Grandma*) Can you coach Mary—help her tell me about the hugging homework and how it worked out?

G: (*To child*) OK, Mary. Why don't you just go and read aloud what we have on that paper? Start with the first day—that's Tuesday.

Because the child (C) is very young and somewhat immature, the therapist knows that much of the actual homework and its recording had to be instigated by her grandmother. However, the therapist wants to reinforce Mary's importance and therefore suggests that she present the report, while at the same time, the therapist also highlights grandmother's coaching role.

T: (*To Grandma and child*) You did a *great* job with the hugging homework.
And (*to child*) I can see from the emojis you picked that getting these long hugs really made you feel better—did I get it right?

C: Hmm. Yeah.

T: Great—so, can you show me again from these faces (*pointing to a facial expressions of emotion poster*), which kid feels the way you feel when you are hugging?
And (*to Grandma*), what did we learn? That you, Grandma, can make Mary feel better!

So, let's look here (*motioning toward The House of ER poster*). When one person helps another to feel better, which room are we talking about?

G: That one with the people.

T: *Right!* One thing to do, or one tool in that room, as we know, is to give and get hugs.

And what other tools in this room? How else can you help Mary to feel better?

Questions like these should be repeated, with the goal of helping the young patient and the parent to articulate their understanding of the progression from being sad, to using one of the tools from The People Room of The House of ER, and the desired affective outcome. The goal is to make the process of interpersonal emotion regulation more explicit.

The questioning now builds on the grandparent–child pair's experiential knowledge of interpersonal mood repair via the successful previous *homework* assignment. Because of this, the lessons learned can be expected to have personal meaning, to be more likely retained in memory, and more available to recall. After establishing the value of interpersonal mood repair, the therapist moves to the next step, which is exploring how to expand Mary's network of social regulators.

T: (*To child*) So, Grandma is one of the people in The People Room. Is there somebody else in The People Room who could help you to feel better when you don't feel good?

(*To Grandma*) Can you put on your coaching hat? Can you help Mary to figure out who are other people that could be in The People Room?

After some back-and-forth, Mary and her grandmother agree that Grandma's sister Karen, who lives nearby and visits them every day, is a person Mary would feel comfortable asking for hugs. Therefore, the therapist proposes a twofold homework assignment: The grandparent–child pair will keep up the hugging sessions. Then after Grandma explains the homework to her sister, Mary will ask her Aunt Karen for hugs. Here is one likely series of remarks from the therapist:

T: OK, let me summarize this again. One of the things we now know is that Mary feels much better if she can get a hug, or she feels that she is not alone when she is upset.

Right? And you [Grandma] are great at helping Mary. But it is a good idea to also have other people to whom Mary can turn. So, Aunt Karen is one of these people.

(*To child*) Mary, can we try something with Aunt Karen? This is like an experiment, something that we try, but we don't know how it will work. That is why it is called an experiment.

(*To Grandma*) Can you put on your coaching hat?

The idea is this: Can you sit down with Mary and Aunt Karen, explain what we are doing, and see if Mary can try to ask her for a hug, just like she did here? And Mary and Aunt Karen then could practice like we did here.

So, when Mary is with her aunt the next 3 days, she could ask Aunt Karen for a hug, and some extra ones if she feels sad. And you would be the coach, reminding everyone when it is time for the hugging session and *also writing it down*.

(*To Grandma*) But first, let's try out how you can explain this to your sister. Let's practice.

I will play you, you will play your sister, and Mary can watch and tell us if we are doing a good job of explaining things. This is called role play. OK? Here we go.

As already introduced in Chapter 6, in connection with Davey's situation, role play is used in CERT to practice behaviors and actions that the parent or child is asked to undertake outside of the treatment setting. The therapist engages in role play with Grandma to maximize the likelihood of Grandma's success at enlisting her sister in the project to help the young patient; namely, the therapist models for Grandma the content of what to say to her sister Karen. By asking Grandma to role-play her own sister, the therapist can uncover possible reluctance (as implied next), which can then be discussed and resolved. Note that while the child's participation is not required in this role play, the therapist finds a task that can keep her engaged during the adults' interactions.

T: (*To child*) Mary, Grandma and I will try out what we just talked about.

I will play your Grandma. Can you pay attention, and when we are done, let me know if I did a good job at playing your Grandma?

T: (*To Grandma*) I will now play you, while you are Karen. So, here we go!

Karen, you know that Mary and me have been going to counseling to help Mary feel better. And we found that it really helps her to get hugs when she feels sad. We were thinking that you also could be the person Mary can ask for hugs.

G: (*Role playing her sister*) Yeah, but why does she have to ask?

T: (*Role playing Grandma*) 'Cause we can't always tell when Mary is sad.

G: (*Role playing her sister*) Hmm, don't know about that.

At this point, the therapist stops the role play and asks grandmother why her sister would likely question the treatment in real life. Apparently, Aunt Karen is mistrustful of all health care personnel, so the therapist offers to meet with her as well. Because the offer to meet appears to satisfy the grandmother, the therapist moves on to question her and Mary about their understanding of the task and its goal (e.g., "Can you tell me your understanding of what the homework is and why you will be doing it?") and their ability to carry it out (e.g., "Can you think of something that might stand in the way of the experiment with Karen? Will you be able to do it?"). Also, the therapist refers to The House of ER (see the previous dialogues) and confirms with the young patient that she understands carrying out the homework involves tools from The People Room.

Note that the homework in this instance will achieve multiple goals. It will reinforce Mary's deployment of a social–interpersonal mood regulatory response (continued hugs with Grandma), help her be more effective at using social regulators (verbalize her need for intervention), and expand her repertoire of social regulators (enlist her aunt). The homework will be on the top of the agenda at the next session: Its successful completion will lead to subsequent attempts to mobilize another person besides Aunt Karen as a regulator, which will afford Mary greater flexibility in interpersonal regulatory responding. Furthermore, because the therapist's case formulation already identified interpersonal mistrust as a key feature of Mary's social–psychological development, increasing the number of emotion regulators is one small step toward Mary gaining ease with and trusting others.

Let's assume that the homework is not executed, which will prompt the therapist to obtain information as to what barriers were encountered. Practical issues could have been at play (e.g., Aunt Karen was away the entire week) as well as some misunderstanding of the task (e.g., confusion about who was to initiate the experiment). The culprit could have been a failure to follow The Rules of Coaching: Mary may have been reluctant to ask her aunt for a hug, which caused her grandmother to lose her temper, after which things went downhill, leaving Grandma remorseful. Such a lapse in coaching needs to be viewed as expected during the process of learning new skills; that is why the sixth rule of coaching states that "coaches are made, not born." Given the just noted scenario, the therapist could say:

T: I see what happened! You spent a bit of time setting up this homework and when it was ready to go, Mary got upset and couldn't ask her aunt for a hug and wouldn't tell you why, so you got upset and a little angry and that ended things!

I understand how you felt. You were angry because you put a lot of time into this, and then Mary wouldn't go along. And then of course, like you said, things don't work out when a person gets really angry.

But coaching is very tough. Because coaching means learning to do some new things. And that's why we have The Rules of Coaching. They can help.

Let's read (*pointing to the poster*) what the sixth rule is: "Coaches are made, not born!" This means a bunch of things—like it is OK to sometimes not be a perfect coach!

Note that although Mary herself failed to follow at least one rule of being a good team player, given her age and maturity level, the therapist judged it more appropriate to work on the grandmother's failure. It is important that the therapist accept such instances of coaching failure in a factual and uncritical manner. Referring to The Rules of Coaching and framing matters from the perspective of learning and skill acquisition helps to diffuse possible self-blame or potential negative affective ramifications of the failed homework before a new attempt is requested.

To strengthen Mary's interpersonal mood repair response domain, the therapist will continue to reinforce her use of both her grandmother and her aunt as mood regulatory agents. The treatment plan also includes the next developmentally important goal as helping Mary to transition from physical hugs as the primary means of interpersonal mood repair to also using language to capture more symbolic forms of interpersonal support. Thus, the therapist will teach Grandma to verbalize emotionally supportive statements while hugging Mary, such as:

> *You are very important to Grandma; she is here to help you feel better. And Grandma can help in many ways. We can talk, we can do things together.*

Or

> *One thing we know helps you to feel better is to hug—that shows that you can count on Grandma to feel better!*
>
> *We can also talk about why you feel sad and that can help, too.*

By capturing in words the essence of supportive interpersonal interactions, concrete acts such as hugging can be supplemented (or eventually replaced) by more symbolic processes such as the sharing of concerns. In turn, mastering such developmental milestones will make it increasingly possible for Mary to eventually benefit from the emotion regulatory input of nonfamilial agents.

Updating her treatment plans and case formulation, the therapist makes a note to start thinking about expanding the scope of Mary's regulatory responses and about which other domain would be most suitable. The therapist also makes a note to be on the lookout for information about whether Mary's interpersonal mistrust plays a role in the stressful events she experiences as depressogenic, an issue that can be addressed later in CERT's coping skills module (see Chapters 9 and 10).

Chantel, Age 9

The approach used to strengthen Chantel's interpersonal mood repair repertoire involved introducing a new response in that regulatory domain. Chantel, a 9-year-old girl with a younger sibling, was accompanied initially by both her parents; in later sessions, her mother was always present, while her father only attended work permitting. Chantel has had trouble adjusting to the birth of her sibling Abe a few years ago and the fact that the parents have been spending quite a bit of time with him due to some behavioral issues. The parents are concerned that Chantel has become chronically sad and had crying spells owing to worries that her parents may die. Her current symptoms seemed to have been triggered by Chantel's recent meeting of relatives from her father's prior marriage for the first time. Recognition that those relatives did not have contact with her father for a long time apparently prompted fears of separation. Family context includes the following: Her mother uses a wheelchair (the result of an injury many years prior) and has been struggling with depression, and her father is a very busy professional. It also soon became clear to the therapist that Chantel's mother was spending little time with her. A separate interview with the mother revealed that her own depression played a role in her withdrawal from Chantel; she felt inadequate to meet Chantel's needs due to her physical handicap.

In the previous session, Chantel and her mother were introduced to CERT and to getting and giving a hug as a way for Chantel to feel better. Because that intervention served as a successful *in vivo* demonstration of how a given response can alter the course of an emotion, it was assigned as homework. The present session, which included both parents, started with setting the agenda and proceeded to reviewing homework. The therapist expected positive reports. Indeed, there was general agreement that Chantel always felt better after Mom gave her a hug and that Chantel was increasingly able to ask her mom for a hug when she felt upset.

The therapist was considering how to further strengthen Chantel's social–interpersonal mood repair response domain when Chantel unexpectedly verbalized a major concern: "Mom and Dad don't love me. They love my brother [Abe] more." She was adamant that her mother ignores her in favor of Abe and became visibly sad and upset. The parents didn't agree; they opined that their greater involvement with the younger child was a minor stressor for Chantel.

Although Chantel's complaint, and the resultant upheaval, interrupted the discussion of homework, the therapist decided to address it because the complaint mirrored a maladaptive cognitive response, which worsened Chantel's usual level of sadness. She is also concerned about these recurrent and acute episodes of dysphoria. But the intensity of Chantel's affect mitigated against the likelihood that the therapist could bring about change by focusing on an adaptive cognitive strategy. Instead, she thus chose to alter the behavior of her mother (a key regulator of Chantel's mood). The therapist knew from the prior session that the mother did not spend much time with the young patient. The therapist expected that increasing her mother's availability to Chantel would lessen the child's negative mood and reinforce the mother as a competent regulator of her daughter's distress. To underscore the importance of access to parents, the therapist also included Chantel's father in the plans and proceeded as follows:

T: OK, I think that Chantel is saying that she feels unloved and sad because you [Mom and Dad] are so busy with Abe.

And if you remember, we talked before about ways in which children can feel better when they feel sad.

One of these ways is to "give and get hugs"—at which you did a very good job. Another way is for children to be with and do things together with important people in their lives. So, we are talking about The People Room in The House of ER (*pointing to poster*). It's about how other people can help us to feel better.

At this juncture, the parents interject and profess their love for Chantel, while the young patient insists that the parents don't love her. Rather than mediating a parent–child dispute, the therapist redirects attention to the goal of helping Chantel to feel better and proposes an experiment, one that will increase the mother's time with Chantel and thereby support the child's use of interpersonal regulation of dysphoria, reinforce the parental (P) coaching role, and diffuse the parent–child conflict. Here is the experiment:

T: I think that one way in which Chantel can feel better when she feels bad is to spend time with Mom and Dad—to do things together. Right?

P: Right!

T: OK, so what would happen if we tried something different, an experiment?

Can we come up with some ideas of what you [Mom] and Chantel could do together once a day—for 15 minutes—and things that you [Dad] and Chantel could do for 15 minutes. And because you guys have so many things happening, maybe we could try this as you [Mom] with Chantel one day; and then Dad and Chantel the next day.

This is part of the coaching we talked about earlier. So, I am going to ask Dad and Mom to alternate as the coach for this experiment. This would mean keeping a record of the tasks on which we agree and writing down when they get done.

(*To parents*) Is that OK with you?

After some back-and-forth, the family listed several tasks and activities they used to do, which included sports, as well as playing cards and board games, and singing. Keep in mind that the mother's use of a wheelchair presented some constraints on the type of activity to be assigned. Following some discussion, the family decided with the therapist that on alternate nights Chantel would sing songs with her father and play a brief card game with her mother. The coaching parent would signal when it was time for the task and then keep time. These activities were scheduled for 15 minutes per day. Because the young patient was chronically in a depressed mood, the therapist did not pair the intervention to mood severity.

As relayed at the following session, the parents noted improvement in their child's persistent sad mood. In this case, mobilizing social agents (her parents) were essential both for improving Chantel's mood and modifying the context of family interactions. The results of the assigned homework also brought about a major change in the mother's view of herself as she recognized that her presence was sufficiently powerful to help Chantel feel better. In turn, this recognition became a crucial turning point in treatment because it had a positive effect on the mother's willingness to undertake the role of coach and energized her actual coaching performance.

The therapist's evolving treatment plan at this stage included the goal of encouraging more symbolic forms of interpersonal mood repair (such as the verbal sharing of concerns and provision of emotional support), as well as exploring whether other people could serve as additional social regulators when Chantel was despondent. Importantly however, because Chantel's parents were her key social regulators *and* the key causes of her despondency, one of the therapist's goals was to explore with Chantel other regulatory domains. Given the evidence that Chantel had maladaptive cognitions, which she was able to verbalize, the therapist eventually focused on The Thinking (Cognitive) Room of The House of ER (see the later discussion in this chapter).

As treatment progressed, there were recurrent and multiple issues that centered on Chantel's relationship with her parents, highlighting a major theme in her life. Thus, the emerging case formulation included the proposition that the slightest perceived potential threat to her key attachments was a salient depressogenic stressor for Chantel. This issue was to be addressed during the coping skills phase of Chantel's therapy.

The Behavioral Regulatory Domain

A host of behavioral responses, ranging from fairly simple acts (e.g., jumping jacks, taking care of a pet, washing a car) to complex planned actions (building a model airplane), can serve the goal of mood repair. One advantage of behavioral regulatory responses is the extent of control that is vested in the young patient. For example, engaging in physical exercise to alleviate dysphoria gives the youngster leeway regarding "what, when, how, and how much." But alongside the extent of autonomy and control they allow, behavioral responses may be constrained by contextual factors. For example, certain sports require specialized venues; walking or jogging as an activity presupposes a safe neighborhood; children and adolescents do not have control over material resources that may be needed for some behavioral responses.

Behavioral regulatory responses are particularly appropriate for young patients who do not have reliable social agents capable of acting as mood regulators. Furthermore, given that some form of behavioral activation has been shown to be more effective than cognitive change in countering clinical depression, the behavioral regulatory domain should be considered for young patients with severe mood problems.

Because practically any planned action sequence can serve the goals of mood repair, there is a near limitless choice of adaptive behavioral responses. The major issues in strengthening behavioral regulatory responses concern feasibility, duration, and effort expended. Be sure to confirm feasibility if the preferred response requires some specialized venue (e.g., a swimming pool). And be sure that both the duration of the regulatory response and the physical and mental energy expended exceed some minimal threshold.

The following vignettes illustrate two approaches to strengthening a young patient's behavioral response repertoire: identifying another response (tool) in the regulatory domain that has been shown to be favored by the child, and reinforcing a previously helpful adaptive response. Note that in the former case, the child's preference for behavioral regulation had been confirmed in the prior CERT session and the therapist merely seeks to provide him with another response in that domain. In the second example, however, the therapist takes a chance in deducing that a past behavior on the part of the child did indeed function as a potential regulatory response, which he seeks to reactivate.

Pete, Age 9

Recall that jumping jacks helped to attenuate Pete's negative mood during an initial CERT session. Its role in mood repair and its effectiveness were then reinforced via homework that called for increasing the frequency of jumping jack episodes during the day and the number of jumping jacks Pete did each time. The homework was successful in providing Pete with better control of his dysphoria. At that point in his treatment, the therapist could have chosen to explore other forms of physical activity (e.g., push-ups, bicep curls) for mood repair. But the therapist wanted to provide the young patient with a greater range of behavioral regulatory response options. This decision reflected the fact that, although feeling better, Pete was severely depressed when he started CERT and that research has shown that behavioral interventions are especially helpful for such patients. Thus, the therapist introduced the idea of new behavioral regulatory responses after his mother coached Pete to report on the success of the prior homework, as next illustrated. Note that the therapist continues to support the coaching team, reinforces the parent's and child's knowledge of mood repair principles, and explains his reasons for what is being proposed:

T: I am happy to see that the jumping jack homework really helped! So (*to child*), you did the jumping jacks with Mom's help, and it looks like that helped you to feel better.

P: He did really good. He did a lot.

T: (*To Mom*) And your help was important. You are getting a lot of practice at being a good coach!

(*To child*) And you have been a *very good* player on this team!

(*To Mom*) Which coaching rule was most important for you when you were helping Pete with the homework? (*Pointing to poster on the rules of coaching*)

P: Hmm, I guess Rule 4. I really had to tell him how good he was doing!

T: (*To Mom*) That's great—like being a cheerleader, right?

(*To child*) And what about you? Which rule (*pointing to relevant poster*) helped most?

C: I dunno.

T: Well, OK. I am guessing it was the first rule. But here is an easier question.

Let's look at this [The House of ER] poster. What room do jumping jacks belong in?

C: Dunno—doing stuff?

T: Yes, the behavioral room: *things that you can do* to feel better when you are sad and upset.

OK, so we know that one thing that you can do is jumping jacks and that really helps. And we will make sure that you continue to do them.

But it's a good idea to have more than one way to get out of feeling sad.

(*To parent*) Thinking as a coach, what other things could Pete do to feel better when he feels sad? [Some examples may have to be provided from The House of ER poster.]

For example, maybe he could get involved in some project when he feels bad?

C: Do my baseball card collection?

P: Yes, that's really important to him! He really likes that.

As the parent–child pair converges on this as a mutually agreed on activity, the therapist seeks to gain a fuller understanding of what is entailed in maintaining such a card collection before it can be assigned as homework. In this instance, the homework involved sorting and cataloguing the collection and making up a list of new cards to be acquired: tasks in which the child would engage for at least 20 minutes anytime he was feeling dysphoric at home during the following week. The parent-coach was to help by monitoring the child's mood for sadness or dysphoria and initiating the behavioral response (reminding the offspring to implement the homework), and both members of the parent–child team were to record the results together. The therapist's regulatory focus for this child and his emerging case formulation were influenced by the fact that Pete had several neurovegetative depression symptoms (indicative of greater severity), that he had a familial history of mood disorder, and that multiple environmental stresses predated the onset of his current depression. Thus, a working hypothesis was that Pete's depression might be a classic example of a "diathesis–stress" etiology, in which innate vulnerability interacts with problems in managing depressogenic environmental triggers: As discussed in later chapters, this formulation eventually informed the personalization of the coping skills module for Pete.

As an alternative approach, the therapist could have continued to ask for other examples of what Pete (or a friend of a similar age) can do so that his sadness does not get out of control. After a discussion of several options with the parent–child pair, they could then decide the response that would constitute a preferred homework assignment. Regardless of which approach is selected, review and discussion of task completion would then be part of the next session's agenda. Its outcome will determine the therapist's next move: to further extend the behavioral domain for Pete or to enhance response flexibility by focusing on another regulatory domain.

Mike, Age 13

A different approach was needed for Mike, a slightly overweight 13-year-old only child, living with his father and paternal grandmother. The father was increasingly concerned about his offspring's mood over the past 4–6 months, and described him as hard to live with because he has been irritable, unfriendly, morose, and oppositional. He believes that his son has low self-esteem and has also complained of frequent generalized somatic symptoms.

Additionally, Mike has become increasingly disrespectful to his grandmother. Mike agreed that he has been feeling miserable, stating that nothing is fun any longer. He called himself "fatso." He recently stopped engaging in various previously favored activities, like video gaming and walking his dog. However, he has been doing reasonably well in school. Family context included the breakup of his parents' marriage a few years back, which his father believes was the original trigger for Mike's mood and behavior problems. Mike's mother has recently remarried and his stepfather appears to be punitive, which seem to be more proximal causal factors.

In the first session, the parent–child pair was introduced to the principles of CERT, and Mike responded reasonably well to behavioral regulation, which was illustrated via sit-ups. However, his comments conveyed that he did not like physical exercise. Furthermore, Mike's relationship with his grandmother suggested that this was not the best time to pursue social–interpersonal regulatory responses. And he did not impress the therapist as favoring cognitive tasks. Moreover, Mike's diffuse somatic complaints, like headaches and bellyaches, were possible surrogates for negative affect, which raised the question as to whether he might be having some trouble in naming his emotions. In light of these factors and because the therapist did not have a clear picture of the extent of Mike's dysphoria, the homework assigned at the first session involved hourly monitoring of Mike's dysphoric affect over the weekend, and pre-school and after-school hours monitoring on weekdays. The first homework was only partially completed (due to practical reasons), did not provide enough information, and was therefore reassigned.

After structuring the current session, the reattempted sadness-monitoring homework was reviewed and discussed. The entries showed that Mike has consistently sad, dysphoric mood, not tied to any particular trigger or time of day. Given the persistence of Mike's dysphoria, the various factors just noted here, and historical information that Mike stopped engaging in fun activities (potentially adaptive regulatory responses), the therapist decides to explore whether a prior behavior could be reactivated that might counter sad affect. Therefore, the therapist directs the conversation to previously rewarding activities in which Mike has stopped engaging, honing in on Mike's pet dog (Jumpy) and the times Mike took responsibility for walking and exercising him. Because taking care of pets (and other living things) involves planned action, it could serve as an adaptive behavioral mood repair response.

The therapist establishes through a series of questions that Mike had liked taking care of and doing things with Jumpy in the past. Then she explores if interacting with Jumpy could serve as a behavioral regulatory response to dysphoria. Note that the therapist does not address why Mike stopped interacting with Jumpy. The discussion might proceed along the following lines:

T: (*To child*) So, from what I just heard, you and Jumpy were a good team. And you always liked it when you took him outside, especially when you took him for a run. It could be fun. Right? (*To Dad*) Do you also remember that?

P: Sure, he took care of Jumpy—don't know why he quit doing it.

T: (*To child*) Was there one special thing you used to like to do with Jumpy?

C: Dunno—stuff.

T: OK, how about doing stuff again with Jumpy?

C: Dunno.

T: Doing stuff like taking him on his walks. I bet that Jumpy would like that!

C: Yeah, I guess.

T: And maybe that can also help you to feel better.

More than likely, such a young patient will not be enthusiastic about the therapist's suggestion or readily willing to change his ways. Therefore, the parent's support must be sought. The idea is to negotiate until the young patient and parent are ready to undertake even the smallest amount of activity. For example, if the therapist proposes the homework with Jumpy for a week but notices reluctance, then a new proposal can be made: "for just a few days." And by proposing the homework in the context of an experiment, the therapist acknowledges a patient's or parent's reluctance. In the dialogue to follow, note that as the therapist continues to negotiate with the parent–child pair, she reinforces the parental role as coach, calls attention to The Rules of Being a Good Team Player, verbalizes the reason for the homework, and locates the strategy in the relevant room of The House of ER. Picking up from the prior dialogue:

T: (*To Dad*) Can you put on your coaching hat? Could we figure out a plan for Mike to do things with Jumpy again?

(*To child*) This would be like a team—Dad would help out—could you give it a try?

C: Dunno.

T: Let's try something with Jumpy. Just for a few days. It would be like an experiment. Like 4 days.

We do an experiment because we want to find out something. Here, we want to determine if Jumpy can help you feel better when you feel bad. Does this make sense?

(*To Dad*) So, what do you think about Mike taking Jumpy out for at least 30 minutes—and could he do this four weekday evenings and one weekend evening *and* any other time Mike feels especially bad?

As the coach, can you help him do that?

P: Sure, what exactly?

T: OK, let's review what that would mean. Like keeping track of which day Mike will be following this routine and reminding him to do so when Jumpy is ready to go out.

(*To child*) Being a good coach, Dad will remind you and then you don't have to worry about forgetting.

Dad also can help you to remember to mark down on this sheet (*provides a copy of Form 5*) how you were feeling before and after walking Jumpy. You did a good job with this sheet during the past week.

C: OK, for a few days.

At this point, the therapist works through the details of the homework with parent and child and makes certain that they understand the task at hand and see no hindrances to its completion. The therapist then returns to previously introduced CERT concepts and reinforces them as follows:

T: Good! (*To child*) OK, you remember that we talked about the rules that help a kid to be a *good team player*?

Let's look at the poster here (*pointing to the poster showing the rules for players*). Which rule did you just show? Can you try to figure it out?

(*To Dad*) What do you think?

P: That he will try something again as we plan?

T: Yes, Mike just showed how a kid can follow the first and second rules that help to be a good team player! I am happy to see that because these rules are not always easy to try.

P: Hmm, I agree, that's great.

T: (*To parent*) And you are being a good coach!

(*To parent and child*) So, the idea is that one way to feel better when we feel sad and bad is to get involved in some action. To *do* something that can oppose the bad feeling.

Like walking Jumpy, taking care of Jumpy. Which room in The House of ER does that belong?

As with all homework, the assignment involving Jumpy was one of the first items on the agenda of the next session. Its successful outcome was indicated at that point, with the child feeling better after interacting with Jumpy, which then became the path toward exploring other behavioral responses that could serve the same goal of improved mood repair.

There could have been other outcomes of the homework besides the one just noted here. Let's assume that Mike did not feel better as a result of doing the homework. Thus, the therapist would need to elicit a description of what transpired to decide if the task was implemented correctly. If done correctly, but without the expected mood benefits, the results are discussed as an experiment: In other words, the results show that spending time with Jumpy did not help (which is OK!). Therefore, other behavioral regulatory responses to dysphoria can be explored.

If the experiment was not implemented properly, there could be various reasons for that: Both parent and child skirted some of the rules or Dad failed to perform the coaching role or the child spent only 10 minutes with Jumpy. In each of these instances, the therapist needs to gently point out the features that were not executed correctly, refer to The Rules of Coaching and The Rules of Being a Good Team Player to correct the inadvertent failures (see the prior illustration of this), and ask the parent–child pair to repeat the experiment.

As Mike's treatment progressed, the therapist continued to reinforce behavioral responses. But in her treatment plan, a further goal was to work with the young patient on social–interpersonal regulation, with the father acting as assistant coach, and to eventually use Mike's good school performance to counter his self-esteem problems. As part of her emerging case formulation, the therapist believed that reinforcing the father as a competent regulator of his son's distress would foster closer and more intimate contacts between father and son. In turn, this might remedy some disturbance in the mother–child relationship, which was likely to account for much of Mike's problems. The therapist also noted that the young patient had a rather unpleasant and provocative interpersonal style, which tended to bring forth adverse feedback from others. However, she was wondering whether these displays were related to his depression, rather than being reflections of his basic temperament and/or problems in recognizing his own emotions (emotion naming) and thus confusion about how different feelings may be communicated and regulated. The foregoing issues were to be addressed as treatment moved along and during Mike's coping skills training.

The Cognitive Regulatory Domain

In CERT, cognitive regulatory responses to sadness are described to children as "things that go on in your head" that help you to feel better. The tools in The Thinking (Cognitive) Room include any cognitive process or product that can serve the goal of mood repair, such as visual or other imagery; cognitions that can interrupt, neutralize, or replace depressive ruminations; refocusing of attention away from the source or experience of dysphoria; neutral or positive reappraisals as to the nature and experience of one's sadness and dysphoria; positive personal memories; and pleasant internal sensory experiences (like hearing music in one's head). But because reappraisal (reinterpretation) involves abstract thinking and the ability to generate alternate mental perspectives on a given event or affect state, those regulatory responses are infrequent among younger children and possibly may be developmentally inappropriate as well.

The use of cognition and cognitive processes to repair dysphoric mood has several advantages. It is entirely within the control of the young patient, a characteristic it shares with many behavioral regulatory responses. But, unlike many behavioral responses, it is "portable," not constrained by context, and can be deployed any time and any place. Cognition is private, which may render it particularly attractive for those young patients who are shy. Cognition is instantaneous, and its effects on mood can be observed in real time. Importantly, refocusing of attention (a cognitive response) away from one's distress appears to be particularly helpful when individuals suffer from severe sadness and dysphoria. On the other hand, as already noted, a major drawback of the cognitive regulatory domain is that response implementation is entirely internal to the individual. Thus, the therapist has no direct information about exactly *what* the young patient is thinking or imagining and *how well* he is implementing a given response.

The vignettes to follow illustrate two cognitive mood repair responses, visual imagery and thought substitution, that can help to replace or interrupt maladaptive cognitions and related distress, respectively.

Chantel, Age 9

Let us return to Chantel, whose chronically depressed mood was notably lessened in response to the increasing availability of social–interpersonal regulators (her parents). However, given the complex role of the parents (they are both social regulators of Chantel's mood and potential causes of her dysphoria), the therapist wanted to explore another regulatory domain that could provide Chantel with different regulatory options. Chantel's ability to report on her ruminations suggested that she would be comfortable with cognitive processes. Therefore, the therapist decided to introduce visual imagery in the service of mood repair: Chantel was going to learn to visualize a stop sign as soon as she had distressing thoughts about her parents. For younger children like Chantel, such a visual exercise can be introduced as finding the **magic picture** (or **sign**) that can help them to feel better.

Having had several sessions, the family has become familiar with the CERT model, including its coaching component and the homework assignments. As part of structuring the session, the therapist notes that she would like to check on Chantel's fears of losing her parents. Then, she returns to that topic after a discussion of current concerns and prior homework. She establishes the fact that Chantel still has almost weekly thoughts of parental loss, which leave her sad, and ascertains that the parents and young patient agree these ruminations are problematic.

The therapist then proceeds to establish that the young patient can generate colorful visual imagery.

T: OK (*to child*), it still happens, maybe a few times a week, that this idea comes to your head that Mom and Dad will leave or will die.

C: Yeah.

T: And that makes you sad and upset? Even though you know that is *not* true, it is hard to stop that idea. So, let's see if we can figure out how to stop those ideas. Would you like that?

P: That'd help!

T: (*To child*) I want to ask you something first. Can you see pictures in your head? Like make-believe?

If I say, "Think about a birthday cake," can you close your eyes and see a birthday cake?

C: Yeah—that's easy.

T: Great! Tell me what the birthday cake looks like. What are the colors on the outside? And what colors do you see when you cut into the cake?

If the therapist intends for the child to use visual imagery as a regulatory response, a test such as the one just described should be conducted to assure that the young patient understands the concept of visualization and can implement it. Visual test images can include commonly known and colorful items, such as various fruits, Santa standing before a Christmas tree, flowers, or a fire hydrant. In the present case, the therapist was satisfied that Chantel could implement visualization and continued along the following lines:

T: OK, that's good.

(*To Mom*) Can you put on your coaching hat? Let's see if you can get Chantel to imagine different flowers—and describe them. (*Mom coaches for a while.*)

T: (*To child and Mom*) That was pretty good! How about an apple? Can you imagine in your head a big red apple?

C: Sure, that's easy.

T: OK, good.

For some children, having a *magic picture* to think about really helps them to feel better when they feel bad. One really good magic picture is a stop sign.

Can you make believe that you see a big *stop sign*? It may be easier if you close your eyes. Try to see a big *red* stop sign—like those on a street corner.

Now, I have some questions about stop signs. If you are on the street corner and see a stop sign, what is the thing to do?

What do cars do? What do people do?

C: They stop?

T: (*To parent and child*) Yes, and a big red stop sign is a magic picture because it can stop ideas that make you feel bad.

When an idea pops up into your head and makes you feel sad and unhappy, thinking of the magic picture stops the upsetting idea.

So, we want to see what happens if Chantel thinks of her magic sign, which is a big red stop sign, and she thinks of it right away as soon as she has upsetting ideas about Mom and Dad.

(*To parent*) Can you tell when Chantel has these ideas in her head?

P: Sure—she starts crying and gets really clingy and won't let go! It's when she is already upset about something like Abe.

T: Hmm. (*To child*) Can we practice?

(*To Mom*) Can you be the coach along with me? Can you help Chantel to think about big red stop signs?

Having the child practice visualizing a big red stop sign, with her mother coaching, is the first step to prepare the parent–child pair for the homework. The next step is to have the child think the distressing thought during the treatment session and implement the stop sign imagery in response. Therefore, after several rounds of practice in visualizing the stop sign, and generous positive reinforcement of the parent–child pair for its efforts, the therapist proceeds to the next step.

T: (*To parent*) You are a very good coach and let's see—it looks like you were just following the rules, especially Rule 2, of coaching.

(*To parent and child*) Now, we will do one more thing. We'll see how the stop sign can actually help.

(*To child*) I will ask you to tell me about the last time you had these ideas of Mom and Dad dying. *And* then we will try to make the ideas go away—OK?

(*To parent*) And you and I will try to help her stop those ideas.

(*To child*) Remember the last time you had those ideas? Can you tell me exactly what you were thinking? How did those ideas go?

The ruminations in question are known to cause the child to become dysphoric and upset. Therefore, a few sentences of the child recounting the cognitions should be sufficient to elicit mild distress, at which point the therapist should promptly interrupt the recitation and continue along the following lines:

T: Chantel, you are very brave to talk about this. Because I know that these ideas are upsetting.

(*To Mom*) Don't you agree?

P: For sure!

T: (*To child*) Now, remember your magic picture? The *big red stop sign?*

Try to see in your mind a big red stop sign. Now—can you make your magic picture even bigger? Just look at your magic picture for a few more seconds.

OK, you did a great job. And how do you feel (*pointing to the facial emotion expression poster*)—which face looks like how you feel?

Implementing the visual imagery in question interrupts and replaces the patient's ruminative cognitions and can be expected to reduce distress. At that point, it is appropriate for the therapist to again verbalize the relationship between a regulatory response and subsequent affect (e.g., "You thought of your magic picture, which got rid of the upsetting ideas and you felt better!"); locate the response in the relevant room of The House of ER (e.g., "Thinking of your magic picture to feel better belongs in which room in The House of ER?"); and reinforce the parent's coaching role (e.g., "When Chantel tries this at home, it will be important for you [parent] to help as the coach"). Assigning the stop sign mental imagery as homework (with one parent acting as coach) can take the form of practice sessions two or three times a day (not specifically connected to distress states) and/or implementation as soon as distressing thoughts of parents surface.

As the homework was successful (it was executed and lowered the level of Chantel's distress), the therapist may continue to reinforce the use of the stop sign and/or explore the viability of other forms of visual imagery (e.g., picturing a favorite object, food, or activity) to counter the patient's maladaptive cognitions and related distress about her parents. Directly asking the young patient about her interest in the latter option is a good way to decide on the direction to take (e.g., "Having a different magic picture in your mind may also help you to feel better. Like, seeing in your mind your favorite dress. Do you want to learn to do that—*or* stay with the magic stop sign for now?").

Had the homework not achieved the expected results, the usual procedure is to determine if the task was executed properly and, if not, to then identify features that need to be corrected before the parent–child pair make a repeat attempt.

If, despite proper execution, the task did not yield the expected results, the therapist may consider shifting to another cognitive response. For example, a nonvisual, linguistic version of the magic picture, which is the *magic word* or *magic phrase,* involves the child repeating in his mind a special word or expression to counter the targeted maladaptive cognition. (One young patient was a huge fan of old Beatles songs and a particular line of lyrics became her magic phrase.) The therapist implements mood repair via a magic word or phrase in a manner similar to what was described for the stop sign visual imagery but with one caveat: The child's comfort with verbal content (rather than visual imagery) needs to be established.

Moving forward, the therapist will continue to support Chantel's use of social–interpersonal regulatory responses, as described earlier in this chapter. The therapist also plans to expand the scope of Chantel's mood repair response repertoire by introducing thought substitution as an additional cognitive regulatory response. A version of this is illustrated next as we continue to explore the case of Lisa.

Lisa: Age 12

Lisa was introduced in Chapter 6 in connection with the homework assigned to monitor her sad affect. The homework revealed that the young patient's mood is regularly worse in the morning but only on school days. Her mother complains that Lisa has an especially downcast affect in the morning, making it hard to get her going and prompting daily anxiety that she will miss her school bus.

Lisa's mood on school-day mornings led the therapist to posit that the young patient worsens her baseline dysphoria by maladaptive negative thoughts that concern school. The therapist therefore decides to introduce a cognitive regulatory response called *thought substitution,* which involves replacing a troubling thought sequence with a neutral or more pleasant sequence of ideas.

But first, the therapist confirms via contextual mapping how the mornings unfold. Note that as the session proceeds, the therapist repeatedly summarizes and frames her goals. This makes them more understandable to the child and parent, reinforces the parent–child coaching relationship, reiterates previously learned concepts about mood regulation, and refers to The House of ER.

T: OK. (*To child*) Can you help me to get a better idea of what happens in the mornings? So, Mom says she found you this morning sitting on your bed and you looked pretty sad—what was going on just before Mom came in?

C: Nothing.

T: All right. So, you were just sitting?

C: Yeah.

T: (*To child*) Do you remember what was on your mind?
If I were a little person sitting in your head, what would I hear you thinking this morning?

C: Ugh. I hate school.

T: OK. So, was it like "Ugh. I hate school; I don't want to go."

C: Hmm.

T: I have a hunch you were thinking that some bad things may happen in school. Tell me about one bad thing that was on your mind.

C: I don't have time to finish my animal project. I am gonna fail.

T: Hmm—OK. So, you are sitting on your bed and you think about going to school, and you think something like "I won't be able to do my animal project and I'll fail" and you feel sad, like really sad.
And this happens on many school days?

At this point, the therapist asks for more information and learns that in one of Lisa's classes, the assignment was to compose an essay about a favorite topic. Lisa has had a longstanding passion for elephants, and she planned to write an essay focusing on the current fate of these animals. The therapist also learns that while much of the text has been finished, Lisa wants the final product to look like a graphic novel. However, the therapist believes that, given her history of learning disability and attention difficulties, Lisa is unlikely to finish the graphic part of the project on time.

While the therapist wonders if a practical problem-solving approach may be appropriate (see WWW.Solve: Solving a Problem, Poster 4 in Appendix B), she decides to focus the current session on helping Lisa improve her affect in the morning by replacing her negative cognitions with a series of positive thoughts about her project. To construct such a list, she asks Lisa why her project is important, what is so special about elephants, and whether any of the other children have a similar project. After the therapist obtains this information, she summarizes it for the child and parent and then continues along the following lines:

T: (*To child*) My goodness, there are *lots* of good things about your project!

(*To parent*) Can you put on your coaching hat? Now, can you help Lisa make a list of all the important things about elephants—one by one—and why her project is special?

(*To child*) Why don't you again list for Mom and me all the special things about elephants and your project?

While the child enumerates her project's characteristics, her mother writes them down. The therapist encourages Mom to prompt Lisa, if needed. After the list is finished, it is reviewed by the young patient to be sure that nothing significant was left out; the therapist may then proceed further:

T: Hmm, this is a very good list. It shows all the positive things about elephants and also shows why your animal project is so special!

So (*to child*), in the morning when you start thinking about how you hate school and how you will fail, instead I would like you to look at this list and think about all the special parts of your project and why it is so important for you to finish it.

(*To parent*) And can you help as the coach?

You could make sure that the list is next to Lisa's bed. It may be easiest if Lisa looks at the list and goes through each item. Maybe she could even read the items aloud to you?

Let me explain the idea: We replace an upsetting idea with ideas that make you feel better.

(*To parent*) Can you put what I just described in your own words? I want to make sure that I explained everything correctly.

P: I guess—It's like replacing the negative with a positive so that you don't get upset by the negative.

T: Yes, that's a pretty good summary. (*To parent and child*) So, if we use thinking to feel better, where does that fit in The House of ER?

Throughout the treatment, it is important to keep checking with parents and the young patient, as appropriate, about their understanding of a specific idea or concept, which the therapist has verbalized. Asking for feedback (as just illustrated) can prevent a potential misunderstanding and maintains the family's active involvement. As the parent provides an accurate summary of what the therapist has explained, the dialogue may continue as follows:

T: (*To child and parent*) Now, let's practice. Mom will watch so that she can help you do this at home.

(*To child*) Think back to this morning. Can you make believe that you are back in your room? And now, let's make believe that I am also in your room.

You are in your room and feeling pretty miserable, and I ask you: "What's on your mind?" Tell me all the ideas that would be on your mind.

C: I don't wanna go to school—I can't do my project; I'll never finish it; I'll fail!

T: Now, right away, start reading the different reasons why elephants are really important and why your project is so special—read it aloud—all the reasons.

(*To parent*) Can you coach Lisa—start with the first idea on the list?

In the beginning and at the end of the process described here, the young patient also can be asked to rate her own sad affect via any of the strategies that already have been introduced, such as using verbal labels (e.g., *feeling very sad; not sad; in between very and not sad*), designating a number on a predefined numeric severity scale like a sadness thermometer, or putting beads or marbles as quantitative indicators of magnitude into a bin prelabeled with the target emotion.

Then, the therapist can verbalize the link between the child's current affect state (decreased dysphoria) and her regulatory response (thinking of the positive features of her animal project) and proceed to locate the response in The Thinking Room of The House of ER. Thereby, the therapist opens the door to discussions of how the given tool (thinking of the positive) also can serve to replace other negative maladaptive cognitions. Plus, other tools in The Thinking Room also can counter the negative cognition (failure) under consideration and repair dysphoric mood.

The therapist's plan to strengthen Lisa's adaptive regulatory response repertoire involves an ongoing emphasis on cognitive strategies, which eventually will include more abstract processes like neutral reappraisal (the affect-free reinterpretation of potentially depressogenic triggers or stimuli). The therapist is additionally considering an exploration of Lisa's comfort level with social–interpersonal regulatory responses to ensure her access to an array of mood repair response strategies.

As the therapist considered Lisa's background and the onset of Lisa's depressive episode in her case formulation and treatment planning, she was impressed: Despite her developmental challenges, Lisa had a history of good adjustment and good school performance until her abrupt mainstreaming into regular classes and the withdrawal of professional psychological support. Thus, her case formulation increasingly pointed to the need to teach the family to practice more assertive proactive planning and intervention to minimize future discontinuities in Lisa's educational settings, along with improved problem-solving approaches.

Potential Problems in Response Implementation

As illustrated in the prior sections of this chapter, children master the targeted regulatory responses as a function of the therapist's repeated interactions with the parent–child pair during the treatment sessions and ongoing homework completed by the child outside the sessions. However, the learning process is jeopardized when mood repair–focused homework *fails to achieve its goal* because of *how* the young patient and parent-coach go about it. Such implementation problems need to be identified via detailed questioning of what was done and how, and then they need to be corrected.

If the assigned homework was not completed, do not automatically assume that generic noncompliance was at play (discussed in Chapter 3). Instead, an incomplete mood repair homework might reflect a specific type of implementation problem, the inadvertent failure of the child and/or the parent to adhere to some aspect of The Rules of Coaching and The Rules of Being a Good Team Player (as in the example of Mary, provided earlier in this chapter). On the part of the young patient, not using words to express feelings and exhibiting a reluctance to follow through with the entire response sequence (not adhering to the third and fifth rules of being a good team player) tend to be the most frequent issues. On the part of the parent-coach, the most common issues that hinder implementation of a homework assignment are getting frustrated with and criticizing the child (not adhering to the fourth rule of good coaching) and insufficient planning for the execution of the homework. Such departures from the rules guiding the coaching team need to be addressed without criticism and as temporary setbacks during the process of learning and mastering new skills.

Implementation issues should also be considered if an emotion regulatory response homework was executed correctly, but its affective consequences fell far short of expectations. For example, in the behavioral regulatory domain, a key issue is the duration of the response or effort that has been put forth. Recall that several of the interventions that were described involved forms of exercise. Their affective consequences can be expected to be more notable the longer the response or the greater the physical effort that was mobilized; thus, if a physical activity was carried out only for a few minutes, its affective consequences may not be detectable. If the behavioral response involved more complex action sequences (e.g., completing a project), an implementation issue may arise if the young patient and parent had problems gathering all the necessary components for successful task completion.

Regarding homework in the social–interpersonal regulatory domain, a key piece of implementation is how the child goes about summoning the adult who is to be the regulator. Recall that infants and toddlers signal their need for regulatory help by crying and fussing. However, with the advent of language, children are expected to verbalize their distress and need for assistance. Thus, a school-age or older child who fails to use language to recruit a regulator may not be very effective at socially mediated mood repair. Probing whether the young patient recognizes that summoning adult regulators is likely to involve verbal requests was illustrated with Mary and her grandmother.

Implementation problems are the most difficult to identify and correct when it comes to homework that targets the cognitive regulatory domain because of the unique features of cognitive processes, which were already noted. A cognitive regulatory response homework assignment may fail because the child has been unable to implement its visual, verbal, or reasoning components. While every effort should be made to obtain from the young patient a narrative of what difficulties were encountered and then correct them, the therapist may consider refocusing efforts on a different cognitive modality (e.g., visual rather than verbal) or a different regulatory domain.

Preventing Sadness and Dysphoria

While CERT's goal is to help the young patient to mobilize adaptive regulatory responses to sadness and dysphoria, at times it may be appropriate to intervene to reduce the child's exposure to depressogenic triggers or aversive stimuli. Such an approach is particularly appropriate when it is known that certain upcoming social interactions and task demands will predictably trigger dysphoria or worsen existing mood. Preventive interventions typically involve changing the context that gives rise to the distress or modifying task demands that appear to be depressogenic.

The therapist may consider changing the features of a specific situation if it is associated with intense emotions and chaotic interpersonal interactions that are likely to prevent learning; if a contextual element is causally related to a symptom; or if the depressogenic situation is inappropriate. From the perspective of contextual mapping (see Chapter 3), modifying a depressogenic trigger means focusing on the antecedents of the episode of distress.

To illustrate such a proactive approach, we return to 9-year-old Pete, who responded well to using a behavioral regulatory response (jumping jacks): It helped to decrease his dysphoric affect. The therapist therefore moved on to incorporate another behavioral response, taking care of his baseball card collection. But his father complained again about the child's irritable and dysphoric affect in the morning. The therapist thus planned to have Pete resume jumping jacks shortly after he got up in the mornings. However, contextual mapping revealed that the mornings were associated with some chaos and conflict for the parents (and multiple offspring) and were not the optimal time to practice mood repair responses.

Indeed, it appeared that the morning conflict predictably elicited Pete's distress. Thus, defusing affective features of morning interactions was likely to be beneficial for both the young patient and his parents. Because the family was already familiar with the mood repair model of CERT, the therapist responded to the information derived from contextual mapping of a recent morning as follows:

T: OK—we'll work on Pete being irritable and cranky in the morning.

So, let me summarize part of what both of you told me. In the mornings, you [parent] are usually in a hurry—you seem to be quite rushed with the all the kids. And, of course, you also rush Pete, but when you do that, he gets very crabby. It goes like that in a bit of a circle. Right?

P: Yeah, pretty much the case.

T: (*To parent*) I wonder what would happen if you were not so rushed in the morning?

Could we go through and list all the things you have to do in a typical morning?

In this exercise, the therapist prompts the parent for details of the morning routine, based on which the therapist and parent jointly produce an itemized list. One useful next step is for the therapist to review the list, ask about each item, and ascertain whether or how each could be done on the previous day. Here is an example of how the therapist might handle such a situation:

T: Let's see what we have here! This *is* quite a lot to do!

Can we go through the items one by one and decide which one of these 12 different things could be done the night before?

Let me see—would it be possible in the evening (*reviewing the following items one by one*):

. . . to put out the clothes for the three kids for the next day?

. . . to put all the breakfast stuff on the table, like the cereal, the bowls, etc.?

. . . to have Pete take his shower?

. . . to get the other children's lunch boxes ready?

. . . to have your own lunch prepared?

What do you think?

P: Hmm. I don't know—but, yes, we could try something different.

T: Well, let's try an experiment to see if we can help Pete be less crabby in the morning.

The experiment is for you [both parents] and Pete, together, to try and get these five things done in the evening, so you have more time in the morning.

But you [father] have to be the coach—start the evening tasks and remind everyone of what to do. Does that make sense?

What do you [parents] think?

(*To child*) And you would be an important part of this activity. For example, you can be a good team player by helping Mom and Dad in the evening to get the breakfast table ready. Could you do that?

And what about helping to make your lunch for the next day to take to school? Could you help with that?

As with all homework assignments, each step needs to be reviewed, with an emphasis on whether the task is doable and which member of the coaching team will do what. After this is accomplished, the parent–child team should be asked to verbalize their understanding of the task and the reasons for it. And then, the intervention should be positioned in the overall scheme of CERT by a statement such as the following:

T: Before we move on, I wanted to say something about this plan we just worked out.

This is really a good example of how we can cut down negative feelings by changing things around us, like parts of our environment. This is important because things can mount up without us realizing all the pressures—and trying to reduce pressures that cause negative feelings is one way to manage things better!

Modifying contextual features to lessen the aversive affective stimulation to which the child is subject is a proactive and preventative intervention. While it is easiest to implement changes within the context of the family, it also should be given consideration in extra-familial contexts.

Modifying depressogenic task demands is another way to reduce a child's exposure to adversity that may intensify depressive symptoms. Recall Lisa and her animal project that was associated with distress and maladaptive cognitions. While the therapist initially focused on teaching Lisa to engage in a different form of cognition in the early morning to improve her mood, she also believed that the parameters of Lisa's project were unrealistic in light of her learning disability; thus, the project was likely to function as a depressogenic trigger. Therefore, in a later session, the therapist focused on changing the scope of Lisa's animal project to alter its depressogenic potential. The therapist proposed to Lisa that she ought to divide the project into two phases and recommended that the graphic part be delayed for the second phase.

As previously noted, modifying contexts or tasks can be conceptualized as a form of problem solving, as pictured on the CERT poster WWW.Solve: Solving a Problem (see Poster 4 in Appendix B). The process involves identifying <u>w</u>hat the problem is, <u>w</u>ho can help solve the problem, and <u>w</u>ays to solve it. For Lisa, the problem was getting the project done by the date it was due; the person who could solve it was primarily Lisa, with help from her coaches, and the best way to solve it was to cut down the scope of the project by deleting the graphic parts (to be taken up later as a separate initiative).

Summary and Next Steps

The alleviation of sadness and dysphoria is the key to CERT because when these affects endure and become intense, they instigate the full depressive syndrome and continue to maintain it. Treating sadness and dysphoria essentially involves achieving better mood repair by strengthening the needed skills. Strengthening the child's adaptive mood repair response repertoire enables the young patient to manage his dysphoric emotions better so that those affects do not take over. This constitutes a crucial phase in the process of recovery from depression.

Helping a child to become more skillful at mood repair starts with strengthening adaptive responses in her preferred regulatory domain(s) and eventually in other domains as well. CERT emphasizes both within-domain and across-domain response mastery so that the young patient's mood repair response repertoire becomes more diverse and more broad-based. This will enable him to respond well to a variety of depressogenic challenges.

As illustrated throughout this chapter, progress in achieving and maintaining satisfactory mood repair is dependent on the continuous reinforcement of the parent–child coaching relationship, its rules, and relentless practice in real life via homework assignments. In turn, the rules that guide the coaching relationship provide the parent–child pair with a new model of relating to one another, which often translates into improved parent–child interactions in other areas of daily life.

Typically, it takes several sessions for a child to begin to master a given mood repair response and thereby manifest lower levels of dysphoria. The present chapter illustrated approaches to strengthening regulatory responses in each of the three functional domains. For any given child, a sequence of such strengthening interactions comprises much of CERT across multiple sessions; by the end of treatment, the child usually achieves mastery of several regulatory responses. Throughout this process, the young patient's domain preferences and the therapist's formulation of the given case together guide the therapist's decisions about which regulatory responses to strengthen and how.

At some point during CERT, most patients will encounter new stressors, which may result in increased sadness and distress. Along with attending to whatever issue was being worked on, such depression symptom relapse may necessitate a return to regulatory response strengthening exercises. As noted several times in the present chapter, relapse in either symptoms or mood repair responding is part of the journey of recovering from depression and should be framed as opportunities to identify functional areas in which additional attention or learning is needed.

The sharp-eyed reader may have noticed that little attention has been paid here to maladaptive mood repair responses, the regulatory responses that maintain or exacerbate sadness and dysphoria. While assessing the child's history and based on observations during CERT, the therapist will encounter many examples of maladaptive mood repair responses (e.g., having tantrums, starting fights or arguments, withdrawing from contact, verbalizing distressing thoughts). It is useful for the therapist to be aware of such responses. However, the aim of CERT is not to reinforce maladaptive responses by focusing on them. Instead, the goal is to replace maladaptive responses with adaptive regulatory strategies.

It is more than likely that the young patient's increasing control over his sad and dysphoric emotions will be associated with improvement in overall well-being and, consequently, reductions in the nonaffective features of depression (e.g., negative self-esteem, sleep problems). But because the nonaffective symptoms of depression may be treatment targets for some young patients, they are discussed in the next chapter; these symptoms may be addressed alongside or after affective symptoms have been attenuated.

Chapter 8

Treatment of Nonaffective Symptoms

As discussed earlier in this book, the contextual emotion regulation therapy (CERT) model posits that problems in regulating sad, dysphoric affect constitute the key feature of depression. Thus, the CERT therapist can expect that the successful treatment of sadness and dysphoria will also result in improvement in nonaffective symptoms of depression. Indeed, clinical experience suggests that once a young patient achieves a favorable emotional equilibrium, other symptoms of depression tend to fade or remain at levels that do not typically impair functioning. However, there will be young patients who may need treatment of their nonaffective symptoms.

This chapter addresses suicidal ideation and behavior, sleep disturbance, and self-deprecation or worthlessness, which are the most likely nonaffective depression symptom targets in younger age groups. As I discuss, these nonaffective symptoms of depression can function as mood repair responses. If so, they are amenable to various CERT interventions introduced in previous chapters. When nonaffective symptoms present as traditional manifestations of depression, they can be treated via evidence-based traditional interventions; I provide several examples of these as well.

Suicidal Thoughts and Behaviors

Suicidal thoughts and behaviors can manifest as thinking about wanting to kill oneself, having a specific suicide plan, or having made a suicide attempt. Thinking repeatedly about wanting to die, or thoughts of death, also are of concern and carry as much weight toward a depression diagnosis as do explicit forms of suicidal behavior (American Psychiatric Association [APA], 2013, 2022). However, it is questionable whether recurrent thoughts of death should be regarded as evidence of suicidality (Kovacs & George, 2020) particularly because as many as 68% of a large sample of depressed youngsters reported such cognitions, while far fewer (48%) had suicidal ideation and 12% had a history of suicide attempts (Liu et al., 2006). Ideation and attempts are far less likely in pediatric population samples (e.g., 14.3% lifetime rate of ideation among 9- and 10-year-olds; Lawrence et al., 2021), although the rates appear to be on the rise.

Symptom Verification and Contextual Mapping

Suicidal thoughts and actions may come to attention at the initial assessment, if the family reports them during therapy as concerns, or if the child endorses the suicidal ideation item on the self-rated Children's Depression Inventory (CDI), which is to be completed before each treatment session (see Chapter 5). Whether reported by parent or child, the therapist must put suicidality on the session's agenda. For example, the therapist may say:

> (To parent–child pair) *You just listed several issues. I would like to start with some questions about [child] talking about killing himself.*

Or

> (To child) *I see that you checked here [on the CDI] that you have been thinking about killing yourself—I have some questions about that and so we will put this on our agenda.*

The suicidal symptom must be evaluated so the therapist can decide if the child may be managed as an outpatient or needs inpatient hospitalization. If the child can be managed as an outpatient, then the evaluation has to focus on the nature of the symptom as illustrated here: The resultant information will indicate the best intervention.

Chapter 5 listed the questions to be asked during the assessment of suicidal thoughts and actions. If there are persistent suicidal thoughts and related actions, ideation not within the young patient's control, consideration of highly lethal and accessible suicide methods, and a notably dysfunctional family environment, the child needs *immediate clinical attention,* most likely within an *inpatient* setting (see Spirito & Esposito-Smythers, 2006). If the therapist does not feel qualified to conduct the assessment and determine the best course of action, the child and family should be referred for an immediate psychiatric evaluation by someone with experience in this area.

If the child can be treated as an outpatient and there is a need for further information, the in-session assessment may be supplemented by homework monitoring of the child's suicidal ideation and/or behavior. Such an assignment is easily accommodated by CERT's coaching model and may be presented by the therapist (T) as follows:

T: OK, we have some idea of what is going on when [child] is saying that he wants to kill himself. We will talk about what to do—all right? But we also need to keep an eye on these ideas to make sure they do not get out of hand.

(*To child*) I would like you and Mom to do the following as homework: She will check with you as your coach about having ideas of killing yourself.

How about this: She will check after you come home from school and later in the evening. And the two of you will write down what was happening when these ideas came to you. And if you have thoughts of killing yourself any other time, you will tell her right away, OK?

Do you think you will be able to work with Mom on this homework? And you [Mom], can you put on your coaching hat for this homework?

OK! Let's practice this.

Although concerned, some parents may feel ill at ease talking about and dealing with suicidal behavior. Indeed, the therapist needs to be prepared for some degree of parental (P) discomfort when the homework involves monitoring suicidality. Here is an example of the most common objection:

P: I don't know about this homework. Isn't it [monitoring suicidal ideation] like putting ideas in [child's] head? Like you are making him think about it?

T: Actually, it is important that you brought this up because some people think that if you ask about suicidal ideas or actions, it's as if you put these ideas into the other person's head.

But there is no evidence that this happens, no evidence at all. Kids and grown-ups can think about killing themselves for many different reasons but not because someone put the idea in their heads.

And, we need to *know* if [child] has such ideas so that we can make sure that they do not get out of control and he is safe. There is no other way to know, except by asking.

After the therapist has verified the symptom and its recency, contextual mapping will help to determine if it is a regulatory response to sadness and distress, in which case several CERT strategies are appropriate (as illustrated in the text that follows). During contextual mapping, pay particular attention to the affective precursors of the suicidal ideation or threat.

The possibility that suicidal symptoms serve to regulate or manage distressing emotions has long been recognized (e.g., Zlotnick et al., 1997), and the association of these variables has been empirically supported (e.g., Hatkevich et al., 2019; Neacsiu et al., 2017; Tamás et al., 2007). Typically, there is a buildup of sadness and dysphoria to which the young patient automatically responds with suicidal thoughts or threats, which then maintain the despondent affect. Thus, suicidal ideation functions as a maladaptive cognitive regulatory response to dysphoria.

However, contextual mapping may reveal that suicidal symptoms and affective distress occurred in separate time frames. Suicidal symptoms may have emerged as impulsive reactions to a problem or confrontation, but without marked changes in baseline dysphoria. They may be driven by a pessimistic and negative cognitive style rather than affective distress. In these instances, suicidal threats may be best viewed as traditional manifestations of depression and approached via traditional intervention strategies.

Regardless of how the suicidal symptom is interpreted or the form of intervention is to be used, the outpatient management of a child with suicidal thoughts or behaviors requires the involvement of dependable adult caregivers who can provide monitoring and oversight, if indicated (as discussed in Chapter 5). If the young patient's parent is facing considerable stress, has limited resources and insufficient social support, and/or is suffering from depression or some other form of mental disorder, monitoring and supervising a suicidal child may be too demanding. Thus, other interventions should be considered (e.g., Spirito & Esposito-Smythers, 2006).

Suicidal Symptom as a Mood Repair Response

After it has been established that the young patient's suicidal symptoms represent maladaptive mood regulatory responses, the goal is to replace them with adaptive strategies, which will help the child to decrease her dysphoria and then resolve the triggering situation. The best strategy is for the therapist to identify a regulatory response that the child already successfully implemented for mood repair, or one that is consistent with the child's preferred regulatory domain, and present it to the parent–child pair for their consideration.

To illustrate a CERT approach when suicidal ideation is a response to despondent affect, we return to 10-year-old Davey, the young patient who was bullied in school (see Chapter 6). By way of background, recall that although the parents listed a history of suicidal thoughts at the intake assessment, suicidal ideation was not a pressing concern at that time.

In earlier sessions, the therapist had focused on improving Davey's ability to manage upsurges of sadness and unhappiness, such as those provoked by the bullying in school; and progress continued to be made. Recall that Davey's initial successful mood regulatory response to the school-based provocation was a cognitive one (visualizing his tormentors without their pants on), and he continued to demonstrate his facility with using it. To expand Davey's regulatory repertoire, and because interpersonal conflicts seemed to trigger most of Davey's dysphoric episodes, the therapist eventually introduced him to a response from the interpersonal regulatory domain, "talking to a parent," which also was successfully implemented by Davey.

As part of structuring the session of interest, the therapist asked the parents whether anything of import had transpired since the last session. They expressed their concern over the recurrence of Davey's suicidal ideation and threats. The therapist put this concern on the agenda and returned to it soon thereafter. After symptom verification (i.e., confirming its problematic nature) and contextual mapping (e.g., the circumstances of the ideation), she established that Davey did verbalize threats to kill himself (which he confirmed) twice over the last 2 days. It was confined to ideation, was of concern, and there appeared to be a confluence of affective triggers, which led to pent up dysphoria and distress.

The next dialogue picks up as the therapist, speaking to the child (C), summarizes the information and confirms that the symptom was a response to dysphoria.

T: Let me summarize what I am hearing. You guys were having a family dinner yesterday and you got upset with your sister. After some fighting, you started to yell that your parents don't love you and that you should be dead and that you want to kill yourself—so it sounds like that is what happened. Yes?

C: Hmm.

T: You know, kids *can* have such ideas, especially when they are sad, or unhappy, or angry.

C: Yeah.

T: That can happen, and so I am wondering—which feeling went along with thinking that you want to kill yourself this last time?

C: Dunno. I was mad. Yeah, like sad, upset.

T: You had this thought during dinner and once later after dinner—in the evening.

So, tell me about this last time, in the evening.

C: Uhmm. Upset—bad—I was feeling bad.

T: So, you were feeling bad. And what was going on? What were you thinking?

C: Nothing.

T: Hmm, that's hard to believe because you are a thinking sort of a fellow!

C: Well, Susie [his disabled sister] got me upset and this new kid is picking on me—and he keeps on me and it was like Susie started picking on me at dinner and she's been acting up.

T: OK. It sounds like different people were picking on you—like kids at school and then your sister and that got you sad and upset.

And all that together made for a lot of bad feelings and then you just had the thoughts about killing yourself. Is that how it went?

C: Hmm.

T: Well, I understand. You know when kids feel sad and upset and think about killing themselves, this can mean a bunch of things: Like they feel really bad and can't stand the feeling or they can't figure out what to do about some problem.

Which fits what was going on with you?

(*To parent*) What do you think?

P: I think he was real upset! It wasn't clear why—he just couldn't settle down. He already was acting kind of off when he came home from school. I was thinking that maybe something happened there?

C: It wasn't my fault.

T: (*To child*) And the feeling got too much, and you thought about killing yourself. That's how it went?

C: Yeah.

T: And how did you feel then—after you started thinking about killing yourself?

C: Bad.

Having confirmed that the suicidal threats served as maladaptive responses to dysphoria, the therapist works with the parent–child pair to identify the trigger and an adaptive regulatory response. The dialogue picks up as the therapist again summarizes the new information and proposes an intervention.

T: (*To parent and child*) It sounds like Davey thought about killing himself because he felt really bad when he believed that both Susie [the sister] and kids in school were picking on him. He thought that they don't like him.

(*To parent*) Can you put on your coaching hat?

(*To child*) Let's talk about what can help you to feel better when you feel bad—or feel sad. You feel bad about yourself and get the idea that you want to kill yourself.

(*To parent*) Can you help Davey to remember when we used The House of ER? In which room did we find stuff that helped Davey to feel better?

(*To child*) What helped you to feel better when you were sad and upset?

P: We had to interrupt it. Davey thought of a funny picture and that helped to make sure that it didn't get out of control.

T: Yes! So, we know that thinking of a funny picture, like Davey did, can help him to feel better. And all of you did a great job with that.

What are some other ways to stop feeling bad, some other ways to interrupt feeling bad and to stop thinking about killing yourself?

C: Dunno—maybe talk to Mom or Dad?

T: Yes, that's another tool in The House of ER, which you already used. Talking is a tool in The People's Room in The House of ER.

Good. You are right. And do you remember—you used it a few weeks ago when you got upset about stuff that happened in school.

(*To parent*) Can you tell me again how that homework went—talking about being upset?

At this juncture, the therapist wants to make sure that both parent and child recall the use of interpersonal regulatory responses that helped to attenuate Davey's sad and upset emotions. From this point onward, the intervention is straightforward. The goal is to replace suicidal ideation as a response to distressing emotions by mobilizing an interpersonal regulatory response; namely, talking to parents about *what* upset Davey. That response can be practiced by having the parent–child pair and the therapist role-play the most recent scenario of suicidal ideation, with the therapist helping to identify the interpersonal triggers (perceived negative view of Davey), which can be alleviated by attentive listening on the part of the parent.

Monitoring of suicidal thoughts also can be assigned as homework, along with implementing the regulatory response that was practiced in the session. Given the problematic nature of the target symptom, the therapist may also ask the parent to call the therapist and report on progress before the next session. The success of the monitoring homework and its discussion should be prioritized on the agenda of the next treatment session.

Suicidal Symptom as a Traditional Feature of Depression

If contextual mapping indicates that the young patient's suicidal thoughts and threats were not triggered by an episode of dysphoria or distress and are better conceptualized as traditional symptoms of depression, the therapist may consider various non-CERT therapeutic interventions. Verbal or written *contracting for safety* or the *no suicide contract* (e.g., AACAP, 2001) is one approach when facing a young patient with suicidal thoughts and actions. Contracting for safety essentially means that the young patient agrees (contracts) to not engage in suicidal acts and to inform caregivers or other key adults of such intents once they arise.

However, there are concerns about the contracting for safety approach. On the one hand, the so-called no suicide contract may be experienced by the child and the family as therapeutic. But Garvey and colleagues (2009) concluded that there is limited evidence, at best, that safety contracts prevent actual suicides. Supportive data are particularly sparse regarding adolescents and close to nonexistent when it comes to younger children. The foregoing statements are not meant to discourage the therapist from contracting for safety, but rather to increase awareness of the limits of such an approach and prevent a false sense of security.

Another potentially relevant intervention is dialectical behavior therapy

(DBT). DBT has long been known as particularly effective with suicidal adults suffering from borderline personality disorder and has been modified for young suicidal patients (Katz et al., 2004; Rathus & Miller, 2002, 2015). Reports indicate favorable outcomes over comparison conditions (reviewed by Spirito & Esposito-Smythers, 2006). However, according to a meta-analysis, while DBT reduces suicidal behavior (i.e., attempts), it has no discernible effect on suicide ideation (DeCou et al., 2019). Nonetheless, the therapist may find that some DBT techniques focused on suicidal thoughts and actions are appropriate and useful.

Finally, partly based on the proposition that suicidal behavior in depression is an expression of hopelessness and related cognitive distortions, versions of individual cognitive-behavior therapy (CBT) have been proposed as the interventions of choice (e.g., Daniel & Goldston, 2012; Spirito & Esposito-Smythers, 2006; Stark et al., 2006). Overall, these interventions seek to remedy a variety of cognitive and behavioral deficits (e.g., biased interpretations, insufficient coping skills) that are believed to culminate in suicidal thought and actions. From among the various CBT strategies, those that focus on cognitive restructuring may be particularly useful because they target inappropriate thoughts and beliefs that presumably perpetuate suicidal behaviors and depression.

Sleep Disturbance

Good sleep quality and appropriate sleep duration are critical to all areas of functioning, ranging from being able to pay attention to mounting an adequate immune response to infection (e.g., Beebe, 2011; Imeri & Opp, 2009). Disturbed sleep, one of the most prevalent symptoms of depression (reviewed by Tsuno et al., 2005), manifests as insomnia or hypersomnia. Insomnia or loss of sleep means that the young patient has trouble going to sleep or has disturbed sleep and wakes during the night. Hypersomnia means excessive sleep: The young patient sleeps far more than what is typical for his age. Among depressed children and young adolescents, sleep disturbance typically manifests as sleep loss (rather than excessive sleep). For example, in one study of young, depressed patients, 54% had insomnia, 9% had hypersomnia, and 10% had both types of sleep problems (Liu et al., 2007).

Patients' complaints of disturbed sleep have been supported by evidence of extensively altered sleep architecture (atypical brain EEG), underscoring the physiological concomitants of this symptom (reviewed by Palagini et al., 2012; Tsuno et al., 2005). Altered neuroendocrine and homeostatic regulatory processes (e.g., Harvey et al., 2011; Tsuno et al., 2005) that characterize depression may be at the root of some patients' sleep disturbance. Intrusive cognitions (thoughts or images) that arise as the individual tries to go to sleep may be another source of sleep loss. Sleep loss also may be instigated by disruptions in evening routines and related behaviors or aspects of the environment.

When sleep loss is due to intrusive thoughts or images, they may be countered by helping the child to deploy cognitive regulatory responses (see the section "Sleep Disturbance due to Interfering Cognitions"). Irrespective of the putative cause of sleep loss, the therapist may undertake sleep hygiene training, a widely used nonpharmacological intervention that has been associated with good sleep quality (LeBourgeois et al., 2005). Sleep hygiene training involves encouraging behaviors that support good sleep quality, appropriate sleep duration, and daytime alertness (LeBourgeois et al., 2005).

Symptom Verification and Contextual Mapping

If the parent and/or the child report a sleep problem, verify its problematic nature and its type (i.e., trouble falling asleep, trouble staying asleep, or sleeping too much). Contextual mapping then can help to identify whether the young patient's sleep disturbance is due to intrusive cognitions or images.

During contextual mapping of sleep disturbance, consider the following: Does the young patient get trapped at bedtimes in "thinking rather than sleeping"? Does he have worries and concerns that stop him from sleeping? Is something in the environment keeping the young patient awake? Given that difficulty falling asleep is the most likely sleep disturbance, queries along the following lines should be helpful:

> T: (*To child*) Think about yesterday (or the day before). When you went to bed in the evening and closed your eyes, were there things going through your head? Like different ideas or pictures? Can you tell me about them?
>
> Is there some idea or picture that keeps you up when you go to bed?
>
> Is there something that stops you from sleeping?
>
> Are you worried about something? Does that stay on your mind when you go to bed? Does that make it hard to go to sleep?
>
> When did this [idea/picture] start—how long ago? Does it happen every night? Many nights? Just a few nights?

If the young patient's sleep problems cannot be explained by intrusive thoughts or images, or there also is sleep continuity disturbance, a sleep hygiene assessment may be warranted. The goal of the assessment is to identify the component of good sleep hygiene practice that may have been breached. Introduce the sleep hygiene assessment by saying something like this:

> T: (*To parent*) I would like to ask you a few more questions about [the child's] sleep and about what goes on before he goes to sleep. These things are important because they affect how well we sleep.
>
> So, let's start by thinking about [child's] sleep over the last few days.

Inquire about the areas listed next, focusing on those relevant to the given patient.

Activities around Bedtime

- *How close to bedtime does the child eat and/or drink? What is eaten, drunk?*
- *Does the child go to the bathroom before going to sleep?*
- *Is the child physically active before bedtime (e.g., running around, playing with siblings or adults)?*
- *Does the child watch TV or use electronic devices around bedtime?*
- *Once the child goes to bed, does he engage in any activity besides trying to go to sleep?*

Sleep Routine

- *Does the child nap during the late afternoon?*
- *Is there a bedtime routine (e.g., brushing teeth, getting clothes ready for the morning)?*
- *Is there a set time to go to bed?*

Sleeping Arrangement

- *Does the child have his own bed? If "no," how many individuals share the bed?*
- *Does the child have his own room? If "no," how many individuals share the room?*
- *Is the child's bedroom separated from the rest of the living space?*
- *What are others in the household usually doing when the child goes to bed?*
- *When does each individual in the family go to sleep?*
- *Do others stay up late? What do they do?*

After the assessment is completed, the therapist can segue into implementing the appropriate intervention.

Sleep Disturbance due to Interfering Cognitions

If the child has trouble falling asleep because she keeps ruminating about some concern, then various techniques can be used from The Thinking Room of The House of ER (e.g., thought substitution or interruption, visual imagery) to stop the cognitions.

In the case of 12-year-old Lisa (see Chapter 7), sleep disturbance was noted by her mother as a symptom of depression when the young patient started CERT, but it was not the most pressing issue at that time. In fact, as Lisa's depression began to lift, the sleep difficulty, along with other nonaffective symptoms, also improved. However, sleep disturbance reemerged as a concern during the later phase of treatment.

Recall that Lisa had notable emotional challenges as her mainstreaming from learning disability support classes was not handled well. Her mother was concerned that the recent sleep disturbance signaled a relapse into depression. However, contextual mapping of the complaint revealed that Lisa had trouble going to sleep specifically because she was preoccupied with the start of another school year and her school placement. The dialogue that follows picks up after symptom verification and contextual mapping. Note that the therapist reframes the mother's concern about "relapse" as an occasion for further skill acquisition, recalls the parent–child pair's past success in recovering from depression, and proposes an intervention that builds on cognitive skills that already have been mastered by the young patient.

T: (*To child*) OK. Let me summarize what seems to be going on.

For the past week or so, when you go to bed and it's "lights out," you cannot fall asleep.

And there haven't been any changes at home, like no specific thing that could have caused this.

But we just figured out that you can't fall asleep because your mind keeps going. You keep thinking stuff like, "What if I have trouble with keeping up with the new courses?" "What if kids make fun of me?" "It was easier in my old classes."

(*To parent*) OK, I understand that you are worried that the sleep problems mean that Lisa is again getting depressed. But it is not unusual for some symptoms to show up again and that gives us a chance to see where we need to do a bit more work.

P: All right. But how can we get her to sleep?

T: (*To parent and child*) Well—it looks like there are these ideas that go around in her head that make her upset or anxious and they interfere with going to sleep.

Recall that previously Lisa's maladaptive cognitions involved worry ruminations that she would not be able to finish a class project. The intervention for it was *thought substitution,* which involved Lisa focusing instead on positive features of her project on elephants. It took several sessions, diligent coaching by her mother, and practice until the thought substitution intervention helped Lisa to better manage her dysphoria. This suggested to the therapist that a less complex cognitive response be tried for Lisa's sleep problem. She chose *thought interference* that involves engaging the child's mind in some simple activity to counter the worrying thoughts. The therapist continued as follows:

T: Do you remember when Lisa had some problems because she was worried about her elephant project?

P: Yeah.

T: (*To parent and child*) Thinking back to the elephant project, what helped Lisa *not* to get upset?

C: Mom and me went through all the good parts of my project and we talked about it—about the good parts.

T: (*To parent and child*) That's right! So, you used your thinking to feel better. Do you remember which room this is in The House of ER?

C: Yeah, the room with thinking—the room about "what is on your mind."

T: Yes, you are right. And you did a very good job with it! So, I want to tell you about another way to use your thinking.

I'd like you to pay attention to your breathing. And then start to *count* very quietly each breath like this: one, breathe in; two, breathe out. (*Therapist demonstrates.*)

(*To Mom*) Can you try also because I will be asking you to do the coaching?

What we are doing here is this: We are using our thinking to focus on relaxing, which is what happens when we breathe slowly.

And we already know that Lisa is good at using her thinking to get things done.

At this point, the therapist asks the mother to be the coach and to run through multiple breathing cycles with Lisa. After further discussion, the breathing exercise is assigned as homework to be done when Lisa goes to bed, with her mother coaching. The coaching time interval is set initially as 1–2 minutes, to be followed by up to three further 2 minutes of breathing exercise intervals, as needed.

Reporting on the homework becomes a top item on the next session's agenda. If the outcome is satisfactory (the child can go to sleep more easily), the homework may be continued. If the task was executed correctly but Lisa's response was not sufficiently satisfactory, the therapist may elect to lengthen the exercise interval and/or add sleep hygiene modifications to the nightly routine.

Sleep Disturbance as a Traditional Feature of Depression

If the young patient's sleep loss appears to reflect the disruptive effects of depression on neurovegetative functions and/or result from some feature of the environment, sleep hygiene training should be considered.

A full sleep hygiene training protocol includes multiple goals, namely:

- Avoiding late afternoon naps.
- Restricting the intake of caffeine (including soft drinks) or other stimulants before bedtime.
- Limiting large meals to several hours before bedtime and substituting light snacks.
- Avoiding any activating or arousing physical or mental activities close to bedtime (e.g., no exercising, avoiding TV, scary or violent films or videos).
- Introducing physical activity several hours before bedtime (vigorous aerobic activity for at least 30 minutes several hours before bedtime can promote sleep).
- Having a bedtime routine (e.g., a set of personal health behaviors every evening, such as brushing teeth, showering, preparations for the morning, conjoint activity with a parent).
- Maintaining a stable sleep schedule (going to bed around the same time every evening) and sleeping in a quiet environment. If the family's circumstances permit, it is preferable to have the depressed child sleep alone.

Sleep hygiene training has to be personalized based on the results of the young patient's sleep hygiene assessment and delivered in a psychoeducational context: The therapist explains why she is selecting a given goal and underscores the importance of normalizing sleep in the process of recovery from depression. It also may help to remind the parent–child pair that the "bed is for sleeping" and discourage other activities (e.g., watching TV, use of digital devices, eating) in bed.

Because sleep hygiene training is personalized, it may focus on limiting exposure to potentially arousing stimuli near bedtime (TV or internet) for one child, while for another, noise-reduction strategies (e.g., earplugs) may be indicated given the night activities of others in the household. Some patients may benefit from engaging in physical activity several hours before bedtime, while for others establishing a uniform nightly routine may be the most useful. If siblings keep awake a young patient because they have different bedtimes, the therapist can propose having the same bedtime for all the children "to see how that may help." If the child sleeps in a noisy part of the apartment or family's living space, the therapist could explore with the parent the feasibility of changing the sleeping arrangement or, if that is not feasible, then consider noise-reduction options.

CERT's coaching model is particularly appropriate when it comes to implementing sleep hygiene training. The goals and interventions to restore sleep should be presented as experiments. Practicing the interventions should constitute homework, be feasible, and make sense to the parent–child pair. The outcomes should be reviewed in the upcoming treatment sessions.

Self-Deprecation and Worthlessness

As described by Harter (2006, 2012), a person's overall view of oneself as competent or worthwhile can be parsed into self-judgments about areas of functioning that include cognitive or intellectual elements (e.g., school performance), social–interpersonal functioning (e.g., quality of friendships and peer relations), and physical characteristics (e.g., athletic ability, looks). Negative views of oneself range from statements that are mildly critical or disparaging to those mirroring a total negation of the self, including: "I am stupid," "I am not smart enough," "I don't know how to do anything right," "Nobody likes me," "I am ugly," "Nobody wants to be my friend," "Mom doesn't love me." Worthlessness, the more severe form of this cognitive symptom, is a global devaluation of the self, manifest in statements such as "I am no good," "My parents would be better off without me," "I am a burden on my family," among others.

When self-deprecation or worthlessness represents maladaptive cognitive responses to dysphoria, they are amenable to modification via various CERT strategies. Alternatively, self-deprecatory statements may reflect a traditional symptom of depression, likely deriving from negative cognitive biases and ruminative tendencies. Self-deprecation also may signal the exacerbation of chronically low self-esteem. In the latter instances, the therapist may turn to any of a variety of commonly used cognitive and behavioral treatment strategies.

Symptom Verification and Contextual Mapping

If self-deprecation is identified as a target symptom, the first step is to confirm how problematic it has been. Then, contextual mapping will help to determine if the symptom represents a mood regulatory response or if it is better conceptualized as a traditional symptom of depression.

Negative self-statements often come to the forefront and are likely to function as maladaptive cognitive regulatory responses during emotionally heated family (or other interpersonal) incidents. Other affective triggers of negative self-statements include receiving adverse feedback about academic or social performance or physical appearance. Thus, during contextual mapping, be particularly mindful of the affective precursors and consequences of self-deprecatory statements. If self-deprecation is a response to dysphoric affect, then the therapist may utilize an adaptive CERT cognitive regulatory response as a corrective intervention (one approach is documented below).

For some young patients, self-deprecation is better regarded as a traditional depression symptom, likely to mirror negative cognitive biases or traitlike low self-esteem. For example, self-deprecation may emerge as a young patient compares himself to his friends and concludes that he is greatly deficient in most respects. In such a case, the therapist may consider a variety of commonly used cognitive or behavioral interventions (e.g., Stark et al., 2006; Weisz, 2004). However, to correct traitlike low self-esteem and entrenched cognitive biases may require more lengthy treatment than is typical for CERT and may necessitate that the therapist renegotiate her contract with the family.

Self-Deprecation as a Mood Repair Response

To counter self-deprecation as a maladaptive mood repair response, the therapist may select any of the tools in The Thinking Room of The House of ER as an intervention. To illustrate this approach, we return to Chantel (age 9) who has had problems adjusting to the birth of a sibling, Abe, and felt unloved because her parents spend more time with him owing to his behavioral issues. As discussed in Chapter 6, Chantel's therapist focused on strengthening the young patient's interpersonal regulatory responses, particularly those involving the parents as regulators. At the same time, however, the therapist wanted to expand Chantel's cognitive regulatory response repertoire.

Recall that Chantel disrupted one of her early CERT sessions by announcing unexpectedly that her parents didn't love her. The statement "My Mom [Dad] doesn't love me" typically mirrors the cognition that "I am unlovable" or not good enough to be deserving of love. The therapist intervened during that session by ensuring that Chantel has greater access to her parents as affect regulators. At a later date, the complaint "My parents don't love me" reappeared in the context of a family conflict about Abe. By this time in treatment, Chantel's depression had much improved and the therapist also recognized that Chantel's low self-esteem was related to jealousy of her younger sibling. Changing her approach, the therapist focused directly on Chantel's negative cognitions and sought to replace them with more adaptive cognitive responses (the *magic sign*), which Chantel mastered easily.

In the session of interest here, her mother related another incident involving Chantel complaining that she wasn't loved. The therapist expected that the verbalization reflected a mood repair response and that, given Chantel's past success with cognitive regulatory responses (recall her visualizing her magic sign), Chantel would be willing to try another response in that same domain to counter her negative thoughts about herself.

After confirming that the verbalizations in question represented a mood repair response, the therapist introduced the CERT intervention. Note in the following how the therapist links the current task to prior tasks and reinforces the coaching framework. The dialogue picks up as the therapist summarizes the results of contextual mapping:

T: Let me see if I got this right. The other day, you [parents] were going to take Chantel to a get-together with her friends but Abe started to act up and so you didn't leave until much later, at which point Chantel got very upset and started crying and saying that you don't love her. And it took a little time to get her to calm down.

P: Yes, that's about it.

T: (*To child*) So, you had the feeling that Mom and Dad don't love you.

C: Yeah.

T: I see, but can you tell me *why* you think that they don't love you?

C: Dunno—Abe is more special.

T: So, you felt upset and then had the idea that your parents don't love you? Because you are not so special as Abe. Did it go something like that?

C: Guess.

T: So, you are thinking that Mom and Dad don't love you *because* you are not special—I guess that thinking *two* things like that made you feel even worse.

Did you feel more sad and more upset as those ideas were on your mind?

C: Yeah. They were only caring about Abe.

T: (*To child*) So, you think that you are *not* special—that can make you feel pretty sad and bad.

C: Hmm.

T: (*To parents and child*). Do you remember a while back Chantel learned a special thing to do to feel better when she feels bad?

It had to do with putting a new idea in the place of an idea that upsets you.

P: Sure (*to child*), remember? That was your *magic sign!* The *stop sign*.

C: Yeah, I guess.

T: (*To child*) Thinking that Mom and Dad don't love you because you are not special makes you feel bad—right?

So, how about thinking about things in another way? If the idea in your head is "My mom doesn't love me," what idea can replace it?

P: That I love her?

T: Yes, that's a good start.

(*To child*) What are things that Mom and Dad did in the past, things that helped you feel special?

(*To parent*) Mom, can you put on your coaching hat? Let's make a list. So, what things can you think of?

P: When we read together.

C: Yeah.

T: (*To child*) Oh—that's good. Anything else?

C: When Dad and I sing together.

T: Here is an idea, Can we make a list of things you and Mom and Dad do together, the things that help you know that they love you.

We already have two things on the list: "When we read and sing together." Can we think of another thing to put on the list?

C: Dunno.

T: How about getting a hug?

In general, such lists should have at least three items; three items are relatively easy to memorize and recall. Because the list will help to replace upsetting ideas, it is likened in this case to the magic sign, which Chantel used successfully to counter dysphoria. The list is compiled in the session, and the homework involves Mom helping Chantel think of the items on the list whenever she vocalizes the cognition that she is unloved. To maximize success, the therapist continues to reinforce the value of coaching and explains the rationale for the homework.

T: (*To parent*) How about putting on your coaching hat when it looks like Chantel is getting upset about Abe, when she is beginning to think that she is not special and therefore you don't love her? It seems to happen when Chantel doesn't get something, when something gets held up due to Abe.

P: Yes—it kind of looks like that.

T: So, when Chantel starts talking like that, can you take several minutes or more from what is going on and spend time with her to review the list?

Can we practice right now? Let's start with this: Let's help Chantel read aloud each item and tell us about the last time that interaction or behavior happened.

Note that this exercise is a form of cognitive restructuring, but rather than having the young patient debate the validity of her negative self-statements, the goal is to substitute an adaptive cognitive response. Following the usual procedures, the results of the homework are reviewed in the next treatment session and the therapist then determines whether it should be continued as planned, modified in some way, or passed up for an alternative response.

What if the parents report that they were not be able to interrupt some activity in which they were engaged to intervene with Chantel in their coaching roles? If that turns out to be the case, the therapist can modify the assignment to include a daily review of the list that is not dependent on Chantel's dysphoric episodes. The therapist also has the option of using any response (tool) from the cognitive domain of The House of ER as well as exploring other regulatory domains to help Chantel.

With regard to her evolving case formulation and related treatment plans, the therapist made a note about the recurrence of negative self-statements whenever Chantel perceives Abe as being favored. Sibling rivalry appears to drive these displays, which suggests the need to eventually consider interventions on some level other than mood repair mastery.

Self-Deprecation as a Traditional Symptom of Depression

If the young patient's self-deprecatory statements appear to reflect a traditional depression symptom, the therapist can turn to a wide array of intervention strategies, many of which have been described in the literature, ranging from simple behavioral tasks to complex cognitive restructuring.

One behaviorally anchored task that is worthy of note is called the *graded task assignment*; it can be particularly helpful to counter negative self-statements of younger patients or those whose self-deprecation is severe or pervasive. This intervention is based on the notion that, when objective evidence is presented in a certain way, the patient will start to recognize that her negative self-statements are untrue. Success is highly likely because every task consists of multiple components, which can be identified, and tackling the simplest possible component, followed by the next simplest and so on, helps the patient regain gradually the sense of mastery and competence that underlies self-esteem (Beck et al., 1979).

Recall Mike, age 13, described in Chapter 7, for whom the therapist sought to interrupt episodes of dysphoria with the behavioral strategy of taking his dog Jumpy for walks. Let's suppose that Mike declined that behavioral experiment stating that he was no good and could no longer take care of Jumpy. Given such a scenario, the therapist can reconceptualize the act of taking Jumpy for a walk as a graded task assignment (Beck et al., 1979). The key to a successful graded task assignment is to work with the young patient and parent to jointly define the task and then break it down into the smallest workable components, with the initial steps or components being so simple that anyone can implement them.

For example, the task of taking Jumpy for a walk would be reframed by the therapist along the following lines:

T: OK(*to child*), I understand that taking Jumpy for a walk seems like a lot.
So, let's try something else. Let's all of us figure out the many steps that are involved in taking Jumpy for a walk, starting with getting the leash.
Let's make a list. (*To parent*) Can you put on your coaching hat and help Mike with starting this list? Do we agree that the very first step is "finding the leash"?

Then the therapist guides the young patient and parent along the process of breaking down the task, from the first step, which is to find the leash, to the next step, which is calling Jumpy to come, followed by putting the leash on Jumpy's neck, and then finding the disposal bag to take, followed by checking with one of the parents to come along for the walk, going out of the house, deciding on a route along which to walk, and so on.

After the task breakdown is complete, the therapist asks the parent and child to agree to a homework assignment: to explore how many steps Mike can complete when they get home after the treatment session. As coach, the parent is asked to motivate Mike to engage in the first few steps of the task. For the parent to model the desired behaviors, getting Mike to agree to try the first step of the task can be role-played in the session by the therapist, along with the provision of lots of positive reinforcement. The outcome is to be reported in the next treatment session.

By having Mike implement the initial steps of the graded task assignment, the therapist is gathering objective evidence that can be used to attenuate the child's total self-negation. For example, Mike is more than likely to be able to find the leash and put it around Jumpy's neck: Completion of these steps is evidence that he *can* do *some* things right, based on which Mike has to modify his self-statements. The implementation of more and more steps of the task can be undertaken in further homework assignments, which can help the young patient to recover his self-confidence gradually.

The therapist also may consider other forms of behavioral interventions or cognitive restructuring, depending on the self-esteem domain in which the young patient is lacking. For example, if the perceived deficit derives from lack of friends or alleged peer rejection, social skills training may be the intervention of choice, elements of which the therapist can model in the session. On the other hand, if a child complains that she is "ugly," cognitive restructuring may be the goal, using evidence-based questioning.

Summary and Next Steps

For many depressed young patients, the successful treatment of disordered mood is usually followed by diminution of nonaffective depression symptoms, which therefore do not require additional treatment. However, some patients do need interventions for nonaffective depression symptoms concurrent with or after remission of affective symptoms. And there are still other patients whose nonaffective symptoms, like self-deprecation, may periodically reappear in response to specific and usually circumscribed triggers.

The fact that nonaffective depression symptoms generally become intervention targets after CERT is underway can facilitate their treatment because the parent–child pair has likely become familiar with CERT's guiding principles, and the young patient has by that time gained some mastery over his sadness and dysphoria. The therapist can build on such demonstrated competencies when deciding about how best to approach nonaffective depression symptoms. Concomitantly, as illustrated in this chapter, it is important that the therapist regularly remind the family about the progress that has been made to overcome the child's depression.

In this chapter, I argued that nonaffective symptoms of depression can represent maladaptive regulatory responses to dysphoria; in which case, the therapist may implement various interventions that adhere to the CERT perspective. But, as I also noted, nonaffective depression symptoms may be traditional manifestations of depression; in which case, the therapist may intervene using a wide array of evidence-based techniques. Irrespective of the symptom's presumed origin, and regardless of the intervention selected, the therapist must continuously reinforce the parent–child coaching relationship, as was also documented in this chapter. Furthermore, if any symptoms call for long-term intervention, the family should be advised, and the therapy contract renegotiated.

Now I turn to the final two chapters in this book, which address conceptual and practical issues regarding coping skills training, the last phase of treatment.

Chapter 9

Coping Skills Training

Its Purpose, Components, and Challenges

Coping skills training is the last phase of contextual emotion regulation therapy (CERT) and is implemented when patients no longer manifest a clinically significant depressive syndrome. However, because youngsters recover from depression at different rates, symptom levels will vary from child to child when coping skills training is initiated. The presence of a few mild depressive symptoms should not interfere with coping skills training.

Coping skills training is most likely to be fruitful if it is delivered over an extended time, with sufficiently long intervals between sessions to facilitate the implementation of new behaviors and the consolidation of learned information. Recall that by the time this phase of treatment is reached, the frequency of sessions will have been reduced to once every 2 weeks. Coping skills training should be delivered at that rate for a few sessions and then gradually tapered to one session every 3–4 weeks. After several monthly sessions, the therapist can consider ending treatment, for which the family should be prepared in advance.

The coping skills training phase of CERT requires more self-direction and motivation on the part of the child and parent than did the earlier phases, partly because of the reduced frequency of contacts with the therapist. An additional challenge is that, as the young patient feels better and is no longer depressed, there may be decreased motivation to comply with homework assignments. The last part of this chapter therefore presents some issues families are likely to raise to explain noncompliance with coping skills training, and counterarguments that the therapist may use in response.

The Purpose of Coping Skills Training

The overarching purpose of coping skills training is to reduce the risk of depression recurrence. To prevent recurrence, the child needs to maintain the ability to respond in adaptive ways to dysphoria and depressogenic triggers. The therapist must therefore assure that any expression of adaptive mood repair by the young patient in daily life continues to be generously reinforced.

Ongoing reinforcement of desirable mood repair–related behaviors is the backdrop for the young patient's personalized coping skills training plan. The training plan itself builds on the given child's and family's CERT achievements and includes coping goals that are reasonable and doable for that child and family, and are likely to provide them with sufficient tools to manage future depressogenic triggers.

Components of Coping Skills Training

Coping skills training is best implemented by developing a training plan for the given young patient. The training plan is an informal set of guideposts set up by the therapist. Think of the plan as a way to organize and implement training goals: It addresses what the therapist seeks to accomplish for that patient and how he plans to implement it.

The training plans for all young patients include the continuous reinforcement of the child to practice adaptive mood repair and to strive to maintain generally euthymic affective states (to be on an even keel emotionally). The personalized components of the training plan, by definition, vary from child to child.

During the session that serves to transition to coping skills training (see Chapter 10), the parent and child are asked to think about coping with stressful events and triggers as a process that has two aspects (similar to the coping paradigm proposed by Lazarus and Folkman [1984]). One aspect is to manage the emotions that are triggered by the stressor (we call this *emotion regulation coping*) and, if appropriate, the other aspect is to solve the problem itself (we call this *problem-solving coping*). The extent to which coping skills training focuses on these two aspects of coping will vary from child to child and the nature of the triggering events they are likely to face.

The Continuous Reinforcement of Successful Mood Repair

The ongoing reinforcement of successful and adaptive mood repair ensures that the child does not forget the emotion regulatory responses that enabled him to overcome depression. But because the young patient is no longer depressed, there may be relatively few instances of sadness and dysphoria that call for regulation. However, states of euthymia mirror good emotion regulation, which then provides the therapist with the opportunity to address the topic.

During the earlier phases of CERT, the therapist and coaching parent were the primary reinforcers of the child's adaptive responses to dysphoria. A major goal during coping skills training is to broaden the basis of reinforcement by putting in place a system, acceptable to the given family, to reinforce the offspring's freedom from dysphoria or adaptive regulatory attempts. Thus, reinforcing a child's sensible mood-related behavior becomes a family affair.

Consequently, throughout coping skills training, the therapist needs to monitor the young patient's emotional well-being and be attentive to instances when the child displays adaptive emotion regulation as well as instances of euthymia.

To accomplish these goals, coping skills training sessions (just like all prior CERT sessions) need to have an agenda. The agenda should include a progress report of the young patient's emotional well-being since last seen, including instances of euthymia as well as dysphoric mood, and the ways in which dysphoric experiences were managed.

The most common "emotional report card" during coping skills training is one indicating that the child has been doing well and that there were no instances of dysphoria or sadness worthy of report. The second most common report card is that there have been a few instances of dysphoria in response to some trigger events, most of which the child handled reasonably well. The least likely emotional report card is one indicating that the child's regulatory responses to dysphoria were solely or mostly dysfunctional.

If the child has maintained her emotional equilibrium, or was able to adaptively regulate experiences of dysphoria, the therapist should offer extensive praise and reaffirm the importance of these accomplishments. The therapist also may discuss how parents can positively reinforce competent emotion regulation of the offspring using tools such as praise, recall of past achievements, or traditional behavior modification techniques (e.g., objective or symbolic rewards).

Importantly, after positively praising an example of emotional equilibrium or adaptive emotion regulation, the therapist needs to explore how the *family* can remain mindful of the importance of these processes in daily life and ways in which they can maintain the reinforcement of the offspring's adaptive mood repair responses. The narrative examples in Chapter 10 illustrate how the therapist uses the family's progress report to model *in vivo* the reinforcement of the young patient's competent mood repair and to plan a reinforcement system that the family can maintain.

If the progress report indicates one or more instances of problematic mood repair, those events need to be explored and contextually mapped, if warranted. If the information suggests a poorly executed regulatory response, the steps used to master it originally will have to be repeated (see Chapter 7). Concomitantly, it is important for the therapist to communicate to the parent–child pair that the child's problematic mood repair experience does not signal a failure or relapse into depression but is a temporary "reset" on the road to staying depression-free. In Chapter 10, I provide examples of how to implement such features of coping skills training.

The Personalized Training Plan

Building on the family's CERT achievements, the personalized training plan specifies the emotion regulation coping and problem-solving coping goals that are appropriate and achievable for the given patient. The training plan also is shaped by and includes content derived from the therapist's case formulation, which can be expected to impact coping success, including the young patient's depression history, mood repair–related vulnerabilities, and family context. Vulnerabilities that may negatively impact regulatory responses include personality traits (e.g., extreme shyness), comorbid conditions (e.g., a diagnosis of attention-deficit disorder), or hypersensitivity to specific depressogenic events (e.g., interpersonal loss). Family context may involve the (in)ability of parents to function as coaches.

The personalized training plan involves an overview of the family's CERT accomplishments that the therapist conducts with the parent–child pair, along with issues raised by the child's depression history, which sets the stage for the specific training goals. Then the team can turn to implementing emotion regulation coping training goals and/or problem-solving coping training goals.

Overview of CERT Achievements and Related Issues

The therapist prepares herself for this aspect of coping skills training by reviewing her own records and case formulation and specifying the content to be covered about the following topics:

- The child's and the family's key CERT achievements, with an emphasis on regulatory responses that "worked"
- The context of the child's depression
- The child's vulnerabilities relevant to emotion regulation
- Stressors and trigger events to which the child may be sensitive

As part of this overview, the therapist also generates a tentative list of training goals specific to the given young patient. Components of the overview and the training goals have to be finalized via discussions with the parent–child pair. At that point, the therapist has the option of presenting her summary to the parent–child pair along with the emotion- and/or problem-solving coping goals she recommends and then seek their feedback. However, that approach may fail to engage younger patients. Therefore, we developed an approach that seeks to make the discussion of mood repair achievements and training goals more fun and more personally relevant. Specifically, the therapist *engages the parent–child pair in a dialogue of the family's CERT experience and potential future regulatory goals using the vehicle of guided discussions of select film clips.* As described further in Chapter 10, the therapist watches with the parent–child pair several film clips that display dysphoric emotions and ways to manage them (the clips are described in the sections "A Vehicle to Address . . . " and "The Film Clips' Key Features . . . " that follow). The therapist then poses a series of questions that invite the parent and child to reflect on the characters in the film clip and their circumstances, and how some features of the clip may resemble what the child and parent experienced and learned. To prepare for this component of CERT, the therapist must be familiar with the recommended film clips to answer the following questions:

What specific content do I want to address with this child and family and which clip is the best vehicle for that?

Which "discussion point," and in which video clips, can I connect with the content I want to cover?

Chapter 10 includes multiple examples of how the film clips can be used to probe the child and parent for information about their CERT experiences.

Emotion Regulation Coping Goals

Starting with the child's regulatory achievements in CERT, emotion regulation coping goals can include the following ways of strengthening her response repertoire: modifying an existing regulatory response, adding a new response within the young patient's preferred regulatory domain, introducing a response from a new regulatory domain, and focusing on a regulatory mechanism. Strengthening the young patient's mood repair response repertoire should help her to continue to manage the affective challenges of daily life in adaptive ways. Chapter 10 includes examples of implementation for various young patients.

Problem-Solving Coping Goals

Problem-solving coping goals include helping the parent–child pair to recognize salient stressors that are amenable to some solution and teach them proactive or reactive ways to intervene. As illustrated in Chapter 10, proactive responses are implemented prior to an anticipated stress or trigger event and can potentially prevent the event or the child's exposure to it while reactive responses are implemented after the onset (or completion) of the stressful event and can mitigate its impact on the child and/or reduce the likelihood of its recurrence.

A Vehicle to Address Overviews and Training Goals: Guided Discussion of Film Clips

The guided discussions of a family's CERT achievements (CERT overviews) and coping skills training goals have to be tied by the therapist to segments/clips from four animated films. These clips display depressed and unhappy protagonists and how they resolve their distress and were identified by a group of clinicians involved in the development of CERT. The clips are from the animated films *The Lion King, Beauty and the Beast, Babe,* and *Dumbo.* The segments' approximate locations on a disc, videotape, or DVD are noted below and should be pre-cued before use.

Each film clip illustrates a story sequence involving: (1) a particular context that gave rise to stress; (2) which, in turn, elicited sadness, depression, or distress in the protagonist; (3) which appears to overwhelm the protagonist but; (4) is then resolved by recourse to adaptive mood repair responses.

After viewing the selected clip together with the young patient and parent, the therapist engages them in a dialogue about relevant aspects of the clips' content, including the relationship of stress, depression, and coping; the importance of sadness regulation; the context of the protagonist's depression; the responses that facilitated recovery from it; and the rooms in The House of ER that reflected the protagonist's regulatory responses. Importantly, the therapist poses questions, which challenge the parent–child pair to identify commonalities between the clip's contents and the family's experience with depression and its regulation, while calling attention to responses that worked for the young patient. Other questions direct attention to a regulatory response enacted by a protagonist that the therapist has tentatively identified as a training goal or explicate the connection between what the child learned in CERT and a proposed training goal.

The guided discussions can also make explicit concepts and processes that were implicit during the earlier phases of CERT. For example, recall that throughout CERT, the therapist either named the emotion to be regulated or guided the patient to its proper identification (e.g., selecting the appropriate facial emotion expression from a poster). However, a child's behavior during treatment may have indicated that emotion naming should be one of the topics in the guided discussion.

To help the therapist *align* the contents of a film clip with the topics to be covered for a given young patient, the sections that follow provide information about the range of topics that can be addressed and identify some features that may influence the therapist's decisions about which clip to use for a given child. Along with a description of each film clip, a list of "discussion points" and a series of prototypical questions are also provided. Chapter 10 includes several examples of how the clips serve to implement coping skills training with young patients and their parents.

General Topics That Can Be Addressed via the Film Clips

The clips from *The Lion King, Beauty and the Beast, Babe,* and *Dumbo* each depict an affect episode that poses a challenge to the depressed protagonist, illustrate responses from the four emotion regulatory domains, and portray the consequences of the regulatory responses that were implemented by the protagonist.

The list offered here includes a range of topics that the therapist can address with the parent–child pair after having viewed the clips; the list is not exhaustive and the therapist may identify additional areas that can be discussed:

- Causes or triggers of sadness, dysphoria, distress
- Context of depression
- Symptoms of depression
- Sad feelings versus clinical depression
- The relationship of stress to coping, sadness, and depression
- How failure to regulate sad emotions can lead to depression
- Emotion naming, emotion identification
- Examples of affect regulatory responses in the three regulatory domains
- Multiple forms of a given regulatory response
- The variety of adaptive mood repair responses and their consequences
- The variety of maladaptive mood repair responses and their consequences
- The role of a coach in emotion regulation
- The role of peers in interpersonal/social emotion regulation
- The relationship between the portrayed regulatory responses and The House of ER
- Contextual mapping (antecedents, consequences) of a symptom or complaint
- Clues to the emotional state of another being and their importance
- Problem solving versus emotion regulation in response to dysphoria

Decide Which Clips to Use

Almost all the topics just listed can be addressed with any of the four film clips. But therapists typically use no more than two clips to jumpstart the discussion about past CERT achievements and future goals. In deciding which clips to use with a given child, consider the areas to be addressed with that child and select the clip that best facilitates the discussion. Consider the child's age, cognitive sophistication, and personal depression experience. In general, *Dumbo* and *The Lion King* are the most suitable discussion vehicles for younger children because of the simplicity of the story lines and the singularity of the affect experiences. *Babe* is ideal as the backdrop to discuss severe depression, while *Beauty and the Beast* is very suitable to discuss how the failure to problem-solve *or* to adaptively self-regulate a strong emotion can have negative consequences.

Here are some specific examples of decision-making steps. Let us assume that the therapist wants to revisit emotion naming and its importance with a given child and parent. As the annotations to follow suggest, any of the four clips can be used to address that topic. However, the *Dumbo* and *The Lion King* clips are likely to be more appropriate for younger children because of the simplicity of the story line and the straightforward emotion being portrayed. On the other hand, the *Babe* and *Beauty and the Beast* clips may be more suitable to discuss emotion naming with older children because both the emotions and stories are more complex.

The clips illustrate a variety of mood repair responses, different ways of implementing them, and taking (or not taking) advantage of mood repair opportunities. For example, each clip portrays the protagonist engaging in social–interpersonal mood repair. If the therapist wants to underscore the importance of peers in interpersonal mood repair and the various forms that their interventions can take, then he may select *The Lion King* and *Dumbo* because those clips show multiple responses in that domain. The clips from *Babe* and *The Lion King* include scenes in which others seek to interrupt the protagonists' dysphoria by getting them to sing and dance. Those clips can be helpful with children whose interpersonal regulatory responding has been constrained to being physically soothed or hugged. The *Babe* clip also can help to discuss the consequences of a maladaptive behavioral regulatory response: Running away to the cemetery (rather than dealing with the presumed rejection) made Babe even more despondent and unhappy. While both *Babe* and *Beauty and the Beast* can serve to discuss how the failure to problem-solve or to engage in adaptive mood repair leads to depression, the latter may not be the most meaningful to younger children because of the complexity of the affect experience being portrayed and the content itself, which is a love story.

A young patient's depression history or presenting complaint also can point to some film clips as particularly appropriate. If the themes of loss and separation are salient for a given child, *The Lion King* and *Dumbo* are the best clips to view because they both portray protagonists who are exposed to such traumatic events and become depressed. If the therapist wishes to underscore the importance of external regulatory resources, the *Beauty and the Beast* clip is a good choice: The Beast is angry and upset and does not react to his friends who try to get him to settle down and act differently. This is an example of not taking advantage of social regulators to manage one's sadness at being rejected (which then has adverse consequences).

The therapist may decide to use a single film clip in several sessions, either to address a given topic repeatedly or to address different topics, or multiple clips in one session or in several sessions. Multiple clips may be particularly useful to cement a better understanding of some aspect of emotion experience or regulatory response. For example, all four clips portray social–interpersonal regulation of dysphoria but using different mechanisms; the four clips depict different causes of sadness; the *Dumbo* and *Beauty and the Beast* clips specifically deal with the role of cognition in depression and two clips (*Dumbo* and *Babe*) also illustrate the negative roles peers can play in the etiology of depression. Thus, the use of the film clips in coping skills training is limited only by the extent to which they mirror topics that are relevant to a given patient and the imagination of the therapist.

The Film Clips' Key Features and Associated Discussion Topics

The therapist should be fully familiar with each clip before attempting to use it and be prepared to answer questions about it. The discussion topics identified for each clip are not exhaustive; the therapist may identify further areas that are relevant to a given young patient. Accompanying the discussion topics, the text that follows includes prototypical probes that may help the therapist jumpstart the discussion (in italics), and commentary that may prompt responses by the parent–child pair (in brackets after the probes). Chapter 10 contains multiple examples of how a therapist can personalize the probes for a clip.

The Lion King

Emotion: Dysphoria, sadness, mourning, bereavement, loneliness

Scene: Begin at the beginning of Scene 12 (Timon and Pumba) and continue through Scene 13 ("Hakuna Matata") until after the song is finished.

Time: Approximately 5 minutes

Background: After just losing his father, Simba the lion cub lies in the desert with buzzards circling overhead. Timon (the meerkat) and Pumba (the warthog) befriend him. Timon comments that Simba looks "blue" and that "he's depressed." Trying to cheer him up, Timon and Pumba sing "Hakuna Matata." Despite his initial reluctance, Simba joins in and begins to feel better.

Discussion topics:

Identification of emotions:

How is Simba feeling?

How do Timon and Pumba know what Simba is feeling? [Note the sad face, head held down, the dragging legs and paws.]

Symptoms of depression:

Timon said that Simba is depressed. We talked about how being really *depressed means more than just feeling bad.*

What are some of the things Timon sees that make him think Simba is depressed? [Simba looks sad, doesn't seem to have energy, doesn't look like he's interested in anything.]

Causes or context of sadness/depression:

What happened to make Simba so sad and so depressed?

What are some things that make kids sad?

And some things that make them get depressed?

What are some things that make you sad?

Problem solving versus mood repair:

Simba is in a very sad situation. Is this a problem he can solve?

So, what happens?

Timon and Pumba try to help him to feel better. They know that they cannot solve Simba's problem of losing his father. But they can help Simba feel better. How *do they help?*

The House of ER; domains of emotion regulation:

Simba's friends are trying to cheer him up. What room is this in The House of ER? [The People (Social–Interpersonal) Room; see Poster 3 in Appendix B.]

What else are they doing? What does Simba do with his friends? [He starts to sing "Hakuna Matata" and dance with Timon and Pumba.]

In The House of ER, what room does that belong in? [The Things to Do (Behavioral or Action) Room.]

So, Simba comes to feel better because his friends help him and because they get him to do *things together with them. That shows how you can put together tools from two rooms in The House of ER.*

What helps you to get over feeling sad and miserable? What works best *for you?*

In what room of The House of ER does that [the response] belong?

Who helped you to feel better? Are there others [besides the person named] who could help if you feel sad?

Emotion regulation mechanisms:

How did Simba feel in the beginning? And how did he feel at the end? [Timon and Pumba helped Simba to feel better by talking to him, and by singing and dancing.]

And it looks like they were also *having* fun. *So, doing fun stuff can help so that feeling miserable does not take over. What are some fun things that kids can do to feel better?*

Do you think any of them [the just cited responses] would help you?

Beauty and the Beast

Emotion: Rejection, upset, anger

Scene: Begin near the end of Scene 8 (Gaston) where the Beast is by the fireplace and continue through Scene 9 (Invitation to Dinner) until the Beast leaves Belle's doorway.

Time: Approximately 2½ minutes

Background: The Beast has a terrible temper and knows that others think he is ugly. He desperately wants to win Belle's love but is discouraged because he believes that Belle will never see past his ugliness. The Beast's friends, Mrs. Potts, Lumière (the candlestick), and Cogsworth (the clock), try to encourage the Beast to behave like a gentleman and emphasize the need for him to control his temper. Although things do not go smoothly at first, at the end of the movie, the Beast's physical size helps him save Belle from wolves, and Belle also comes to see his inner kindness, which makes her come to love him.

Discussion Topics:

Identification of emotions:

How did the Beast feel in the beginning?

He seemed upset and cranky—how could his friends tell he was cranky? **[Pacing, shouting, angry or annoyed facial expression.]**

How did he feel at the end? He seemed angry—how can you tell?

Was there a feeling before that? **[Establish that the Beast probably felt rejected and unhappy because Belle turned him down.]**

The Beast was upset that Belle did not like him. What *feeling goes with that? How is that different from being angry?*

Causes or context of sadness/upset:

Let's look at what happened here. How did the Beast end up being so angry? **[The Beast wants Belle to fall in love with him, but doesn't think that Belle will ever like him, so he asks her to dinner, already upset and expecting to be turned down.]**

Also, he was pacing back and forth in front of the fireplace. Do you think that put him in a good mood or bad mood?

What else was going on? **[The Beast was talking to his friends who sought to help him to regulate his mood and to approach Belle in a more positive way.]**

How do you think things would've turned out if the Beast had listened to his friends?

The House of ER; domains of emotion regulation:

Let's go back again to the start. So, the Beast wants to spend time with Belle, but she turns him down at first.

How does he feel at first? **[Rejected, unloved, upset.]**

But right away—another feeling comes—what feeling is that? **[Anger.]**

That is because he thinks *that everyone is against him, right?*

So, when some kids feel sad and down, they may think that there is nothing they can do or that everyone is against them, which leads to an opposite feeling, anger, *which makes them* act *in angry ways.*

Does that help them to feel better? [No, it actually makes the feeling worse.]

His friends were there to help; they were trying to take care of the Beast. That means the Beast had the chance to use tools from which *room in The House of ER?* [The People (Social–Interpersonal) Room; see Poster 3 in Appendix B.]

So, when the Beast's friends get him to think differently about things, does he feel better? [Yes.]

How does that work? And where does that belong in The House of ER? [The Thinking (Cognitive) Room.]

Did you use tools from The Thinking Room to get over your depression? What *tools worked for you?*

So, this film is another example of how tools can work together from two rooms in The House of ER.

Babe

Emotion: Dysphoria, sadness, hopelessness, exclusion

Scene: Begin in the middle of Scene 12 (Beware of Bad Cat) when Babe's "mother" (the dog) leaves the room and continue through Scene 13 (If I Had Words) until the Boss stops dancing and Babe goes and eats.

Time: Approximately 8 minutes

Background: Babe is a little pig who gets "adopted" by Boss, Farmer Hoggett, who takes him home and puts him among the other animals. Fly and Rex (who are dogs) become his foster mother and father, respectively. Babe comes to believe that he is special and does not realize that he is a pig. So, Duchess (the cat, who is mean) tells Babe that Farmer Hoggett wants Babe only to eat him. Babe becomes upset and depressed, he runs away, ends up in the cemetery, and lies down among the graves. When Farmer Hoggett, Fly, and Rex (the foster father) find Babe, he is severely depressed, does not want to live, is anhedonic, and has no appetite. Farmer Hoggett has to find a way to keep Babe from dying, which he does!

Discussion Topics:

Identification of emotions:

Before he ran away, how was Babe feeling? How can you tell that he was feeling sad and miserable? [Note the nonverbal communication, speech tone, downcast eyes.]

Symptoms of depression:

How can you tell that his depression was more *than just feeling sad?* [Hopelessness, wanting to die, psychomotor retardation, anhedonia, lack of appetite.]

Causes or context of sadness/depression:

What made Babe so miserable? What made him think that Farmer Hoggett didn't love him? [The "stress" was a set of lies made up by the cat.]

Can this happen to kids also? That something which really makes them feel bad may not *be true?*

Problem solving versus emotion regulation coping:

Let's think about what happened here. Babe had a very bad thing done to him—one big stress. *He is told that Boss wants to get rid of him.*

Is that a problem he could have tried to solve? Was there anything that Babe could have done to solve the problem before *he started to feel so sad? Did he try?* [Get more information; discuss the situation with Farmer Hoggett.]

So, Babe gets very *depressed.*

What could Babe have done so that his sad feelings didn't get out of hand? Which tool from which room in The House of ER might have helped him?

The House of ER; domains of emotion regulation:

What helped Babe feel better? [Farmer Hoggett stayed with him, sang him a song, and did a dance.]

So, Farmer Hoggett helped and took care of Babe. In what room in The House of ER does that response belong? [The People (Social–Interpersonal) Room; see Poster 3 in Appendix B.]

How *did Farmer Hoggett help Babe to get over his sadness?* [Singing and dancing]

So, by doing *things, the farmer helped Babe.*

The Farmer helped Babe, and your mom [or dad] helped you when you felt sad.

Do you remember one thing Mom [Dad] helped you with as your coach?

What are some other things people can do to help a kid manage feeling sad?

Would these other things also work for you*?*

Dumbo

Emotion: Sadness, friendlessness, being teased, shame and guilt

Scene: Start at the beginning of Scene 7 (Mrs. Jumbo in Solitary Confinement) and continue through the beginning of Scene 8 (Dumbo Meets a New Friend)

until the mouse says "Dumbo the Great" and he and Dumbo walk out (with the clowns talking in the tent).

Time: Approximately 5½ minutes

Background: After going on a rampage against Dumbo's tormentors, Dumbo's mother has been locked away. The other elephants blame Dumbo and humiliate him. Dumbo feels miserable, he misses his mother, and believes that he is all alone. But he has a friend in Tim (the mouse). Dumbo is able to overcome his own anxieties and enters into a friendship with Tim.

Discussion Topics:

Identification of emotions:

What is Dumbo feeling at the beginning of the clip?

How can you tell he is feeling sad? [Tears, drooping ears, downward glances.]

Causes or context of sadness/depression:

What did the other elephants do to make Dumbo feel sad? [Made fun of him; tormented him. He was not in the in-group.]

Are these things that also can make kids feel sad?

Was there a time when kids made fun of you? Has that happened to other kids you know?

What about not having friends? Can that be a reason for feeling sad and miserable?

Stress and depression; problem solving versus emotion regulation coping:

We saw that Dumbo has had more than one tough thing or stress happen in his life, which makes him sad and depressed. What were those things? [He is being tormented or bullied; his mom is locked up; he is thus separated from his mom and isolated; at the beginning of the story, he does not have friends.]

What are the most serious problems? [The grown elephants make fun of him and his mother being locked away.]

It's hard for Dumbo to do something about these two big problems—right?

And why is that? [He is just a baby elephant. He has no control over the other elephants or friends to help him figure out what to do.]

What is one thing Dumbo is doing that will help him? [He is making friends with Tim.]

Can you think of ways in which friends can help a kid with problems in school/or with other kids?

When kids help you to feel better, what room is that in The House of ER?

The House of ER; domains of emotion regulation:

Tim also helped Dumbo to think about things differently.

Do you remember that Dumbo felt terrible about his ears?

But what did Tim say about them? **[Although the other elephants thought Dumbo's ears were silly, Tim thought that his ears were pretty cool!]**

So, when Dumbo thought that his ears were big and stupid, he felt pretty miserable.

But, when he thought his ears are "cool," did he feel better?

So, let's see: He feels bad, but then changes his mind about his ears and feels better! (Looking at The House of ER poster)

When he changed his ideas, where does that belong here? **[The Thinking (Cognitive) Room; see Poster 3 in Appendix B.]**

And how did this change come about? It was his friend who helped him—right?

So, that's an example of feeling better because he used which room *in The House of ER?* **[The People (Social–Interpersonal) Room.]**

This is a good example of how things work together from which two rooms *in The House of ER?* **[The Thinking Room and The People Room.]**

Can you come up with another example of using your thinking to stop feeling sad?

At the end of the film, do you know what happens with those ears that all the other elephants made fun of? Dumbo learns to fly with them and becomes the star of the circus!

Challenges

The personalized training plan, noted in the beginning of this chapter, is at the heart of coping skills training. And as the case examples in Chapter 10 illustrate, homework assignments are the core components of training plans. Thus, it may not be a surprise that noncompliance is the single biggest challenge during coping skills training. Clinical experience suggests that compliance with treatment recommendations invariably declines as the young patient's mood and functioning improve. Once the youngster is less depressed, both the parent and child may be less motivated to undertake and complete homework assignments or continue with treatment. At some point, it may be useful for the therapist to acknowledge that people are generally less motivated to do "extra work" when the child is feeling better and underscore that this phase of CERT therefore is challenging.

Noncompliance during coping skills training can involve partial completion or total noncompletion of the assigned homework. The therapist needs to explore the context of noncompliance because the alleged reasons for it could point to problems that can be remedied.

The following section lists three reasons families commonly provide for noncompliance and how the therapist may respond. Homework noncompliance is also briefly discussed in Chapter 3.

Reason 1: Homework was going to take too much time; it was inconvenient; it interfered with the family's activities.

Response: Acknowledge the burden of homework or task assignments. Probe to establish more precisely if noncompliance was due to the time it would have taken to complete the assignment, its complexity, or its lack of overt fit with the child's daily life. Break down the assignment into subcomponents. Once a parameter has been identified that likely made the task burdensome (e.g., its length or its multiple parts), changing that parameter may help to assure task completion.

Reason 2: Parent and child forgot the homework.

Response: Acknowledge that it is easy to "forget" the assigned tasks, especially given the lengthy time intervals between treatment sessions. Identify strategies that can help the pair to remember. Encourage the parent and child to generate possible solutions, such as putting a reminder into the parent's smartphone calendar and/or having the therapist send a reminder text to the young patient and parent.

Reason 3: It was unclear how the task was going to help since the child already is feeling better and no longer depressed.

Response: Acknowledge that the motivation to act requires a clear goal and that the tasks can indeed appear to be somewhat removed from [the child's] daily life. Use the sports analogy introduced at the start of CERT to remind the parent–child pair of the importance of practice. A player must practice even when it is out of season to remain fit in the future. So, doing [the task] is helping [child's name] to be prepared to handle his feelings in the future. It also may help to acknowledge that you (the therapist) may have not provided a sufficiently clear explanation of how the homework assignment was going to further the child's well-being.

Summary and Next Steps

The coping skills training phase of CERT focuses on prevention, which is not ordinarily a part of the psychotherapy of depression. Coping skills training is initiated when the young patient is no longer suffering from depressive symptoms. This can present a challenge because some families may find it difficult to motivate themselves to continue treatment when the young patient is feeling and doing well. But it is an important phase of CERT because it seeks to prepare the child and family to manage certain stressful events and difficulties that are likely to occur. Importantly, the training revolves around those stressful events or triggers that are known to be depressogenic for the given child. Being prepared for such events, and knowing what to do to decrease their impact, lowers the chances of the child becoming depressed.

This chapter reviewed the reasons for and components of coping skills training. It also introduced tools that have been found useful in presenting the goals of training to a young patient and parent(s). The next chapter addresses how to transition to this phase of CERT and provides examples of how to implement specific training goals for given young patients.

Chapter 10

Implementing Coping Skills Training and Ending Therapy

As the young patient becomes increasingly successful at mood repair and continues to recover from his depressive symptoms, the therapist can start to remind him and his parent(s) of the impending transition to Phase III of CERT. Important content to be communicated about Phase III includes that it will involve further tapering of the frequency of sessions, reviewing what has been learned, and a shift to future-oriented mood repair–related coping.

Chapter 9 highlighted several ways in which coping skills training differs from the prior phases of CERT. There are further differences. While the symptom-reduction phases of CERT are primarily reactive and the overall goal is to be palliative, coping skills training is mostly proactive and the overall goal is preventative. Also, the therapist engages in far more didactics and psychoeducation during coping skills training than in the earlier phases of CERT. The shift in emphasis and in the therapist's style can render coping skills training a challenge for some patients and parents.

Prepare the Family

Remind the parent–child pair of the impending change in the frequency of contacts and the focus of sessions several weeks before the anticipated transition. Decide whether multiple reminders are needed. Use the reminders to answer any questions about Phase III of CERT. The following prototype reminder for therapists (T) may be helpful:

T: Well, we've been making very good progress and [child] is feeling and doing much better—and you [parent] have been a great coach. So, we are ready to move into the next phase of CERT. We talked about this when you first started.

This phase will mean some changes. One change is the time between sessions. We will continue to meet once every 2 weeks a few times and then once a month, or once every 6 weeks several times—we can decide together how many times when we get to it.

Another change is that in this part of CERT, we will focus on *coping.*

Coping means, first of all, to keep doing things that you know have been helpful.

And, at the same time, to be prepared so that even when things get rough and even if [child] sometimes feels sad or unhappy, those feelings will *not* take over.

It's OK to feel sad and unhappy sometimes but we want to make sure that [child] won't become depressed again. This means that we will be talking a lot about the future. That is another difference.

The final big difference is that we will be talking about ways of dealing with sadness and depression although [child] is *not* depressed and has been doing great. But we want to prevent [child] from getting depressed in the *future,* which takes some work.

Introduce Coping Skills Training

Introducing coping skills training to the parent–child pair serves as the transition to Phase III of CERT. The introduction should be initiated the first time a session is devoted mostly or entirely to coping and can be delivered in one or multiple sessions. Depending on the given child's training plan, the therapist can decide on the extent to which she elaborates on the various themes and may elect to defer some details until a particular theme is handled later on.

The introduction should address the following:

- Definition of stress and coping
- Goals of coping skills training
- Emotion regulation coping versus problem-solving coping
- The child's training plan
- Expectations of task completion and compliance

Here is a prototype narrative that can be used and altered as needed:

T: (*To parent/child*) Let me tell you more about this last part of treatment. If you remember, when we first met, we talked about how stress can get children (and parents) feeling down, blue, or cranky, and when those feelings take over, they can lead to being depressed—which is more than just being sad.

Stress is when things get to be too much to handle. Stress can be one big thing or many little things that add up, or a process that goes on for a while.

Coping is being able to manage things so that even if there is stress, and [child] feels sad or upset, those feelings do *not* take over.

This part of CERT is called coping skills training. Basically, we will be talking about what you [child] and the family can do to make sure [child] continues to feel OK—like he is now.

What we did together for the past few months is one way to cope—we paid attention to feelings and tried to manage them so that they don't take over.

Another way to cope is to try to solve the problem that caused the upset in the first place, if that is possible. We will also talk about this.

So, how will we do this?

First, we'll try to make sure that [child] keeps doing what we know worked for him. That means we'll continue to pay attention to how [child] handles his feelings day to day.

At the same time, we will review key things you and [child] learned since we have been working together *and* talk about goals for the future to be sure that [child] will continue to handle any sad and upset feelings. For example, one goal will be to prepare for stresses that may come up.

We will watch some film clips together that show how sad and upsetting feelings come about and what can be done about them, and we will use these clips to review what both of you learned about being sad and depressed and how to get better.

Just like before, we will have homework—the homework will help you [child] to try out in real life some of the things we will be talking about—like a new way to manage a feeling or a way to solve problems.

(*To child*) With Mom [Dad] being your coach, I will count on you to do homework. Also like before, I will make sure that you understand the homework and can see why it is important.

At this point, the therapist may turn to the need for the ongoing reinforcement of adaptive mood repair, addressed in the "The Continuous Reinforcement of Successful Mood Repair" section of Chapter 9 and in the discussion that follows. Alternatively, she may continue to elaborate on problem-solving coping versus emotion regulation coping. Here is one example of how the therapist can proceed by elaborating on the two categories of coping:

T: So, let's talk about stress. What are some stresses for children? [Have parent and child generate items. Conclude by summarizing.]

Yes, stress can be things at school, like having many tests, or a new and tough teacher. It could be children teasing, or parents, siblings having fights and arguments, or your friends moving away, or people getting sick in the family.

So, when you have a stress or problem that makes you feel sad or unhappy or miserable, you can *cope* in two ways:

. . . by trying to manage your feelings.
. . . by trying to solve the problem.

For example, let's say you [mother] have another child about to start school and you need extra money for clothes. But you start worrying that the money you have coming in every month may not be enough.

At that point, you could try *to feel better* by telling yourself not to worry or by talking about the situation with friends, or praying, so these are ways to regulate emotions or ways to feel better. In The House of ER, these approaches are in The People Room and The Thinking Room, right?

Or, you could try to *fix the problem*. For example, you could try to plan your budget differently, or try to get a temporary part-time job, or you could ask your parents to help out, or you could see if there are clothes other children in the extended family have outgrown that may work.

So far, we have worked mostly on how to handle feelings. We worked on how to feel less sad and upset.

But sometimes, what gets us sad and upset is a problem that can be solved.

The poster here (*pointing to the WWW.Solve poster*) shows some steps that can help to solve a problem—the phrase "WWW.Solve" is just a way to remember what questions you want to ask yourself when you try to solve a problem. So,

. . . the first *W* stands for *what* is the problem.
. . . the second *W* stands for *who* can help to solve the problem.
. . . the third *W* stands for *ways* to solve the problem!

After you put together the answers to the three *W*'s, you will have a plan for what to do to solve the problem or the steps you can take to find a solution to the problem; WWW.Solve is a *way* to remember what to do when you face a problem.

If problem-solving coping is not a primary goal for the given patient, the therapist can conclude by noting that there will be a further discussion of this topic at some future time. But if problem-solving coping is a training goal for the patient in question, then the therapist may elect to continue further. As illustrated by Davey's case in the section "Problem-Solving Coping" near the end of this chapter, the most meaningful way to discuss this topic is to identify a stressful event from the young patient's history that would have lent itself to problem solving.

Continue to Reinforce Adaptive Mood Repair

Adaptive mood repair should be self-reinforcing. In other words, the child eventually should engage in adaptive ways of responding to dysphoria because the outcome is desirable. However, for most young patients, maintaining a consistent pattern of adaptive emotion regulation requires the utilization of new skills and extra mental or behavioral effort, which can be bolstered by the provision of external reinforcement.

The progress report by the parent of the child's well-being since the last contact is likely to provide examples of the child's mood repair attempts. If the young patient maintained an essentially euthymic affective state (was mostly on an even keel emotionally), that can be interpreted as mirroring good self-regulatory skills. Such reports create the opportunity to continue to reward the child's emotion regulatory competence as part of the family's daily life via an agreed on reinforcement system.

As responding becomes self-reinforcing, expect a gradually decreasing use of the external reinforcement system, and that is acceptable! The important point is that the therapist has reemphasized the centrality of mood repair, the family has learned what reinforcement is and how to use it, and consequently, the external reinforcement system can be reactivated by the family as needed.

If the progress report reveals one or more instances of failure to regulate sadness and dysphoria, review the context, the child's response, and decide if remediation is warranted. Correcting the misapplication (or nonapplication) of a previously mastered regulatory response may temporarily interrupt the flow of a young patient's coping skills training, but it is a minor hurdle and to be expected in some recovering patients.

Following are some examples of how the therapist may respond if the progress report reveals no interim evidence of dysphoria, or just a few versus multiple examples of poorly regulated episodes of sadness. The first example is one possible approach after the parent reports that she did not recall any instances of the child experiencing distress or dysphoria since he was last seen:

> T: So, let me summarize what has been going on. Over the past few weeks, [child] has been doing well—and when it comes to emotions—he has been like other kids. There have been no problems with him being sad or upset.

That is wonderful!

And you and [child] really worked very hard to get here. You made a *great* team.

Being emotionally on an even keel is a big achievement. So, do you think we could set up a system, some way to remind [child] and the family about how well [child] is doing?

For example, what do you think about a "brownie points" system—where [child] could earn a certain number of points at the end of the day if his feelings stayed on the even side?

Feeling sad or upset would also be OK as long as [child] was in control. We can decide how many brownie points that would be worth.

Or, can you think of other ways to reward [child] for being on an even keel *and* for using his tools from The House of ER well?

If a brownie points–based paradigm is acceptable to the parent–child pair, the therapist can continue to help devise a reinforcement system. For example, evidence of euthymia or adaptive regulatory response deployment both are worthy of brownie points, which could be awarded by parent–child agreement at the end of the day. The therapist also can help negotiate the reward amount between parent and child. Part of the negotiation should involve the eventual value of brownie points (or other rewards) to be traded in for tangible or intangible items of value to the young patient (e.g., desired athletic wear, a particular privilege).

If the parent–child pair appears reluctant to commit to a daily reinforcement system, the therapist can offer other temporal frames (e.g., weekend reviews). Regardless of the type of reinforcement, the therapist's responsibility is to help devise a system with well-defined component pieces, simple rules for implementation, and agreed on value exchange. The fundamental goal is to keep the child and parent mindful of the importance of successful mood repair and the fact that positive external reinforcement is one way to maintain a desired behavior.

Here is an example of how to respond to a progress report, which revealed both regulatory success and failure (the text pertaining to regulatory success is also applicable when only success has been reported):

T: Let me see if I got this right. A few times over the past few weeks, things happened at school that usually would make [child] be very upset or sad and a few times [child] got really upset— but it sounds like those displays did not last long.

I can see that this was upsetting to you [parent] as well. But, this can happen with any kid—that sometimes feeling sad and upset takes over—and we will talk more about that later.

But what's really important is that, while [child's] feelings got out of control a few times, the other times when [child] felt upset, [child] remembered what helped her before. And she used those tools and didn't fall into being sad. She did really well!

(*To child*) That was a great job, and I am really proud of you and I can tell that Mom feels the same way.

What can we do so that everyone in the family keeps track of how well [child] is doing? Because she is doing a terrific job using what she knows helps her to stay on top of sad feelings.

For example, what do you think about setting up a whiteboard for [child], and noting or putting a big star on it each time she handles feeling sad or upset well?

As in the previous example, the therapist should help devise a system for the family that is acceptable and doable. This includes negotiating both the timing and nature of the reinforcement. While the ideal timing is to reinforce a desirable behavior when it occurs, practical considerations (e.g., a parent's work schedule) may dictate otherwise. And while the examples provided so far included observable and tangible rewards with potential "exchange" values, verbal or symbolic reinforcement should also be considered.

The progress report may also reveal that when the child had faced a depressogenic trigger, she had not been successful at deploying the learned regulatory responses. The therapist needs to decatastrophize those experiences, emphasize their isolated nature, and call attention to the fact that much of the time, the child was in reasonably good emotional equilibrium. Consider feedback along the following lines:

T: I see that you [parent] are concerned because of this incident when [child] had a "meltdown" and [child] could not get her upset feeling under control.

Many kids find that there may be times when they are overwhelmed with how they feel, although they have been able to handle the same feeling before. And that is OK!

Think about it like this: It's been several weeks since I have last seen you—that's lots and lots of days—right? And this incident we are talking about happened only once (or twice) in all that time. So, that means that [child] was emotionally OK most of the time.

When emotion regulatory failure is of concern, it may be helpful to (1) focus on a reinforcement plan for the days when the young patient is generally euthymic (see the prior example) and (2) explore what led to regulatory failure, determine if remediation is warranted, and if so, implement a remediation plan. (See Chapter 7 for examples of handling problems in regulatory response implementation.)

It is important to remind the parent–child pair that the road to consistently adaptive mood regulation is like the road to recovery from depression: There are ups and downs. A few isolated instances of regulatory failure should be expected, and the family can be reassured that such events do not mean the child is relapsing into depression. As in the earlier phases of CERT, failure needs to be reframed as a new learning opportunity on the road to more effective mood repair responding.

Present the Personalized Training Plan to the Child and Parent

Table 10.1 presents an overview of key components of planning personalized coping skills training. More details about training plans, integrated with case formulations, can be found in Appendix C. In the remainder of this chapter, four young patients introduced earlier in this book—Mary, Davey, Chantel, and Pete—will serve to illustrate how to implement the components of coping skills training. Lisa and Mike, the remaining two young patients whom we first met in Chapters 6 and 7, respectively, appear briefly in this chapter in support of some features of coping skills training.

After the parent–child pair is introduced to coping skills training and the need to reinforce adaptive mood repair has been discussed (see the previous two sections of this chapter), it is time to explain the *personalized* portion of the training plan. Presenting the personalized training plan to the young patient and the parent(s) sets the stage for the remainder of CERT and serves to frame expectations. The presentation can include all the components of the plan, as shown in Table 10.1 and illustrated by the case of Mary and her grandmother here. Alternatively, the therapist may focus the presentation initially only on the part of the training plan that will be the target in the current or next session, as illustrated by the case of Davey and his father; the remaining parts of the training plan can be addressed in subsequent sessions.

As described in Chapter 9, *the personalized training plan is a set of child-specific targets related to mood regulation: It reflects the therapist's clinical judgment as to what actions are most likely to support the child's ability to maintain consistently adaptive mood repair and thereby remain free of clinical depression.* As can be seen in Table 10.1, the training plan builds on what the young patient has already learned in CERT and the mood regulatory responses that have been shown to work for him. The plan therefore includes existing regulatory competencies that can be broadened or further developed and new directions in mood repair responding based on the therapist's clinical judgment and case formulation. In deciding on a young patient's training plan, be sure that the goals are limited in number, reasonable in scope, and achievable within the time frame under consideration.

To illustrate how the personalized aspect of coping skills training can be **presented,** we return to Mary, the 8-year-old patient, and her grandmother (see Chapter 6).

TABLE 10.1. Planning Personalized Coping Skills Training: An Overview of Key Components

- Identify the child's mood repair strengths (and vulnerabilities) and preferred adaptive regulatory responses (as manifested during CERT, per film-clip–based discussions).
- Consider the resultant information in light of the child's personal characteristics, family and social contexts, and overall resources. Based on these considerations, decide which **emotion regulation coping goal or goals** are indicated and the specific ways in which the goals will be implemented for the given child. The goals include the following:
  - Strengthen a preferred emotion regulatory domain (expand the scope or alter the form of responses already used, encourage the deployment of additional responses in the domain).
  - Venture into a new emotion regulatory domain (introduce and reinforce responses from a hitherto mostly underutilized or unexplored but relevant mood repair domain).
  - Explore emotion regulatory response mechanisms (learn about attention refocusing and instigating positive affect as the mechanisms in a variety of regulatory responses and how this knowledge can help to identify new ways to repair dysphoric mood).
- Identify the depressogenic, stressful events that were implicated in the child's depression (based on history, as manifested during CERT, per film-clip-based discussions).
- Consider the nature of the stressful events and the likelihood of their recurrence, along with the child's mood repair strengths (and vulnerabilities), personal characteristics, family and social contexts, and overall resources. Based on this information, decide if **problem-solving coping goals** are indicated: If so, identify which problem-solving goal corresponds best to the identified stressor and the specific ways in which the goal will be implemented. The goals include the following:
  - Ways to prevent, avoid, or defuse a specific stressor or proactive coping
  - Ways to mitigate the impact of a specific stressor and address it's causal features or reactive coping.

Note. The scope of coping skills training will vary from child to child. See Appendix C for case narratives that include specific training goals for the depicted young patients and that shed light on the considerations shaping the therapists' decisions about those goals.

Mary

In the dialogue between Mary and her grandmother that follows, the therapist enumerates all the training goals in her presentation. Also note that this young patient's training plan closely mirrors her achievements in CERT. It focuses on the use of interpersonal regulators, modestly expanding that domain by encouraging the child to enlist nonfamilial adults and peers as regulators. Further goals include helping Mary and her grandmother to become aware that interpersonal trust is a major issue for Mary, which renders certain events particularly stressful for her, and how such events may be best handled.

T: I wanted to talk about what we will be doing from now on and see what you think about it.

As I mentioned before, we will be focusing on coping—which means managing stresses—but we first want to be sure that Mary continues doing the things that worked for her and kept her free of depression.

One important thing that we will be doing is to look at what Mary and you [grandmother] can do to make Mary even better at being on top of sad and upsetting feelings when they come up. This will mean some changes in the things that have worked for her and also new ways of reacting to being sad that she can try.

And we will also talk about what makes some things especially stressful for Mary and how to deal with them.

We will start with watching some short film clips that show different feelings and ways to manage them. And then we will use these film clips to help Mary and you [grandmother] review what you learned about feelings and what works for Mary so that her sad or upset feelings don't get out of control.

So, going back to what works for Mary, we already know that the tools in The People Room in The House of ER really help her. And, of course, you and your sister have been the major people who worked with her on this.

We will then talk about how people other than the family can help when Mary feels bad and also about the different ways in which others can help a kid feel better.

Let's keep in mind that Mary also started to try some other things—other ways to handle sad feelings. She tried jumping rope, which also worked so that feeling sad did not take over. We will figure out a plan for her to try similar things.

One other thing—we talked about how hard it was for Mary that Mom was in and out of the picture. Because of this, it is hard for her to trust new people or feel comfortable around them, and this has been an issue with new teachers. Meeting new people can be a big stress for Mary. So, we will work on how Mary, with your help, can prepare for meeting new people, like teachers in school and feel OK about it.

The film clips will help us talk about feelings and the different things that can be done to make sure Mary stays free of depression. We will start with a film clip right now and see what you think—OK?

As just illustrated, the first component of Mary's personalized training is to use the film clips to engage her and her grandmother in a dialogue about their CERT experiences and prepare them for Mary's specific emotion regulation coping training goals (see the section "Review CERT Achievements, Issues . . ." below).

Having identified the training goals, the therapist then proceeds to address the first goal, which is to help Mary to strengthen the interpersonal domain of mood repair (see the section "Implement Personalized Training Goals," below).

Davey

Ten-year-old Davey's therapist chose a different approach to introduce the training plan for his young patient because it featured problem-solving coping as a prominent training goal. The importance of problem-solving coping for Davey reflects the fact that his depression was instigated by a specific stressor (school-based bullying), which is likely to recur and could be amenable to problem-solving interventions. Therefore, after having introduced coping skills training to Davey and his father, the therapist immediately segues into working on problem-solving coping (as per the bottom section of Table 10.1) and leaves for a later session the presentation of other training goals. The introduction goes along the following lines:

> T: At this point, I wanted to talk about what we will be doing for the next few months.
>
> As I already mentioned, we call this last phase of therapy *coping skills training*—this means that we want to make sure Davey continues doing all the things that helped him so far *and* will also try new ways of doing things that can help with stress or upsetting feelings in the future.
>
> We could start by going over the things both of you learned in CERT and then talk about new things that he and you can try out, but I think we should start in a different way.
>
> I would like us to focus on problem solving as a way to deal with stressful events that can cause sad and upset feelings. We just started to talk about that.
>
> I think that problem solving is important here because a major issue for Davey's depression is the bullying at school—it is a very negative and repeated stressor.
>
> We can think of bullying as a problem that should be solved or prevented before it actually starts. So, in the next few sessions, I would like us to work on what we call problem-solving coping, which is how the bullying may be prevented or lessened. This is one part of Davey's training plan.
>
> There are a few other things that we can work on later, like how Davey can use or develop more tools from The House of ER or new ways to manage sad feelings so that they don't get the upper hand in the future.

After this presentation, which emphasized one part of Davey's personalized training plan, the therapist moved immediately to work on problem-solving coping, as illustrated in the implementation section later in this chapter. Note that it was only toward the end of the session that the therapist introduced the film clips and used them to support the discussion of problem-solving coping. Thus, Davey's case documents both the flexibility afforded to a therapist in how he introduces and starts to work on the personalized components of coping skills training and the manner in which the film clips can be used.

In summary, as the therapist transitions from presenting the training plan to implementing it, it may be easiest to start with the summary of CERT achievements via the film clips, then move to the mood repair–related components of the plan (maintaining, expanding, or introducing new regulatory responses), and end with the proactive coping segment (anticipating stressful events). However, as just noted, the flexibility afforded to the therapist in the presentation of the training plan also applies to the order in which the therapist may implement its various components. For example, both Mary's and Pete's therapists follow the previously noted sequence (as illustrated in the text that follows in this chapter). But Davey's therapist did not do so; he segued from the introduction of the plan into working on problem-solving coping, bypassing the overall summary of CERT-based achievements (to be addressed later). If a child has stressful events coming up, the therapist may likewise prioritize the proactive coping segment component of the training. Thus, the order in which components are addressed is left to the clinical judgment of the therapist.

Review CERT Achievements, Issues, and Resultant Training Goals Using Film Clips

This component of the personalized training plan is mostly a summary of what has transpired in the given child's treatment: It is the framework for setting the goals of that child's coping skills training. The central feature of the overview is the regulatory responses (and domain) that "worked" for the child, along with issues that can facilitate or hinder the child's mood repair competence and resultant goals for the rest of the treatment. The context of the child's depression also is acknowledged, including stressful events that may reoccur and/or personal vulnerabilities that can undermine mood repair.

Helping the young patient and parent to review the features and context of the child's depression and their CERT experience in overcoming it is one way to facilitate a conceptual integration of what they learned. Presenting coping skills training goals in the context of the child's CERT's achievements links past, present, and future mood repair functioning. Using film clips of characters who are facing emotional challenges, just like those the young patient has faced, helps to normalize the child's experiences. The multiple ways in which the film's protagonists finally cope with dysphoria provide the young patient with a panorama of regulatory responses as they are being implemented; by linking the protagonist's story and the young patient's story, the therapist can easily introduce mood repair–related goals.

As described in Chapter 9, the therapist prepares for this component of coping skills training by reviewing his case notes, specifying the topics and issues to be covered, and identifying the film clips that are most suited to address the given patient's CERT experiences and training goals. While it is best to view each film clip in its entirety, the therapist may focus the guided discussion on particular segments.

Mary

To illustrate how this phase of CERT is implemented, we return to Mary and her grandmother. According to the therapist's notes, the overview will highlight that social–interpersonal regulation was the domain favored by Mary for which her grandmother was an excellent coach; that Mary was learning about features of this regulatory domain, including the fact that interpersonal regulation can take various forms, such as hugging or verbal reassurance; and that the person experiencing sadness can initiate interpersonal regulatory responses. As a training goal, the therapist identified expanding this regulatory domain by introducing peers as regulatory agents, along with possibly adding another domain to enlarge Mary's response repertoire. Mary's clinical history revealed that actual or symbolic losses were important stressors for her. These connect to the issue of trust and thereby have implications for emotion regulation. This issue was to be addressed as part of proactive coping.

The therapist planned to use *The Lion King* and *Dumbo* clips as the vehicles to summarize Mary's and her grandmother's CERT experiences, introducing them along the following lines:

> T: As I just mentioned, we will now watch some film clips—these are from *The Lion King* and *Dumbo*. You may have seen these films; they show different emotions and ways to handle them.
>
> Let's start with *The Lion King*. I'd like you to pay special attention to what happened, what Simba is feeling, and how he handles his feelings. How does he get to feel better?
>
> Afterward, we will talk about this film clip and how Simba and Mary may have some things in common.

After the initial viewing of *The Lion King*, the therapist starts the discussion by posing questions about the identification of depression. This serves as the backdrop or context. Then the therapist steers the conversation toward the examples of social regulation displayed by Simba's friends and their impact on Simba.

This focus links to the fact that social–interpersonal regulation of dysphoria was Mary's preferred regulatory domain; the therapist wants to underscore that interpersonal regulation can be implemented by multiple actors and take a variety of forms. The therapist also enumerates the training goals that naturally follow from Mary's regulatory achievement.

Note in the following how the therapist's questions move from Simba's story to Mary's story, then back to Simba, and so forth, as she addresses two major topics, namely, the nature of depression and the domains of emotion regulation (those topics appear as bold and italicized headings). Note also how the therapist modifies the standardized statements and probes (presented in Chapter 9) to make them relevant to Mary and her grandmother. By structuring the discussion around specific topics and contents, the therapist bridges past achievements and upcoming goals, and prepares to work on specific training targets.

The therapist's probes and statements listed next are guideposts (in italics). Additional prompts to encourage responses from the parent–child pair appear in bold type in brackets. In the actual discussion, the therapist directs some of the probes to Mary and other probes to both her and her grandmother; there is an ongoing dialogue.

Symptoms and causes of depression:

Timon said that Simba is depressed. So, what are some things Timon sees which makes him think that Simba is depressed? **[Simba looks sad, doesn't seem to have energy, doesn't look like he's interested in anything.]**

What about when kids like you get depressed? How do you think people can tell?

What made Simba get depressed? Why does he feel so bad?

The House of ER; domains of emotion regulation:

How does Simba feel better?

What happens so that Simba's sadness does not *take over at the end?* **[Timon and Pumba try to cheer him up—they are his friends.]**

If a kid, like you, is sad, can other people help her to feel better?

In The House of ER (directing attention to poster), *in what room does that belong?*

Let's think back. When you were feeling really sad, what helped you *to feel better?*

In the time you have been coming here, who helped you to feel better? **[Grandma and Aunt.]**

How did Grandma [and aunt] help you to feel better?

Simba did not have a Grandma! Who helped him to feel better? [His friends.]

What does Simba do with his friends? [He starts to sing "Hakuna Matata" and dance with Timon and Pumba.]

In The House of ER, in what room does that belong? [The Things to Do (Behavioral or Action) Room.]

So, Simba gets over being depressed by using tools from two rooms in The House of ER: The People Room and The Things to Do Room.

We also saw in the film that doing fun things is another way to stop feeling miserable.

Tell me again. What were some things that helped you to feel better? [Got many hugs. Talked to Grandma and aunt.]

So, there are many ways in which other people can help you to feel better. What do you think about what Simba did with his friends?

When you feel sad, do you think what Simba did would work for you?

Like singing, listening to a song? How about watching a dance video? Maybe watching with friends? Which friend would be best? How could Grandma or your aunt help with that?

Let's make that one goal, one important thing we will do over the next few weeks.

In continuing the discussion of *The Lion King*, the therapist notes that cheering up Simba was a *group* effort. Therefore, what unfolds onscreen bears some similarities to Mary's Grandma and aunt (and the therapist) forming a "team" to help Mary. In further elaborating on the possible overlap of social and behavioral sadness regulation, the therapist then addresses the idea of behavioral emotion regulation as another training goal. Finally, she returns to the loss experience Simba suffered and notes that another topic to be discussed is that being afraid of losing people can make it hard to feel comfortable with and trust people. The therapist may then proceed to the second film clip, *Dumbo*, to underscore three topics: the role of friends as social regulators of sadness, the various ways in which they can help a child to feel better, and how a loss experience is one of the causes of depression. Alternatively, the therapist may decide to show *Dumbo* during the next treatment session to review the themes and issues that were discussed after *The Lion King*.

Pete

Pete will serve as another example of how to use the film clips to summarize a young patient's CERT experience and introduce mood repair–related training goals. Recall that 9-year-old Pete presented with severe depression and multiple stressors in the prior 12 months. Pete learned to control his dysphoria through regulatory responses that involved action, such as physical activity (jumping jacks), and by taking care of his baseball card collection. The therapist's notes indicated that these were major CERT accomplishments, but that Pete needed to have a wider regulatory landscape: The therapist thus elected to pursue the interpersonal realm because Pete had good relationships with his older brother and sister.

The therapist selected *The Lion King* and *Babe* for the focused discussion because they portray a range of social–interpersonal regulatory responses. The viewing starts with the *Babe* clip because it depicts a very severe form of depression. After having introduced the films (see the prior examples) and watched *Babe,* the therapist starts the dialogue by establishing the story's context: Babe developed severe depression in response to a stressor. The therapist then focuses the discussion on the behavioral mood repair responses portrayed because those attempts echo successful behavioral regulation of sadness by Pete and his mother during CERT. She calls attention to the fact that the behavioral regulatory responses in the film clip involved others, namely, a parent surrogate, and raises social–interpersonal mood repair as a training goal. Note that the therapist selects only those discussion points from among the ones suggested in Chapter 9 that she considered relevant and edits the recommended questions to make them suitable to Pete's case. The following themes were covered in the overview:

Stress and symptoms of depression:

Let's think about what happened here. Babe had a very bad thing happen in his life—one big stress*—he is told that Boss wants to get rid of him. So, he feels sad and miserable. He gets* very *depressed.*

How can you tell that Babe's depression was more *than just feeling sad?* [Hopelessness, wanting to die, no energy or being slowed down, anhedonia, lack of appetite.]

Do you remember when you first came here? How did your depression show?

How were your depression and Babe's depression similar?

Babe felt depressed because he had a big stress—he was told that the Farmer did not love him!

(To child and mother) *If you remember, Pete got depressed because he had not just one but a bunch of stresses like starting a new school and getting used to a new visiting schedule with Dad.*

So, Pete and Babe have something in common; they know what it feels like to become depressed. And they both found ways to get out of the depression.

The House of ER; domains of emotion regulation:

What helped Babe feel better? [Farmer Hoggett stayed with him, sang him a song, and did a dance.]

Yes, Farmer Hoggett really helped Babe. In what room [in The House of ER] does that belong? [The People (Social–Interpersonal) Room.]

How *did he get Babe to feel better?* [Singing/dancing.]

So, tell me again—what were all the things Farmer Hoggett did to help Babe? [Singing, dancing, trying to feed him.]

And where do you think that fits in The House of ER? Which room? [The Things to Do (Behavioral or Action) Room.]

Here, we have a way to deal with feeling sad that puts together tools from two rooms in The House of ER.

And what helped you *[Pete] to get over feeling depressed?* [Jumping jacks and taking care of the baseball card collection.]

You didn't just sit around, you did *things. You put in a lot of work. In which room in The House of ER do those "tools" go?* [The Things to Do Room.]

So, Farmer Hoggett helped Babe, and Mom helped you as your coach—right?

What do you think about having someone who is not *Mom help you to feel better?*

Who else in the family (besides Mom) could help you to do things so that when you feel sad, it does not take over? [My brother and sister.]

And what are some things you could do *with your brother and sister when something makes you feel sad and upset?* [Singing is one thing.]

What are some other things you could do? What about playing games? Solving picture puzzles? [Probe for other viable actions.]

So, one thing we can work on is what your sister and brother could do to help you feel better when you feel sad. This would give you more tools from two rooms in The House of ER.

Then the therapist may turn to *The Lion King* clip to underscore the variety of forms that the interpersonal or social regulation of sadness can take. Having previously introduced the idea of Pete's siblings as regulatory agents, the therapist can return to that theme after watching *The Lion King* and confirm it as a training goal. He can then continue to list the remaining elements of Pete's training plan; namely, how to anticipate stressors and the role of personal vulnerability in shaping one's response to stressful events (see later in this chapter).

The objection could be raised that interpersonal regulation of sadness is not a new regulatory domain for Pete because his mother's actions as the CERT coach exemplify the interpersonal regulation of dysphoria. The objection has some validity. However, the mother's role as coach was unique and had strong enforcement and accountability components that are not characteristics of the interpersonal regulation of sadness in daily life. Therefore, it seemed reasonable to separate her coaching role from her role as an interpersonal regulator, and also to consider social regulation as a new domain and training goal for Pete.

Implement Personalized Training Goals

As already noted, coping skills training addresses both emotion regulation and problem-solving goals and involves considerable psychoeducation and role playing. Emotion regulation coping goals include strengthening (enlarging, improving) an existing regulatory domain, introducing a new regulatory domain, or focusing on a regulatory mechanism. Problem-solving coping goals include learning how to plan and implement reactive or proactive strategies. The specific goals are personalized by reflecting the given young patient's needs. Implementation of specific training goals is now illustrated by two case examples.

Emotion Regulation Coping: Strengthen a Regulatory Domain

As noted throughout this book, each regulatory domain, or room in The House of ER, contains multiple responses or "tools." One of the most reasonable training goals is to strengthen a child's preferred regulatory domain by modifying and/or improving responses the youth already has mastered.

Mary

For 8-year-old Mary, strengthening a regulatory domain included expanding the scope of her social–interpersonal regulatory responses. More specifically, the therapist encouraged Mary to enlist regulators other than Grandma and her aunt, and also to continue to verbalize her affect while enlisting a social regulator. As the next dialogue unfolds with the child (C) and grandmother (G), note that the therapist responds immediately to some hesitancy on the part of grandmother to "buy into" the training goal:

T: OK, we agreed to work on some things that Mary could do so she has more ways to deal *with* being really sad and upset.

(*To child*) This will be something to try, with Grandma's help as coach over the next few weeks.

G: Sure, but she's been doing OK—we had no problems.

T: Yes, and that is great!

But I see that you have some concerns. So, let me explain what I mean because it's important that I'm totally clear about what I am proposing here.

Do you bake?

G: Sure.

T: So, let's say you want to bake a cake for dinner. You have the ingredients. But as you start putting everything together, all of a sudden, you realize that the yeast you have is not good anymore.

So, you could really be stuck. *But* if you have baking powder on hand, you could modify your recipe and still finish the cake by dinnertime. Right?

G: Yeah, I guess.

T: So, being ready to cope with feelings is like that. You want to have more than one way to feel better. It is just like you want to have not only the yeast, but also the baking powder on hand to finish the cake.

(*To child*) Mary, does that make sense—to have more than one way to be sure that feeling sad does not take over?

C: Yeah.

T: (*To child*) When you get sad, you go to Grandma or your aunt and they help you to feel better. Right? And how do they do that? How do they help?

C: Hugs and stuff, and we talk.

T: That's really good!

Now, here is a question. Are there other people who could maybe help Mary feel better when she feels sad?

G: Our minister. He is a good person.

T: Yes, that is a possibility. But how about someone nearer in age to Mary. Are there cousins or friends she is close to?

C: My cousin Helene—yeah.

T: And how old is she? Does she live close by?

G: She'd be about 12, and they live next door.

T: That sounds good. (*To child*) What are things you could do with Helene to make your sadness go away?

C: Dunno. Maybe we could do hair and makeup!

Given the agreement on the type of response, the therapist then engages Mary and her grandmother in role playing, with the goal of rehearsing how Mary can best verbalize what she is feeling and what she needs (e.g., "I feel bad. Could we play, like do hairs, so that I feel better?"). As illustrated in Chapter 7 in the sections on reinforcing a regulatory response, the therapist needs to go over the details of the homework, which should involve role-play sessions with Grandma, followed by how to enlist Helene and inform her of the plan, and specifically naming what Helene can do to help Mary.

A major way in which modifying an existing response (or adding a new response in that domain) during coping skills training differs from how it was handled in the earlier phases of CERT is the additional time devoted to psychoeducation. Picking up the dialogue between Mary, her grandmother, and the therapist, the following is one example of this approach:

T: Good—we now agree on the homework and why this is a good idea. But I would like to talk more about it to be sure we all agree on why this is important.

(*To grandmother*) We talked about how Mary is doing great—she is no longer depressed, and a lot of people would think that this subject is now all well and done.

But it is important to be ready to handle sad and upset feelings that will happen in the future. So, like we talked about it in the beginning, if you want to be a good player, you have to practice and you can't sit around and just wait until the next game, right?

(*To child*) Mary, do you know kids who play sports, a kid who is on a team?

C: Yeah, Trevor. He's on the football team.

T: So, does he practice even if there is no game, like next week or the week after?

C: Yeah.

T: Why do you think he and his teammates do that?

C: They gotta stay in shape.

T: Exactly! Just like you have to stay in shape to handle a game, you have to stay in shape to handle your feelings.

(*To child and grandmother*) So, the goal that we are working on is for Mary to have more than one way to stop sadness or upset from getting the upper hand after these sad feelings start.

(*To grandmother*) You and your sister have done a great job as coaches with helping Mary. But, let's say that you are at work and your sister is busy and something happens that makes Mary sad—this new homework will help Mary get practice with asking Helene, and later possibly other people like your minister, for help to feel better when she feels bad. So, does this make sense?

Davey

Another way to strengthen a regulatory domain is to introduce a new response in that domain. For Davey, this meant a new cognitive mood repair response. Recall that Davey had learned to successfully manage a recurring depressogenic situation by deploying a response that involved imagining his tormentors losing their pants and being exposed in their underwear, which was evidence that he was comfortable with cognitive processes. By introducing a new cognitive response, the therapist sought to enlarge Davey's regulatory options. The therapist presented this training goal to Davey and his parent (P) as follows:

T: (*To parent and child*) If you remember, one of the goals we talked about is for Davey to have more than one way to interrupt feeling sad or bad.

So, let's spend a little time talking about different tools kids can use to interrupt feeling sad or bad.

(*To child*) Do you remember what helped you to not feel bad when kids teased you?

C: Sure, I made them lose their pants so everybody could see their underwear like in my head.

T: Yes, and you did a great job (*directing attention to The House of ER poster*)! So, looking at that, which room was that from? (*Child points to The Thinking Room.*)

Yes, The Thinking Room. We also called it the "what's in your head" room. And you are really good at using your thinking.

So, Davey, let me ask you this. Is there other stuff in The Thinking Room that you could use to stop a sad or upset feeling so it doesn't take over?

C: Dunno.

T: OK, let's think about some other things that've made you sad.

Do you remember when you didn't do so well on one test in school [a specific past incident]. Can you think back to it? Like role play!

C: OK.

T: Let's make believe that this just happened—remember? We have done role playing before.

You just got back your test results and you didn't do so well, and you feel kind of sad. That's OK, but we want to make sure that the feeling doesn't get bigger!

Let's see if you can interrupt feeling sad and bad with something that you can do in your head—can you come up with some *idea*?

P: What kind of idea?

T: Sometimes what works is to replace an idea that makes you feel bad with a new idea.

We are still doing the role playing, right? You just got back a test and you got a bad grade—what is the idea that is in your head?

C: I am stupid.

T: And what feeling goes with that idea?

C: You feel bad.

T: (*To Dad*) Can you put on your coaching hat? What would be an idea that is true, but it would not make Davey feel bad, an idea that could *oppose* the idea that "I am stupid."

P: Hmm . . . he could be thinking that the test wasn't fair. But maybe that would upset him. Maybe that he will do better next time?

T: That's good. How about, "This was only the *first* test in the class, and I know I will do better next time I take a test on this subject."

C: Ah, that's too long.

T: OK, so what about just ending the "idea" this way: "I know I'll do better next time!" Can you try that?

At this point, the therapist can ask the parent–child pair to continue the role play, with the parent coaching. This exercise, which focuses on opposing a depressogenic idea with one that can neutralize it, then serves as homework so that the young patient can develop greater facility with its implementation. The psychoeducational and didactic aspects of this training goal also must be articulated as follows:

T: (*To child*) You went into The Thinking Room (*pointing to The House of ER poster*) and picked a new way to deal with feeling sad.

You already know that making up funny pictures in your head helps when kids make you sad and upset. This is another way to be sure that being sad or upset does not get out of hand.

So, we've been figuring out how you [child] can have several ways of feeling better if you get sad or upset, and we use role playing to practice because you are not depressed—which is great!

Emotion Regulation Coping: Venture Into a New Regulatory Domain

The coping goals of many young patients, based on their CERT experiences and prior histories, may include venturing into a new domain of emotion regulation or mood repair. A child who has at his disposal multiple regulatory responses from different domains may be better equipped to meet emotion regulatory challenges than a child whose responses are confined to a single domain. Additionally, because each regulatory domain has some constraints, access to responses in multiple domains is a logical training goal for young patients.

Chantel

Let us return to Chantel, whose relationship issues with her parents were based on rivalry with her younger sibling Abe. The therapist helped Chantel to deploy adaptive interpersonal regulatory strategies (with the parents as regulators) and a cognitive strategy (her "magic sign") to attenuate sadness and dysphoria.

Nonetheless, the therapist was concerned that the parents could occasionally undermine Chantel's attempts at adaptive interpersonal responses because they were depressogenic triggers as well as key regulators. Also, the intensity of Chantel's affective episodes could interfere with cognitive responding. Thus, the therapist explored the behavioral regulatory domain as a training goal for Chantel.

T: (*To child*) OK, so we want to be sure that, when you get into a spot that makes you feel sad, the sad feelings don't take over. One way to do that is to have more than one way to react when a sad feeling starts.

Do you remember that, a while back, we agreed that what is tough for you is when Mom and Dad have to spend extra time with Abe?

Sometimes, it makes you feel very bad, and you even have trouble using your magic sign. So, let's come up with something else that you could do.

What do you think would happen if you tried to *do* something—taking something from this other room of The House of ER (*gesturing to The House of ER poster*)—from The Things to Do Room? It may be another way not to get stuck feeling bad.

C: I guess, but like what?

T: Well, a while back, we were talking about things you really liked to do. One of the things we worked on is how you guys can spend time together, and you picked singing and making music.

P: Oh, yes, that is true. We all play instruments except Abe. He is too young.

T: OK. (*To child*) What do you play?

C: The piano, since I was little.

T: Do you have a favorite piece?

C: "Für Elise."

T: Here is an idea. I wonder what would happen if, whenever you start feeling sad or cranky at home, you went to the piano and played "Für Elise" for a while?

(*To parent*) What do you think?

P: Well, she likes playing. I don't know, we could try it.

T: This would be like an experiment. Let's try it for homework, OK? During the next few weeks, anytime you feel even a little down or cranky, you'll sit down and play "Für Elise."

As already described in connection with homework assignments, the therapist ascertains that the exercise makes sense to both parent and child, that they recognize how it could help the child to expand her mood repair repertoire, and that they are able to make the commitment to implement it. Finally, a portion of the session should be dedicated to psychoeducation in connection with the need to strengthen emotion regulation coping skills as a way to ward off clinical depression.

Pete

For Pete, the new response domain to be explored was the social–interpersonal regulatory domain. Pete has shown himself to be adept at deploying behavioral responses, such as physical activity/exercise and taking care of his baseball card collection to counter dysphoria or distress. But the therapist was concerned that his response repertoire was limited to a single domain. As noted earlier in the chapter, Pete's good relationship with his two older siblings was one of the reasons that the therapist wanted to explore the social regulation of sadness as a training goal. The quality of the sibling relationships was noted at the intake interview, with occasional evidence emerging during the course of treatment, but the therapist has not yet capitalized on it. This training goal was explored as follows:

T: We have been talking about different things that kids can do when they feel sad and upset so that such feelings don't get out of hand. And there are some examples of them—but certainly not all—on that poster (*directing attention to The House of ER poster*).

And most kids have some favorites—they have one thing that they know works for them when it comes to not letting sadness take over.

So we already know that *one* thing that works for you is *doing* stuff, like when you were doing jumping jacks or taking care of your baseball card collection.

And those are from which room in The House of ER?

C: What you can do.

T: Yes—correct! And these really worked for you.

But it's always a good idea to have several different ways to manage feeling sad or miserable.

When you [child] look here (*again pointing to The House of ER Poster*), is there something from the other rooms that could also work for you?

C: Dunno.

T: (*To parent and child*) What about the People Room? This is when other people help a person feel better when he or she feels sad.

So, for example, would Pete's brother and sister be interested in helping Pete?

Are there things Pete could do with his brother and sister that could make him feel better when he starts to get depressed?

P: Oh yes, sure—of course! They love their baby brother. And they were very concerned when Pete started to get depressed last year.

T: That's terrific. (*To child*) Let's make this one of the training goals for you.

Let's figure out what your brother and sister and you could do together, and as a first step, you could try it out as homework. And Dad will help as coach.

Because it is highly likely that Pete will not be experiencing depressed or markedly dysphoric mood at this point in the treatment, the homework will have to include Pete role-playing feelings of sadness and then having the siblings implement a regulatory response, which has been agreed on in advance by the therapist and the parent–child pair. Once again, psychoeducation about the need for a broad emotion regulatory response repertoire should be part of the session.

Emotion Regulation Coping: Focus on Mechanisms

Under some circumstances, the emotion regulation coping goals the therapist identifies for a young patient and parent may include learning about mechanisms that are believed to account for the effectiveness of some mood repair responses. This goal may be appropriate if the family anticipates notable environmental or contextual changes that may attenuate the young patient's access to his preferred regulatory responses and if the young patient is facing a developmental transition that is likely to impact the forms that some regulatory responses may take.

In Chapter 2, I discussed the fact that although many ways exist through which children and adolescents can repair their sad mood, there probably are only a limited number of mechanisms that are responsible for the effectiveness of most regulatory responses. Based on the research to date, two important mechanisms are attention refocusing and instigating positive affective/hedonic processes.

Consider the range of regulatory responses that have been described so far in this book, like getting hugged and being told that one is loved, doing jumping jacks, organizing a baseball card collection, imagining a humorous scene, playing music with the family, visualizing a stop sign, and countering a distressing idea with an opposing nondistressing cognition. All these responses have some unique features that contribute to their positive outcomes: For example, being touched, being hugged, and getting physical exercise have known physiological correlates that can impact mood.

However, the various responses also share a key mechanism that probably accounts for much of their salubrious effects on dysphoria: Engaging in any of them involves the refocusing of one's attention away from the sadness being experienced. When attention is directed away from one's dysphoric feeling, the affect is allowed to run its course (Teasdale, 1988), diminish in intensity, and no longer overwhelm the individual.

Certain other regulatory responses appear to work because they trigger some form of pleasure experience. Recall Davey's use of mental imagery that involved seeing his tormentors in underwear, which he found very funny. Davey's regulatory response worked not only because it allowed him to refocus attention away from his unhappy feelings, but also because the imagery involved humor, which is a form of positive affect. In a parallel vein, the family involvement in music and singing, which represented an interpersonal regulatory response for Chantel, also had a strong component of pleasure.

Raising the question "How do the tools in The House of ER rooms work?" will allow the therapist to discuss with the parent–child pair the role of attention refocusing as a mechanism of mood repair and how instigating positive affect can facilitate adaptive responses to sadness. Command of such information may enable the young patient and parents to identify other responses in the future that are driven by similar mechanisms.

The conversation about mechanisms should unfold along the following lines:

T: Today, I'd like us to talk about a different way to be prepared to deal with feelings.

Up to now, we focused on specific things to do or to think about so that [child] can better manage sadness and it does not get out of hand—that was a lot of work but now we know what works for [child], like [cite relevant responses]. But there may be situations when [child] cannot engage in [the specific regulatory response].

So, another way to be prepared for sad, upsetting feelings is to think about what makes the different ways of managing the feelings actually work? What is the engine that drives them?

One of the engines is "attention."

Let's think back to when [child] used [magic sign, exercise, other people] to feel better. Each of these meant that he stopped paying attention to how badly he was feeling and *instead* paid attention to [magic sign, exercise, other people].

Can you think of other things that a kid can do or think, alone or with others, that would pull his attention *away* from feeling sad?

As an example, let's assume that when he is dysphoric, a young adolescent's primary regulatory response is to engage in physical chores in the family's house and surrounding property. But, owing to a move, he will no longer have that response option. Knowing that attention refocusing probably was a key ingredient in his attempts to regulate sadness, he and his coaching parent should be able more easily to identify alternate response options in the family's new context that seem to work in the same fashion.

Alternatively, let's assume that social–interpersonal mood repair is another young patient's preferred domain, with her two close friends as the regulatory agents, but that both are moving far away. Questioning by the therapist revealed that the friends helped the young patient overcome sad affect mostly by engaging her in entertaining and fun things to do. For this parent–child pair, knowing that the child's key responses rely, at least in part, on mobilizing hedonic processes makes it easier to select new regulatory activities.

Should the therapist consider mood repair mechanisms with every young patient and parent? The answer is "no" for several reasons. It may be too difficult to engage some families in this dialogue because *mechanism* refers to an abstract concept, which may be viewed by the parent–child pair as far removed from their daily lives. Also, the discussion of mood repair mechanisms is nearly 100% didactics, which may be unappealing to some families. The topic requires a certain level of cognitive maturity on the part of the young patient and some conceptual interest on the part of the parent. In general, therefore, mood repair mechanisms as a topic in coping skills training should be considered only with patients in their early adolescence (or later years) and depending on parental interest.

Problem-Solving Coping

Some young patients' histories may suggest that they are likely to benefit from learning to approach stressful events or processes from a problem-solving perspective. Problem-solving coping can be proactive or reactive (noted in Table 10.1). Proactive coping with depressogenic stressors means taking action before a stressor occurs to prevent, avoid, or defuse it. Reactive problem-solving coping with depressogenic stressors means taking action after the stressor has occurred to mitigate its emotional impact and possibly address its cause.

Davey

If problem solving is a salient part of a patient's personalized training plan, it is best to identify a stressful event from the patient's history that would have lent itself to problem solving and anchor further discussion in that event. This was the approach taken with Davey (the 10-year-old who was being bullied at school), whose personalized plan involved problem-solving coping. Having introduced coping skills training, the therapist immediately focused on problem-solving coping (see the dialogue that follows). Note that the therapist addresses both proactive coping (talking to the principal to prevent such events from happening) and reactive coping (getting a teacher to intervene once the event occurred). As noted earlier, in this case, the therapist introduced the film clips only toward the end of the session to underscore the importance of problem solving:

T: Let's talk about the idea that you can deal with a problem either by solving it or by taking care of how you feel.

The idea is that sometimes when you solve a specific problem, that can prevent a person's depression.

Let's think about a situation, like the time when kids bullied you in school.

And let's see if we can use WWW.Solve if that happens again.

(*To child*) Do you remember when you had a rough time in school with the other kids?

C: Yeah. They were picking on me, a bunch of them, calling me names and stuff.

T: Yes, so let's look at the poster here.

The first *W* stands for *what* is the problem. What is the problem in this case?

P: OK. The kids ganging up on Davey is the problem situation.

T: Yes, and you've done the first step. Bullying is the problem!

The second *W* stands for *who* can help solve this problem.

(*To child*) This is a problem in school. So, *who* can help you solve it?

C: Nobody!

T: What about Mom (or Dad)—could they help? Would it help if they talked to the teacher?

C: Dunno.

P: We tried. It didn't work.

T: Yes, I remember that you talked to two teachers. So, let me move on to the next thing.

The third *W* stands for *ways* in which we could solve this problem.

You talked to two teachers and that didn't work. Can you think of anything else? Maybe talking to the principal?

P: We just figured the teachers would have told him.

T: Hmm . . . but maybe they did not. Maybe each was thinking that the other would do it.

(*To child*) If this happens again, do you think it might help if Mom or Dad talked to the principal?

C: He is real nice.

T: That is good. Can you come up with another thing that can be done to solve the problem of bullying? Some other way to deal with the problem?

(*To child*) Did you ever talk to the teacher when the bullying was about to start or when it was already going on?

C: No, he wasn't in the room.

T: Would that help solve the problem? Talking to the teacher—how do you think that would work?

C: Dunno.

T: You are right. We don't know until we try it out.

So, this is like an experiment. When the kids tease you next time, how about talking to the teacher and then making a note of what happens. OK?

If it solves the problem, that's great! But this is an experiment. If talking to the teacher does not solve the problem (kids bullying), we'll figure out why.

(*To parent*) What do you think? Would it be OK for Davey to do that?

P: Sure.

T: And another thing. The steps in WWW.Solve (*pointing to Poster 4*) can help in many different situations. So, I was wondering, how about another homework?

Can the two of you set up every evening a 10-minute talk time to go through the things that happened to you [child] that day, and discuss if that was a problem situation that could be solved? Can you list them?

(*To parent*) And can you be the coach to help Davey do this?

We will go over the list at the next session and decide in which situations WWW.Solve can be used. For example, I would like us to talk about Davey taking care of his sister. This came up a few times, that as she is getting older it is becoming a bit of a problem for Davey. So WWW.Solve may help—OK?

T: Do you remember, I mentioned that we will also watch some film clips. I have two clips we will watch—one from *Babe* and one from *Beauty and the Beast.*

As you watch the film clip, try to figure out *what* the problem is. Also, how is the unhappy character trying to solve the problem? We will talk about it afterward.

The post-film clips discussion can focus on how Davey's problem was similar or different than the problems *Babe* and the *Beast* had, if there are alternative responses to the same problem, and the pros and cons of each response.

Pete

As another illustration of proactive problem-solving coping, let's consider 9-year-old Pete, who experienced several stressful events prior to his depression. While reviewing their CERT achievements and Pete's depression history, the parent–child pair and the therapist explored whether any one of the stressors is likely to recur and could be problem-solved. With the therapist's guidance, the mother and Pete selected the change in the "parental visiting schedule" as the past stressful event that will most likely be amenable to problem solving. The dialogue then continued as follows:

T: So, we all agree that the change in the visiting schedule for the two parents was a big problem and very stressful for Pete.

The idea is that by using the WWW.Solve steps, we can make sure that if the schedule has to be changed in the future, things will go more smoothly.

(*To child*) So, let's look here (*motioning to the WWW.Solve poster*). *What* was the problem with the schedule change?

C: Everything. All of it upset me.

T: OK. Tell me one thing that was upsetting about it.

C: They didn't tell me!

T: Your parents didn't tell you that this was coming up?

C: Yeah. It wasn't fair.

T: OK. I want to be sure that I get this right. You were not upset because the visiting time changed?

C: Nah, they do that all the time.

T: So, the *real* problem is that your parents didn't tell you about it. And I guess that means you did not have a say in the plans.

(*To parent*) Do you agree?

P: Sure, but we just didn't have time.

T: That's OK, but this problem may happen again.

So, let's go to the next part of WWW.Solve. *Who* can help solve this problem?

As the dialogue has revealed, contrary to the family's initial statements, the stressful event was not the change in parental visiting times; instead, the problem was that Pete was not told about it beforehand and was not included in the negotiations. Going through the remaining steps of the WWW.Solve paradigm, it is clear how the problem at hand can be solved. By making sure that Pete is involved each time there is going to be a change in the parental visiting schedule, this source of stress for Pete could be eliminated. This serves as an example of successful proactive problem-solving coping.

Summary

As the final phase of CERT, coping skills training prepares the young patient to continue to respond in adaptive ways to future dysphoria elicited by depressogenic stressors and triggers so that such affect experiences do not get out of hand. The overarching goal is to prevent (or forestall) a recurrence of clinical depression by strengthening the young patient's mood repair response repertoire, introducing him and the coaching parent to problem-solving coping, and reinforcing emotion regulation coping. Because coping skills training is implemented when the young patient is no longer depressed, role playing and accompanying psychoeducation are critical components of this phase of CERT.

Progress in coping skills training is likely to have its ups and downs, a phenomenon already discussed in connection with recovery from depression. The therapist's general approach is the same in both instances: The child and parent have to be reassured that neither the road to recovery nor the road to the mastery of coping strategies is straightforward and that temporary roadblocks are important opportunities to identify areas where further work is needed. The overall emphasis should always be on what has been achieved, rather than on setbacks.

Ending Therapy

Throughout the entire course of treatment, the parent–child pair should be occasionally reminded that CERT is a time-limited intervention and that after completing its last phase (coping skills training), it will be time to end the therapy. As the sessions are spaced at longer intervals during the last phase, and the family gets closer to termination, it is also useful to mention the remaining time frame. The communication should proceed along the following lines:

> T: Well, this is our ____th session. We are almost done. We have only a few sessions left. We will be focusing on [whatever the remaining goals are], and we will be done in a month [or other appropriate time frame].

At the last session, summarize the child's progress during the first two phases of CERT and during coping skills training. Remind the family of the importance of practicing the skills they learned. It is usually a good idea to ask the parent and child for their own summaries as well. The closing dialogue could go something like this:

T: So, this is our last session! I would like to use this session to tell you how I see all the progress you [child and parent(s)] have made over the past months. I would like to hear your own summaries, too. And, I want to be sure to answer any questions you may have.

If you recall, when we started, the biggest problem was that [child] was overwhelmed by feeling sad and upset, and on top of that [child] also had trouble with [cite other symptoms]. When we discovered that [child] could feel less sad by [fill in the details about the mood repair responses that were mastered], [child] was not so overwhelmed anymore—those feelings were not in control any longer. Other things that [child] learned included ____________. And during the last part of treatment, you [child and parent(s)] also learned ways to be prepared for sad feelings. This means that those feelings won't take over. And things to watch out for include . . .

The summary should include achievements but also make a note of vulnerabilities. It is also important to reiterate the goals of coping skills training and orient the family's attention to upcoming issues. Depending on the therapist's context and practice guidelines, she could ask for a brief "check-in" phone call in 6 months or so to monitor the child's well-being.

Most families will not have trouble with termination particularly because CERT is a short-term intervention and the families had been given periodic reminders. Furthermore, the frequency of contacts was tapered gradually, which itself signals an eventual end. Nonetheless, some families may become anxious and express a reluctance to terminate, while others may become angry, especially if the child has failed to live up to parental expectations of therapeutic progress. In some cases, parents' negative affective reactions to termination may conceal the fear that they will now have to deal with the young patient on their own. Eliciting and empathizing with underlying parental concern are important therapeutic postures at this stage. If warranted, a separate session may be arranged with the parent(s) so that they can voice and then resolve with the therapist's help their own concerns about termination.

One factor that may argue against termination is if the young patient remains intermittently symptomatic with depression. If that is the case, the therapeutic contract should be renegotiated for a limited time to determine the best course of action. Importantly, a careful review of the context of symptom relapses is warranted to determine if they have any features in common that could be remediated. The other factor that may argue against termination is if the child has a comorbid psychiatric condition (e.g., an anxiety disorder), which came to the forefront as the child recovered from depression. If the therapist has the expertise to treat the nonaffective disorder, then it is advisable to negotiate a new contract with the parents about the scope and goal of the extended therapeutic relationship. Or else, a referral may be arranged so that the child continues to receive the needed help.

Appendix A

Questionnaires and Logs

The Feelings and Me Suite of Questionnaires

The Feelings and Me (FAM) suite of questionnaires includes three versions:

Feelings and Me Questionnaire for Adults (Form 1)

Feelings and Me Questionnaire for Children (Form 2)

Feelings and My Child Questionnaire—Parent Report (Form 3)

Content and Phrasing

Each version of the FAM contains 54 core items that are essentially identical and mirror strategies in response to sad and dysphoric emotions. There are 14 further items that are not included in the main scores (see the descriptions that follow). The text of the FAM varies slightly depending on (1) the respondent and the target of the questionnaire (e.g., the respondent is reporting about "I" vs. "my child") and (2) the social context of adults versus youth (e.g., seeking the support of "spouse or partner" vs. "mom or dad"). Furthermore, the reading grade level of the child self-report in Form 2 is suitable for children.

The FAM is organized around stem questions that are followed by possible responses. Each response can be endorsed as "not," "sometimes," or "many times" "true of [me/my child]." The answers are scored on the following scale: 0 = not true of me/my child, 1 = sometimes true of me/my child, 2 = many times true of me/my child. For details on the FAM's development and score characteristics among adults and youth with and without a history of depression, see Kovacs et al. (2009, 2019) and Bylsma et al. (2016).

Types of Scores and Items

To facilitate the computation of scores, each item has an abbreviated name, which is identical across the three FAM forms. If data have to be merged from different respondents, the item names need additional designations to avoid confusion. For example, if the rater wants to compare the FAM results of one parent about herself and about her child, the item names from the version where the parent informs about herself could start with PS, while the item names from the parent version about her child could start with PC.

1. The FAM yields **three major scores** that reflect aspects of a person's regulatory response repertoire when feeling sad and dysphoric: a score reflecting *adaptive regulation,* a score reflecting *maladaptive regulation,* and a *ratio score* reflecting the extent to which a person's mood repair repertoire consists of adaptive responses. (These are described in more detail in the text that follows.)
2. The FAM also yields **six domain-specific subscale scores** that reflect adaptive and maladaptive regulation in each of the three regulatory domains of functioning (e.g., the Adaptive Cognitive Responses Score). (These also are described in this appendix.)
3. An additional score reflects emotion regulation–related **self-efficacy**, which is the extent to which the respondent feels that he has control over his dysphoric emotions. That score is based on the following two items (the scoring algorithm is provided later on):

Item name abbreviation:	*Item:*
HARDFBET	When I feel *sad* or *upset/down,* I have a hard time feeling better.
MKFEELGO	When I feel *sad* or *upset/down,* I can make the feeling go away fast.

4. There are 12 further items that probe regulatory responses to other emotions (anger, anxiety, happiness). These have been designated as **validity items:** The responses can be used in various ways depending on the scorer's interest. For example, the validity items can serve to examine whether certain regulatory responses are specific to sadness.

The validity items are *not* included in any of the noted FAM scores. Starting with the abbreviation of each item's name, they are as follows:

BRTHINGS	When I feel *angry* or *mad,* I throw, kick, or hit things.
FIGHTFFR	When I feel *angry* or *mad,* I have arguments or fights with my family or friends.
GETWILD	When I feel *angry* or *mad,* I get wild or lose control.

THHURTSM	When I feel *angry* or *mad,* I think about hurting someone.
DEEPBRTH	When I feel *anxious* or *nervous,* I try to take deep breaths or breathe slowly.
GETPARH	When I feel *anxious* or *nervous,* I get someone to hold or physically comfort me.
RUNCIRC	When I feel *anxious* or *nervous,* I pace around in circles.
THBRAVE	When I feel *anxious* or *nervous,* I think about being relaxed or calm.
FUNFRND	When I feel *happy,* I do fun things with friends.
THGOODF	When I feel *happy,* I think about how good I feel.
DOSPORT	When I feel *happy,* I do some physical activity such as run, swim, play ball, rollerblade.
BUSYSCWK	When I feel *happy,* I get busy doing projects or other work.

Item Categorization for the Purpose of Scoring

As noted earlier, FAM items are categorized along two dimensions. One dimension reflects the presumed impact of the response on the affect to be regulated; responses that have been shown or are known to maintain or exacerbate **negative affect** are designated as *maladaptive.* Thus, for example, ruminating about how badly one feels is a maladaptive response to depressed affect because it maintains and makes the feeling worse and typically interferes with functioning. Responses that have been shown or are known to alleviate or lessen the negative affect in question are designated as *adaptive.* So, for instance, responding to sadness by keeping busy or turning to some project is an adaptive response because it helps to lessen the subjective feeling of sadness to levels that do not interfere with functioning.

The second dimension along which items are categorized reflects the **functional domain**, or area of functioning, that is primarily utilized in the service of mood repair. The *cognitive* response domain includes the use of attention, thinking, reappraisal, rumination, and other mental activities. The *behavioral/physical* functional domain includes two groups of responses: those that mirror mood repair via somatosensory processes (e.g., listening to music) and those that reflect goal-directed activities (e.g., moving forward with some project). The *social–interpersonal* domain includes the use of interpersonal processes to alleviate depression (e.g., getting social support, discussing the problem). Table A.1 lists the FAM items' classifications.

TABLE A.1. Feelings and Me Questionnaire Items by Functional Outcome and Regulatory Domain

Maladaptive	Adaptive
Cognitive	
• Think about everything being my fault. (THFAULT)	• Make believe that I am a happy kid. (MBELHAPP)
• Think about things being bad forever. (THBADFOR)	• Daydream about good things I want. (DAYDREAM)
• Think about feeling miserable. (THMISER)	• Think about feeling better soon. (THFEELBT)
• Think about what a bad person I am. (THBADPER)	• Try to forget about how I feel. (TRYFORFL)
• Think about many sad things. (THMANSAD)	• Think of something fun or enjoyable. (THSOMEFN)
• Think about why I feel sad. (THWHYSAD)	• Think about feeling happy. (THFEELHP)
• Think about the many times I feel this bad. (THMANBAD)	• Think about projects or things to do. (THINKPRJ)
• Think about people who hurt me. (THPEOPH)	• Think about what to do to feel better. (THFEELB)
• I blame myself for being bad. (BLAMSLFB)	• Think about God or pray. (THGODPR)
Behavioral/physical	
• Throw, kick, or hit objects. (THROW)	• Get busy doing projects, chores, or other work. (BUSYSCWK)
• Eat a lot. (EATNEAT)	• Listen to uplifting music. (LISTFMUS)
• Pick my skin, pull my hair, or bite my fingers. (PICKSKIN)	• Go outside to run or walk around. (RUNWALK)
• Listen to sad or "blue" music. (LISSADMS)	• Watch TV or work on my computer. (TVCOMP)
• Write about how sad I am. (WRITESAD)	• Find some game or other play activity. (FINDGAME)
• Lie down and just feel bad. (LIEBAD)	• Do physical activity such as play ball, ride a bike, swim, run, rollerblade. (DOOUTDR)
• Curl up into a ball or rock back and forth. (CURLROCK)	• Try to sing or dance. (TRYSINGD)
• Stomp my feet, bang my head, hit myself. (STOMP)	• Take care of pets, or plants, or special things. (TAKECARP)
• Go to sleep. (GOSLEEP)	• Take a bath or shower or pamper myself. (TAKEBATH)
• Take pills or drugs, or drink alcohol. (TAKEPILL)	• Read magazines, newspapers, or books. (READMAGB)
	• Get my hands busy with building, fixing things, knitting, drawing, painting, cooking. (DOHANDS)

TABLE A.1 *(cont.)*

Maladaptive	Adaptive
Behavioral/physical (*cont.*)	
	• Houseclean or do physical chores. (CLEANRM) • Treat myself to candy, ice cream, or chocolate. (EATTREAT) • Try to relax my body or meditate. (TRYRELAX)
Interpersonal–social	
• Argue with friends or people I know. (FIGHTFRD) • Go off to be alone. (GOALONE) • Yell and scream at family members. (YELLFAM) • Hide from people. (HIDEPEOP) • Won't let anybody touch me. (NOTOUCHM)	• Look for a friend or other adult to talk to. (LOOKADUL) • Try to call or see a friend. (TRYCALFR) • Talk to my spouse or partner about how I feel. (TALKPARF) • Talk to family (other than spouse/partner) about it. (TALKFAMA) • Try to get someone to hug or hold me. (TRYSOMHG) • Try to sit close to someone or hold their hand. (TRYSITCL) • Try to help others with something they are doing. (HELPFAMD)

Scoring Procedures and Rules

This section provides the algorithms for obtaining the major FAM scores: Maladaptive Regulatory Response (MalAdapt ERR), Adaptive Regulatory Response (Adapt ERR), and Adaptive/Maladaptive Balance of ERR (AMBERR). Note that the AMBERR score is based on the proportion of items endorsed, *not* on the total scores. The remaining score reflects Self-Efficacy with regard to emotion regulation.

Two steps are needed to derive the final scores. First, use the *hand-scoring template* given in Form 4 to determine the numeric value of each response to each item. Second, use the *scoring algorithms* shown below to arrive at all possible FAM scores. The scoring algorithms assume that the respondent answered all the items *or* that no more than 10% of the items are missing from among those required for a given score. Missing items are prorated. But if more than 10% of the items required for a specific score are missing, then that score cannot be computed.

FAM score computations are based on the values of the responses that were endorsed, coded as:

0 = not true   1 = sometimes true   2 = many times true

Maladaptive Regulatory Response (MalAdapt ERR)

Answers are present for all 24 maladaptive items (or 10% or fewer of the 24 items are missing).

Total MalAdapt ERR Score. The potential score ranges from 0 to 48. *The higher the score, the greater is the use of maladaptive mood repair responses and the larger the size of the maladaptive response repertoire.*

- Sum the nonmissing maladaptive items (THFAULT, THBADFOR, THMISER, THBADPER, THMANSAD, THWHYSAD, THMANBAD, THPEOPH, BLAMSLFB, FIGHTFRD, GOALONE, YELLFAM, HIDEPEOP, NOTOUCHM, GOSLEEP, TAKEPILL, EATNEAT, THROW, PICKSKIN, LISSADMS, WRITESAD, LIEBAD, CURLROCK, STOMP).
- Multiply the sum by [1 + (Number of Missing Items ÷ Number of Nonmissing Items)]. This yields a prorated total with mean value substitution for missing items.

Percent of frequency needed for the ratio score:

- Count the number of maladaptive responses endorsed as 1 or 2 [i.e., sum of max(1, item)].
- Divide by the number of nonmissing items.
- Multiply by 100.

Adaptive Regulatory Response (Adapt ERR)

Answers are present for all 30 adaptive items (or 10% or fewer of the 30 items are missing).

Total Adapt ERR Score. The potential score ranges from 0 to 60. *The higher the score, the greater is the use of adaptive mood repair responses and the larger the size of the adaptive response repertoire.*

- Sum the values of the nonmissing adaptive items (MBELHAPP, DAYDREAM, THFEELBT, TRYFORFL, THSOMEFN, THFEELHP, THINKPRJ, THFEELB, THGODPR, LOOKADUL, TRYCALFR, TALKPARF, TALKFAMA, TRYSOMHG, TRYSITCL, HELPFAMD, EATTREAT, TRYRELAX, BUSYSCWK, LISTFMUS, RUNWALK, TVCOMP, FINDGAME, DOOUTDR, TRYSINGD, TAKECARP, TAKEBATH, READMAGB, DOHANDS, CLEANRM).
- Multiply the sum by [1 + (Number of Missing Items ÷ Number of Nonmissing Items)]. This yields a prorated total with mean value substitution for missing items.

Percent of frequency needed for the ratio score:

- Count the number of adaptive responses endorsed as 1 or 2 [i.e., sum of max(1, item)].
- Divide by the number of nonmissing items.
- Multiply by 100.

Adaptive/Maladaptive Balance of ERR (AMBERR)

Total AMBERR Score. The potential score ranges from 0 to 100. *The percentage reflects the extent to which the respondent's mood repair repertoire is dominated by adaptive regulatory responses.* Research suggests that AMBERR scores above 65% characterize normative samples, with a typical 2:1 ratio of adaptive to maladaptive responses.

Compute as follows if both the percent of adaptive and percent of maladaptive frequencies have been calculated and at least one is nonzero:

- Multiply the adaptive percent frequency by 100.
- Divide by the sum of adaptive and maladaptive percent frequencies.

Total Self-Efficacy Score

Potential score ranges from 0 (no self-efficacy) to 4 (high self-efficacy). *The higher the score, the greater is the respondent's confidence in self-managing emotions.*

MKFEELGO – HARDFBET + 2

Feelings Logs

Form 5, the simplest version of the daily feelings log, can be adapted to meet various more complex treatment goals for specific youth. For example, if certain times are most problematic for the child, column 1 can be altered to specify the select time intervals, such as "before breakfast" and "after school," or activities like "during school lunch" or "during music practice." If the child is implementing a specific regulatory response as homework, the therapist may divide the last column into two sections: "How strong was the feeling?" and "Did (the response) help to feel better?"

The next feelings log, Form 6, includes a column for the child or parent to list the place where the feeling or behavior being monitored takes place. This column can be appropriate if the child's mood difficulties appear to be related to specific locations like being at home.

The final feelings log, Form 7, is an example of a daily monitoring log of affect including severity rating and context. It can be adapted to meet various treatment goals for specific youth. For example, if the interpersonal context is particularly important, the therapist may add "Who was there?" to the third column. If the focus is on the use of available regulatory responses, the therapist may add "Did anything help to feel better?" to the last column.

Homework to Do Log

As treatment progresses and the therapist has become familiar with the nature of the young patient's mood difficulties, homework assignments can shift from monitoring of affect and its characteristics to reporting on the outcomes of homework assignments such as behavioral experiments. The columns in the form to be used can be titled in any way to reflect salient features of the goal of the homework. For example, if it is important to know the context of some behavior, one column can be labeled "Where are you?" Or if it is useful to know who initiates the homework, one column can be labeled "Initiator."

FORM 1

Feelings and Me Questionnaire for Adults

Your name: ____
First Last

Your relationship to child:

0. Not related
1. Mother
2. Father
3. Stepmother
4. Stepfather
5. Other parent figure ______________________________

Instructions

This is a list of various things that individuals do or think when they feel sad, blue, or down. A few questions are about *other* feelings. This is *not* a test. There is no right or wrong answer. Please read each sentence and decide how well it describes you. Put an "X" in the one box next to each sentence that fits you the best to show your answer. There is one example for you to try and mark your answer.

Example

	Not true of me (0)	Sometimes true of me (1)	Many times true of me (2)
When I feel *sad* or *down*, I cry.	☐	☐	☐

	Not true of me (0)	Sometimes true of me (1)	Many times true of me (2)
When I feel *sad* or *down*, I:			
throw, kick, or hit objects.	☐	☐	☐
think about everything being my fault.	☐	☐	☐
have a hard time feeling better.	☐	☐	☐
make believe that I am a happy person.	☐	☐	☐

(*continued*)

	Not true of me (0)	Sometimes true of me (1)	Many times true of me (2)
When I feel *sad* or *down*, I:			
think about things being bad forever.	☐	☐	☐
think about feeling miserable.	☐	☐	☐
go to sleep.	☐	☐	☐
think about what a bad person I am.	☐	☐	☐
When I feel *sad* or *down*, I:			
can make the feeling go away fast.	☐	☐	☐
eat a lot.	☐	☐	☐
argue with friends or people I know.	☐	☐	☐
take pills, or drugs, or drink alcohol.	☐	☐	☐
When I feel *sad* or *down*, I:			
look for a friend or other adult to talk to.	☐	☐	☐
pick my skin, pull my hair, bite my fingers.	☐	☐	☐
daydream about good things I want.	☐	☐	☐
treat myself to candy, ice cream, or chocolate.	☐	☐	☐
When I feel *sad* or *down*, I:			
listen to sad or "blue" music.	☐	☐	☐
write about how sad I am.	☐	☐	☐
think about feeling better soon.	☐	☐	☐
try to forget about how I feel.	☐	☐	☐
When I feel *sad* or *down*, I:			
go off to be alone.	☐	☐	☐
think of something fun or enjoyable.	☐	☐	☐
get busy doing projects, chores, or other work.	☐	☐	☐
listen to uplifting music.	☐	☐	☐
When I feel *sad* or *down*, I:			
go outside to run or walk around.	☐	☐	☐
watch TV or work on my computer.	☐	☐	☐
try to call or see a friend.	☐	☐	☐
talk to my spouse or partner about how I feel.	☐	☐	☐

(continued)

	Not true of me (0)	Sometimes true of me (1)	Many times true of me (2)
When I feel *sad* or *down*, I:			
talk to family (other than spouse/partner) about it.	❑	❑	❑
find some game or other play activity.	❑	❑	❑
think about many sad things.	❑	❑	❑
do physical activity such as play ball, ride a bike, swim, run, rollerblade.	❑	❑	❑
When I feel *sad* or *down*, I:			
lie down and just feel bad.	❑	❑	❑
yell and scream at family members.	❑	❑	❑
try to get someone to hug or hold me.	❑	❑	❑
think about feeling happy.	❑	❑	❑
When I feel *sad* or *down*, I:			
try to sing or dance.	❑	❑	❑
think about projects or things to do.	❑	❑	❑
take care of pets, or plants, or special things.	❑	❑	❑
take a bath or shower or pamper myself.	❑	❑	❑
When I feel *sad* or *down*, I:			
curl up into a ball or rock back and forth.	❑	❑	❑
try to sit close to someone or hold their hand.	❑	❑	❑
hide from people.	❑	❑	❑
stomp my feet, bang my head, hit myself.	❑	❑	❑
When I feel *sad* or *down*, I:			
think about what to do to feel better.	❑	❑	❑
think about why I feel sad.	❑	❑	❑
read magazines, newspapers, or books.	❑	❑	❑
try to help others with something they are doing.	❑	❑	❑

(*continued*)

	Not true of me (0)	Sometimes true of me (1)	Many times true of me (2)
When I feel *sad or down*, I:			
think about the many times I feel this badly.	❑	❑	❑
try to relax my body or meditate.	❑	❑	❑
think about people who hurt me.	❑	❑	❑
get my hands busy with building, fixing things, knitting, drawing, painting, cooking.	❑	❑	❑
When I feel *sad or down*, I:			
houseclean or do other physical chores.	❑	❑	❑
won't let anybody touch me.	❑	❑	❑
think about God or pray.	❑	❑	❑
blame myself for being bad.	❑	❑	❑
When I feel *angry or mad*, I:			
throw, kick, or hit things.	❑	❑	❑
have arguments, fights with my family or friends.	❑	❑	❑
get wild or lose control.	❑	❑	❑
think about hurting someone.	❑	❑	❑
When I feel *anxious or nervous*, I:			
try to take deep breaths or breathe slowly.	❑	❑	❑
get someone to hold or physically comfort me.	❑	❑	❑
pace around in circles.	❑	❑	❑
think about being relaxed or calm.	❑	❑	❑
When I feel *happy*, I:			
do fun things with friends.	❑	❑	❑
think about how good I feel.	❑	❑	❑
do some physical activity such as run, swim, play ball, rollerblade.	❑	❑	❑
get busy doing projects or other work.	❑	❑	❑

Thank you for answering!

FORM 2

Feelings and Me Questionnaire for Children

Your name: ____

First Last

Are you a boy or girl?

1. Boy
2. Girl
3. Nonbinary

Instructions

Hi! This is a list of different things that kids do or think when they feel sad, grumpy, or upset. A few questions are about *other* feelings. This is *not* a test. There is no right answer or wrong answer. Please read each sentence, one by one. Think about the sentence and decide if it describes you. To show your answer, make an "X" in one box that fits you the best. There is one example, try it and mark your answer.

Example

	Not true of me (0)	Sometimes true of me (1)	Many times true of me (2)
When I feel *sad* or *upset*, I cry.	❑	❑	❑

	Not true of me (0)	Sometimes true of me (1)	Many times true of me (2)
When I feel *sad* or *upset*, I:			
throw, kick, or hit things.	❑	❑	❑
think about everything being my fault.	❑	❑	❑
have a hard time feeling better.	❑	❑	❑
make believe that I am a happy kid.	❑	❑	❑

(*continued*)

	Not true of me (0)	Sometimes true of me (1)	Many times true of me (2)
When I feel *sad* or *upset*, I:			
think about things being bad forever.	☐	☐	☐
think about feeling miserable.	☐	☐	☐
go to sleep.	☐	☐	☐
think about what a bad person I am.	☐	☐	☐
When I feel *sad* or *upset*, I:			
can make the feeling go away fast.	☐	☐	☐
eat and eat.	☐	☐	☐
fight with friends.	☐	☐	☐
take pills or drugs, or drink alcohol.	☐	☐	☐
When I feel *sad* or *upset*, I:			
look for a teacher or other adult to talk to.	☐	☐	☐
pick my skin, pull my hair, or bite my fingers.	☐	☐	☐
daydream about good things I want.	☐	☐	☐
eat treats like candy, ice cream, or chocolate.	☐	☐	☐
When I feel *sad* or *upset*, I:			
listen to sad music.	☐	☐	☐
write about how sad I am.	☐	☐	☐
think about feeling better soon.	☐	☐	☐
try to forget about how I feel.	☐	☐	☐
When I feel *sad* or *upset*, I:			
go off to be alone.	☐	☐	☐
think of something fun.	☐	☐	☐
get busy doing schoolwork or other work.	☐	☐	☐
listen to fun music.	☐	☐	☐
When I feel *sad* or *upset*, I:			
go outside to run or walk around.	☐	☐	☐
watch TV or work on my computer.	☐	☐	☐
try to call or see a friend.	☐	☐	☐
talk to my mom or dad about how I feel.	☐	☐	☐

(continued)

	Not true of me (0)	Sometimes true of me (1)	Many times true of me (2)
When I feel *sad* or *upset*, I:			
talk to family (other than mom/dad) about it.	☐	☐	☐
find some game to play.	☐	☐	☐
think about many sad things.	☐	☐	☐
do something like play ball, ride a bike, swim, run, rollerblade.	☐	☐	☐
When I feel *sad* or *upset*, I:			
lie down and just feel bad.	☐	☐	☐
yell and scream at my family.	☐	☐	☐
try to get someone to hug me.	☐	☐	☐
think about feeling happy.	☐	☐	☐
When I feel *sad* or *upset*, I:			
try to sing or dance.	☐	☐	☐
think about projects or things to do.	☐	☐	☐
take care of pets, or plants, or special things.	☐	☐	☐
take a bath or shower.	☐	☐	☐
When I feel *sad* or *upset*, I:			
curl up into a ball or rock back and forth.	☐	☐	☐
try to sit close to someone or hold their hand.	☐	☐	☐
hide from people.	☐	☐	☐
stomp my feet, bang my head, hit myself.	☐	☐	☐
When I feel *sad* or *upset*, I:			
think about what to do to feel better.	☐	☐	☐
think about why I feel sad.	☐	☐	☐
read magazines or storybooks.	☐	☐	☐
try to help mom/dad/brother/sister with something they are doing.	☐	☐	☐

(continued)

	Not true of me (0)	Sometimes true of me (1)	Many times true of me (2)
When I feel *sad* or *upset*, I:			
think about the many times I feel this bad.	❑	❑	❑
try to relax my body.	❑	❑	❑
think about people who hurt me.	❑	❑	❑
do stuff with my hands like building, fixing things, knitting, drawing, painting.	❑	❑	❑
When I feel *sad* or *upset, I:*			
clean my room.	❑	❑	❑
won't let anybody touch me.	❑	❑	❑
think about God or pray.	❑	❑	❑
blame myself for being bad.	❑	❑	❑
When I feel *angry* or *mad*, I:			
break or kick things.	❑	❑	❑
have a fight with my family or friends.	❑	❑	❑
get wild or lose control.	❑	❑	❑
think about hurting someone.	❑	❑	❑
When I feel *scared* or *nervous*, I:			
try to take deep breaths or breathe slow.	❑	❑	❑
get mom or dad to hold me.	❑	❑	❑
run around in circles.	❑	❑	❑
think about being brave.	❑	❑	❑
When I feel *happy*, I:			
play or have fun with friends.	❑	❑	❑
think about how good I feel.	❑	❑	❑
do something like run, swim, play ball, rollerblade.	❑	❑	❑
get busy doing schoolwork and other tasks.	❑	❑	❑

Thank you for answering!

FORM 3 **Feelings and My Child Questionnaire—Parent Report**

Your name: ____
First Last

Target of form: ____
First Last

Your relationship to child:

0. Not related
1. Mother
2. Father
3. Stepmother
4. Stepfather
5. Other parent figure ______________________________

Instructions

This is a list of different things that kids do or think they feel sad, grumpy, or upset. A few questions deal with *other* feelings. This is *not* a test. There is no right answer or wrong answer. Please read each sentence. Think about the sentence and decide how well it describes your child. To show your answer, make an "X" in one box that best describes your child. There is one example; please try it and mark your answer.

Example

	Not true of my child (0)	Sometimes true of my child (1)	Many times true of my child (2)
When my child feels *sad* or *upset*, he/she cries.	❑	❑	❑

When my child feels *sad* or *upset*, he/she:	Not true of my child (0)	Sometimes true of my child (1)	Many times true of my child (2)
throws, kicks, or hits things.	❑	❑	❑
thinks about everything being his/her fault.	❑	❑	❑
has a hard time feeling better.	❑	❑	❑
makes believe that he/she is happy.	❑	❑	❑

(*continued*)

	Not true of my child (0)	Sometimes true of my child (1)	Many times true of my child (2)
When my child feels *sad* or *upset*, he/she:			
thinks about things being bad forever.	❑	❑	❑
thinks about feeling miserable.	❑	❑	❑
goes to sleep.	❑	❑	❑
thinks about what a bad person he/she is.	❑	❑	❑
When my child feels *sad* or *upset*, he/she:			
can make the feeling go away fast.	❑	❑	❑
eats and eats.	❑	❑	❑
fights with friends.	❑	❑	❑
takes pills, or drugs, or drinks alcohol.	❑	❑	❑
When my child feels *sad* or *upset*, he/she:			
looks for a teacher or other adult to talk to.	❑	❑	❑
picks his/her skin, pulls his/her hair, or bites his/her fingers.	❑	❑	❑
daydreams about good things he/she wants.	❑	❑	❑
eats treats like candy, ice cream, or chocolate.	❑	❑	❑
When my child feels *sad* or *upset*, he/she:			
listens to sad music.	❑	❑	❑
writes about how sad he/she is.	❑	❑	❑
thinks about feeling better soon.	❑	❑	❑
tries to forget how he/she feels.	❑	❑	❑
When my child feels *sad* or *upset*, he/she:			
goes off to be alone.	❑	❑	❑
thinks of something fun.	❑	❑	❑
gets busy doing schoolwork or other tasks.	❑	❑	❑
listens to fun music.	❑	❑	❑

(continued)

	Not true of my child (0)	Sometimes true of my child (1)	Many times true of my child (2)
When my child feels *sad* or *upset*, he/she:			
goes outside to run or walk around.	☐	☐	☐
watches TV or works on his/her computer.	☐	☐	☐
tries to call or see a friend.	☐	☐	☐
talks to me (or other parent) about how he/she feels.	☐	☐	☐
When my child feels *sad* or *upset*, he/she:			
talks to family (other than parent) about it.	☐	☐	☐
finds some game to play.	☐	☐	☐
thinks about many sad things.	☐	☐	☐
does something like play ball, ride a bike, swim, run, rollerblade.	☐	☐	☐
When my child feels *sad* or *upset*, he/she:			
lies down and just feels bad.	☐	☐	☐
yells and screams at family members.	☐	☐	☐
tries to get someone to hug them.	☐	☐	☐
thinks about feeling happy.	☐	☐	☐
When my child feels *sad* or *upset*, he/she:			
tries to sing or dance.	☐	☐	☐
thinks about projects or things to do.	☐	☐	☐
takes care of pets, or plants, or special things.	☐	☐	☐
takes a bath or shower.	☐	☐	☐
When my child feels *sad* or *upset*, he/she:			
curls up into a ball or rocks back and forth.	☐	☐	☐
tries to sit close to someone or hold their hand.	☐	☐	☐
hides from people.	☐	☐	☐
stomps his/her feet, bangs his/her head, hits him/herself.	☐	☐	☐

(*continued*)

	Not true of my child (0)	Sometimes true of my child (1)	Many times true of my child (2)
When my child feels *sad* or *upset*, he/she:			
thinks about what to do to feel better.	☐	☐	☐
thinks about why he/she feels sad.	☐	☐	☐
reads magazines or storybooks.	☐	☐	☐
tries to help family members with something they are doing.	☐	☐	☐
When my child feels *sad* or *upset*, he/she:			
thinks about the many times they feel this bad.	☐	☐	☐
tries to relax his/her body.	☐	☐	☐
thinks about people who hurt him/her.	☐	☐	☐
does stuff with their hands like building, fixing things, knitting, drawing, painting.	☐	☐	☐
When my child feels *sad* or *upset*, he or she:			
cleans their room.	☐	☐	☐
won't let anybody touch them.	☐	☐	☐
thinks about God or prays.	☐	☐	☐
blames him- or herself for being bad.	☐	☐	☐
When my child feels *angry* or *mad*, he or she:			
breaks or kicks things.	☐	☐	☐
has a fight with family or friends.	☐	☐	☐
gets wild or loses control.	☐	☐	☐
thinks about hurting someone.	☐	☐	☐
When my child feels *scared* or *nervous*, he or she:			
tries to take deep breaths or breathe slowly.	☐	☐	☐
gets me (or other parent) to hold them.	☐	☐	☐
runs around in circles.	☐	☐	☐
thinks about being brave.	☐	☐	☐

(continued)

	Not true of my child (0)	Sometimes true of my child (1)	Many times true of my child (2)
When my child feels *happy*, he or she:			
plays or does fun things with friends.	❑	❑	❑
thinks about how good they feel.	❑	❑	❑
does something like run, swim, play ball, rollerblade.	❑	❑	❑
gets busy doing schoolwork and other work.	❑	❑	❑

Thank you for answering!

FORM 4 Scoring Template for the Feelings and Me Questionnaires

Instructions

Duplicate the scoring template for each Feelings and Me (FAM) questionnaire you have. Take the completed FAM form and assign to each response the value of the answer that was checked by the respondent (0 = not true, 1 = sometimes true, 2 = many times true). Then copy the values (0, 1, or 2) into each of the two open spaces for each item in the scoring template, that is, enter the same number twice in each row. When finished, compute the total scores according to the instructions at the bottom of the template. **Note:** The phrasing of an item may differ somewhat across the three versions of the FAM. The list below is meant to capture each item's essential content.

Enter actual rating (0 = not true, 1 = sometimes true, 2 = many times true) into both open boxes for each item.

When I feel *sad* or *down*, I . . .	Maladaptive			Adaptive	
1. throw, kick, or hit objects.	M	B			
2. think about everything being my fault.	M		C		
3. have a hard time feeling better. **(Self-Efficacy item)** –SE ____					
4. make believe that I am a happy kid.				A	C
5. think about things being bad forever.	M		C		
6. think about feeling miserable.	M		C		
7. go to sleep.	M	B			
8. think about what a bad person I am.	M		C		
9. can make the feeling go away fast. **(Self-Efficacy item)** +SE ____					

(continued)

Note. M = maladaptive response; B = behavioral/physical regulatory domain; C = cognitive regulatory domain; A = adaptive response; S = social–interpersonal regulatory domain; # = actual number of; / = divide by; % = percentage.

Scoring Template for the Feelings and Me Questionnaires *(p. 2 of 4)*

When I feel *sad* or *down*, I . . .	Maladaptive				Adaptive			
10. eat a lot.	M	B						
11. argue with friends or people I know.	M			S				
12. take pills or drugs, or drink alcohol.	M	B						
13. look for a friend or other adult to talk to.					A			S
14. pick my skin, pull my hair, or bite my fingers.	M	B						
15. daydream about good things I want.					A		C	
16. treat myself to candy, ice cream, or chocolate.					A	B		
17. listen to sad or "blue" music.	M	B						
18. write about how sad I am.	M	B						
19. think about feeling better soon.					A		C	
20. try to forget about how I feel.					A		C	
21. go off to be alone.	M			S				
22. think of something fun or enjoyable.					A		C	
23. get busy doing projects, chores, or other work.					A	B		
24. listen to uplifting music.					A	B		
25. go outside to run or walk around.					A	B		
26. watch TV or work on my computer.					A	B		
27. try to call or see a friend.					A			S
28. talk to my spouse or partner (or parent) about how I feel.					A			S

(continued)

Scoring Template for the Feelings and Me Questionnaires *(p. 3 of 4)*

When I feel *sad* or *down*, I . . .	Maladaptive				Adaptive			
29. talk to family other than spouse/partner (or parent or siblings) about it.					A			S
30. find some game or other play activity.					A	B		
31. think about many sad things.	M		C					
32. do physical activity such as play ball, ride a bike, swim, run, rollerblade.					A	B		
33. lie down and just feel bad.	M	B						
34. yell and scream at family members.	M			S				
35. try to get someone to hug or hold me.					A			S
36. think about feeling happy.					A		C	
37. try to sing or dance.					A	B		
38. think about projects or things to do.					A		C	
39. take care of pets, or plants, or special things.					A	B		
40. take a bath or shower or pamper myself.					A	B		
41. curl up into a ball or rock back and forth.	M	B						
42. try to sit close to someone or hold their hand.					A			S
43. hide from people.	M			S				
44. stomp my feet, bang my head, hit myself.	M	B						
45. think about what to do to feel better.					A		C	
46. think about why I feel sad.	M		C					

(continued)

Scoring Template for the Feelings and Me Questionnaires *(p. 4 of 4)*

When I feel *sad* or *down*, I . . .	Maladaptive				Adaptive			
47. read magazines, newspapers, or books/storybooks.					A	B		
48. try to help others (parent, siblings) with something they are doing.					A			S
49. think about the many times I feel this bad.	M		C					
50. try to relax my body or meditate.					A	B		
51. think about people who hurt me.	M		C					
52. get my hands busy with building, fixing things, knitting, drawing, painting, cooking.					A	B		
53. houseclean or do physical chores.					A	B		
54. won't let anybody touch me.	M			S				
55. think about God or pray.					A		C	
56. blame myself for being bad.	M		C					

Totals and subscales (sum all ratings in each column)	M	B	C	S	A	B	C	S
Endorsement counts (number of items > 0 in each column)	#M	#B	#C	#S	#A	#B	#C	#S
Number of nonmissing items	/24				/30			
% Endorsed (100 × Endorsement count ÷ Number of nonmissing)	%M				%A			
Adaptive/Maladaptive Balance of Regulatory Responses (100 × %A ÷ [%M + %A])					AMBERR			
Self-Efficacy (item 9 – item 3 + 2)	SE							

FORM 5

Daily Feelings Log

Day/time	Feeling	How strong was the feeling? (pick a number between 1 = not strong and 10 = very strong)

FORM 6

Daily Feelings Log by Location

Day/time	Place (for example, home)	Feeling	How strong was the feeling? (pick a number between 1 = not strong and 10 = very strong)

FORM 7

Daily Feelings Log by Location and Context

Day/time	Place (for example, home)	What was going on?	Feeling	How strong was the feeling? (1 = not strong; 10 = very strong)

FORM 8

Homework to Do Log

Day/time	What to do? What is the task?	Was it done?	Initiator	Child's feelings after + severity (from 1 = little/ none to 10 = a lot/very strong)

Appendix B

Posters

The Rules of Coaching

A GOOD COACH:

- **Focuses** on the player's abilities and strengths.
- **Works** with the player on new ways to do things.
- **Helps** the player use different abilities to reach goals.
- **Praises and encourages** the player to keep going!
- **Hangs in there** and works with the player even if the coach had a bad day!
- **Learns and practices** because coaches are made, not born.

The Rules of Being a Good Team Player

A GOOD TEAM PLAYER:

- **Will try new ways** to do things.
- **Works with the coaches** on game plans and goals.
- **Uses words** to tell the coaches how he or she feels.
- **Asks for help** when things get tough or confusing.
- **Does NOT give up** even if a game plan doesn't work right away.
- **Practices, practices, practices,** because that's what it takes to reach a goal.

POSTER 3

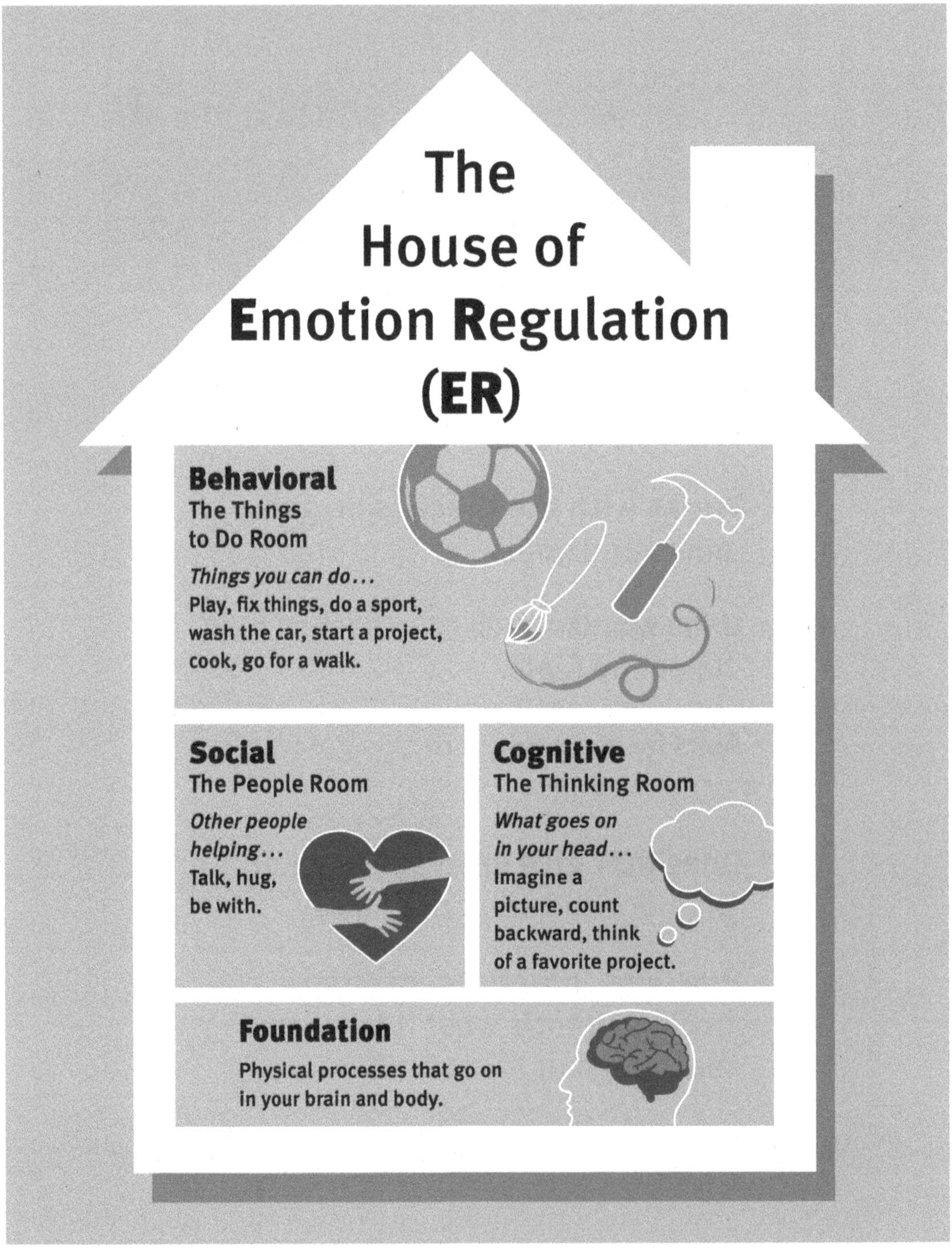
The
House of
Emotion Regulation
(ER)
Behavioral
The Things
to Do Room
Things you can do...
Play, fix things, do a sport,
wash the car, start a project,
cook, go for a walk.
Social
The People Room
Other people
helping...
Talk, hug,
be with.
Cognitive
The Thinking Room
What goes on
in your head...
Imagine a
picture, count
backward, think
of a favorite project.
Foundation
Physical processes that go on
in your brain and body.

WWW.Solve: Solving a Problem

WHAT is the problem to solve?

WHO can help to solve this problem?

WAYS to solve this problem

Appendix C

Case Formulations and Personalized Training Plans for Four Young Patients

Formulation and Plans for Chantel

Nine-year-old Chantel started to develop affective symptoms after the birth of her sibling Abe and has recently become clinically depressed with the added stressor of the following family event. For the first time, she had met relatives from her father's first marriage. Her recognition that they had had no contact with her dad for years induced fears of being abandoned. It also became clear during the initial session that her mother was clinically depressed, and the depression played a role in the mother's belief that her physical disability (she uses a wheelchair) somehow compromised her competence as a parent. As a result, she distanced herself from Chantel. The therapist identified sibling rivalry as a recurrent cause of Chantel's affective instability and shaky self-esteem; it also appeared that any perceived potential threat to her attachment relationships to her parents were salient stressors. The therapist separately identified the mother's depression as needing attention.

The therapist initially focused on interpersonal mood repair strategies (mostly involving Chantel's parents) given that interpersonal issues were at the forefront for Chantel and she appeared to prefer this domain. This also provided her mother with a positive role vis-à-vis Chantel, which, the therapist hoped, could counteract the mother's withdrawal. But since the parents were not only important social regulators but also served as depressogenic triggers, the therapist believed that Chantel's mood repair response repertoire should be expanded. Chantel's ruminations were evidence that she was familiar with cognitive processes. The therapist therefore next targeted cognitive regulatory responses as ways for Chantel to interrupt the negative ruminations and associated dysphoric affect that were prompted by depressogenic triggers.

In her coping skills training plan for Chantel, the therapist wanted to reinforce the young patient's use of both social–interpersonal and cognitive mood repair strategies and added a behavioral strategy as well. She also considered how to capitalize on the family's strengths with regard to their many conjoint activities (like singing and making music) to counter Chantel's sibling rivalry and recurrent negative self-statements. However, the therapist remained open to the possibility that other longer-term interventions may be indicated. Coincidentally, while the mother's effective coaching of Chantel lifted her depression somewhat, she was still referred for individual treatment.

Formulation and Plans for Mary

Eight-year-old Mary was brought for treatment by her 62-year-old grandmother, who has been her caregiver for several years since her mother first abandoned her. Although the mother eventually reappeared, her presence was intermittent and inconsistent. Her prior history of chaotic appearance and disappearance apparently resulted from substance abuse. It was the most recent maternal disappearance that prompted Mary's depression. Her grandmother appeared to be very nurturing of Mary but was a bit overwhelmed by having to take care of an 8-year-old while she herself was so close to retirement. The grandmother appeared to have limited material resources but had access to a wide and supportive social network. Mary impressed the therapist as emotionally needy, cognitively and behaviorally immature, and generally appearing to be younger than her chronological age.

Given Mary's age, presentation, and history, the therapist elected to focus initially on the interpersonal regulation of her sadness, emphasizing physical touch and contact, to which Mary was very responsive. Because the grandmother was the sole person who acted as a regulator for Mary, the therapist sought to expand the range of potential regulatory agents by having the family recruit an aunt. During treatment, the therapist also modeled for Mary's grandmother how to accompany physical comforting of Mary with verbalizations of love and reassurance so that social–interpersonal regulation could also occur symbolically; this was a developmentally important goal. Correspondingly, another goal for Mary was to recognize that she often needs to initiate interpersonal regulation herself (seek help from others). Furthermore, because the therapist wanted to be sure that Mary has a broader scope of regulatory response options, she also focused on having Mary explore the behavioral regulatory domain.

Coping skills training goals included strengthening Mary's existing mood repair response repertoire by expanding the range of people who could serve as social regulators of her sadness. Case conceptualization centered around the fact that repeated maternal abandonment of Mary undermined her trust in others, with potentially negative consequences for the social–interpersonal regulation of sadness. One part of her coping training plan therefore included the goal of developing new relationships (e.g., with new teachers in school) as a way of gradually rebuilding trust in others.

Formulation and Plans for Pete

The youngest of three children, 9-year-old Pete had experienced mild to moderate mood symptoms for several years, starting right after his parents' divorce. During the 8- to 10-month period just prior to his mother seeking treatment for him, Pete developed additional symptoms with clear diurnal variation. They were especially severe in the morning. He presented with a variety of depression symptoms, including social withdrawal, lethargy, anhedonia, worthlessness, and sleep disturbance. There were also multiple recent major life events, including attending a new school. Other stressors included the remarriage of his mother, the difficulties of joint custody, and his parents' financial issues. Additionally, his maternal grandmother had died about a year earlier. There was a very strong family history of mood disorder, with multiple people affected on both the maternal and paternal sides. The family dynamics were unclear with one exception: His two older siblings and Pete got along well and, as related by the mother, they both had expressed concerns about Pete.

When he entered treatment, Pete was extremely depressed with many of his symptoms mirroring a type of depression that had been labeled in the past as "endogenomorphic" and thus presumably driven mostly by biological predisposing factors. The therapist's major goal was to get Pete to engage in action; hence, the emphasis was on the behavioral regulation of his dysphoria. As time went by, Pete impressed the therapist as a shy and quiet child. This impression was reinforced when Pete elected to expand his behavioral mood repair repertoire by working on his baseball card collection, a solitary activity. Pete's symptom presentation, the presence of multiple stressors, and the family history of mood disorder shaped the therapist's goals for Pete's coping skills training.

Given that Pete likely had some predisposition to react to multiple stressors with depression, both proactive and reactive coping became key topics. Additionally, the therapist wanted to capitalize on Pete's good relationship with his siblings and enlist them as social–interpersonal regulators to whom Pete could turn when he experiences sadness and dysphoria. Strengthening Pete's mood repair response repertoire in this manner was important to assure that future experiences of dysphoria do not get out of hand.

Formulation and Plans for Davey

Davey, a 10-year-old, previously a very good student, with a history of asthma, was brought for treatment by his father because of growing sadness and dysphoria, social withdrawal, anxiety, and suicidal ideation. The proximal factor appeared to be increasing bullying at school after Davey decided to dress in all black as some sort of personal statement. Family context included a maternal history of mood disorder several years ago and an intermittent neurological condition, occasional arguments between his parents, and a younger sister, who had autism and whom Davey had to watch for short periods on certain days of the week. The therapist was concerned about the appropriateness of Davey being responsible for his sister and made certain to remain attentive to this issue. Davey's parents, both professionals, worked different shifts, which was occasionally problematic. However, as his mother was able to attend some of the sessions, it became evident that both parents were very supportive of Davey and would make good coaches.

Davey impressed the therapist as very articulate and bright and perhaps even a bit too mature for his age. Given Davey's apparent verbal and intellectual skills, the therapist first explored the use of cognitive regulatory responses to manage his dysphoria. Davey was successful at implementing humorous visual imagery, which not only attenuated his dysphoria but eventually defused some bullying encounters. However, having access to mood repair responses in multiple domains (rather than relying solely on one domain) better prepares a person to respond to a range of depressogenic triggers. The therapist therefore also had Davey implement social–interpersonal regulatory responses by talking with his parents about issues that upset him. This approach became especially useful when Davey voiced suicidal ideation, which was a response to his despondent mood.

No particular individual vulnerabilities or family context characteristics appeared to be implicated in Davey's depression and his father, in particular, was an excellent coach. Thus, the coping skills training goals emphasized proactive and reactive problem solving as they applied to the bullying situation at school, along with further strengthening Davey's cognitive mood repair responses. The therapist also believed that taking care of Susie (the younger sibling) was becoming physically and emotionally taxing for Davey and was a potential source of stress. This was to be presented to the parents as a problem-solving scenario, to be resolved by working with them on alternative child care arrangements.

Appendix D

Manual for Parents

Overcoming Your Child's Depression with Contextual Emotion Regulation Therapy

Introduction

This manual is for parents of clinically depressed children being treated with contextual emotion regulation therapy or CERT. The manual explains clinical depression, and how CERT can help your child feel better. For CERT to work best, you and your child need to actively participate. Helping your child to recover from depression takes a team effort. The team includes the therapist, your child and you, and possibly other family members. The therapist is the head coach of the team, and your child is the key player. Your role is to be an **assistant coach**. This manual describes the ways in which you can be an effective assistant coach in the team effort to help your child. You may find it helpful to reread it from time to time. This manual is yours to keep. Feel free to make written notes in it.

(*continued*)

Appreciation is due to Vincent Ho, MD, and Gretchen D. Clutter for their contributions to the initial version of this manual.

What Is Clinical Depression?

Children who are depressed usually feel miserable and think negatively about themselves. They have trouble with their energy level, appetite, or sleep, and often have problems in school or at home. The symptoms of clinical depression in general, and among youth, include the following:

- Depressed, sad, unhappy mood
- Cranky, crabby mood
- Feeling unloved and friendless
- Feeling worthless, blaming oneself for things that go wrong
- Problems concentrating or keeping one's attention on a specific task
- No longer interested in school or fun activities
- Pessimism and hopelessness
- Thoughts of wanting to die, thinking about or trying to kill oneself
- Low energy, being tired a lot, or being slowed down
- Sleeping or eating much less or much more than usual

Is Clinical Depression the Same as Being Sad?

Clinical depression is not the same as feeling sad, unhappy, or blue. Everyday feelings of sadness or being blue generally don't last more than a few hours or a day or two; a person can usually snap out of it. When a child or adult suffers from clinical depression, he cannot snap out of it. The unhappy feelings last, and sooner or later, they seem to take over. It is like the sad feelings are in control.

Having clinical depression means that the child not only feels sad, unhappy, or miserable but also experiences several of the symptoms just listed and has problems in daily life because of them. Your child may no longer get along with the family, may stay away from friends, do worse in school, and not get homework done on time. Overcoming this type of depression usually requires quite a bit of effort from the depressed person and the family.

How Does Clinical Depression Come About?

Depression usually starts out as a negative emotional reaction to some stressor. A child may start feeling sad and unhappy because of changes at school, such as no longer having a favorite teacher, or being in a class with a new group of kids. Another child may become miserable and cranky when she is not doing well in a new sport. Some children may feel ignored and become upset when a parent starts a new job and has less time to spend with the family. There may be problems between parents, conflict between a parent and child, the death of a relative or friend, or many small issues piling up. Developing a medical problem also can trigger distress.

When faced with stressful situations, like those described, most children and adolescents feel sad, unhappy, or resentful, but they can shake off those feelings. However, some children can't cope with the problem or the negative emotions. The feelings become deeper or go on and on. Feeling sad, miserable, or cranky may eventually take over. When these feelings seize control, they affect the child's attitude toward people, his or her thinking, and some body functions like sleep.

In other words, clinical depression can start when a person has *not* been able to shake feelings of sadness, unhappiness, and crankiness in response to stress. Feeling sad can create further problems, for example, other kids may choose to avoid a depressed girl. This can cause that girl to feel even more miserable. This then triggers new symptoms and additional problems. All these factors together can result in clinical depression.

What Is Contextual Emotion Regulation Therapy for Depression?

Contextual emotion regulation therapy (CERT) is a psychological treatment for depression. Through CERT, children and adolescents can overcome depression by learning ways to better handle sad and upsetting feelings. As a result, kids can keep sad and upsetting feelings from getting out of hand. In other words, CERT helps your child to improve his or her emotion regulation skills. CERT also teaches ways to solve stressful problem situations.

CERT has three phases. In Phases I and II, the major goals are to reduce your child's depressive symptoms and have him or her feel better. In Phase III, the goal is to teach your child skills to prevent the depression from returning. Sessions are most frequent in Phase I. Time between sessions increases in Phases II and III.

What Is Emotion Regulation?

Sadness, irritability, and anger are examples of emotions. When a feeling lasts a while, it is called a *mood.*

A person's (often automatic) reactions to her emotion determine how strong the emotion gets and how long it lasts. In other words, people's reactions to their own sad feelings can make those feelings stronger and last longer *or* their reactions can reduce those feelings; the process of reacting to our own emotions is called **emotion regulation**. In CERT, we pay a lot of attention to how a person "regulates" feelings or moods of sadness, unhappiness, crankiness, or disappointment. Trying to lessen feelings of sadness and distress is also called *mood repair.*

Ways to Regulate Emotions and Repair Mood

One important goal of emotion regulation is *to feel better,* to lessen the feelings of sadness, unhappiness, crankiness. Getting to feel better has much to do with how a person reacts to his own sadness. Most reactions help to reduce sad feelings so that those feelings do not take over. For example, talking to a parent about sad feelings usually helps a child to feel better. But some reactions will make sadness worse. For example, not getting out of bed and avoiding everyone will worsen the sadness. When a child just thinks on and on about how sad and miserable he feels, that also makes the sadness last longer. Mood repair is about learning different ways to react to sadness so that it does not take control.

Learning to reduce sad and upsetting feelings so that they do not take over is the key to your child overcoming depression. For most children, getting to feel less sad and upset goes along with improvements in other depressive symptoms, such as sleep problems or feeling badly about themselves.

There are many reactions that can help kids feel better when they feel sad. In CERT, we identified three categories or groups of responses through which kids can repair their sad mood: (1) by behavior and action (doing things like projects); (2) by getting others like family or friends to help; and (3) by using their thinking and imagination. We consider these three ways as rooms in a house: The House of Emotion Regulation (ER). Each room includes many specific ways of repairing mood or overcoming sadness; think of these as tools.

The Things to Do (Behavioral or Action) Room

The tools in this room are ways of acting or doing things. For example:

- Do something physical like wash the car, play a sport, go for a walk.
- Help with chores around the house, fix broken items, cook or bake.
- Start a project, play a musical instrument, sing or dance.
- Take care of pets or other living things.

The People (Social-Interpersonal) Room

The tools in this room involve turning to other people for help in feeling better. For example:

- Play with, talk to, or be around friends.
- Talk to Mom or Dad (or another adult) about the sad feeling.
- Ask for advice or emotional support.
- Get a hug from Mom, Dad, or another favorite person.
- Help out a favorite grown-up (e.g., a grandparent) or friend.

The Thinking (Cognitive) Room

Cognitive tools are ways to use one's thinking and imagination to feel better. The tools in this room include forming special mental pictures or doing mental exercises that take the mind away from sadness. Other tools include thinking about sadness and its causes in new ways. For example:

- Make a mental picture of something special, interesting, or colorful.
- Think about a favorite project.
- Sing a song in your mind; count backward from 100; repeat a special word.
- Work on a puzzle or study your favorite subject.
- Think about different ways of explaining what made you sad.

The three ways or domains to manage emotions often overlap. For example, if you go out to dinner with friends to lift your mood, this involves tools from the behavioral (the act of going out), social–interpersonal (the contact with friends), and cognitive (discussions about your feelings) rooms. However, for most children and adults, one domain (or regulatory category) is more important. In the example just described, the social–interpersonal context of regulation may be the most important for you, even if you do not do anything special with your friends, or do not discuss your feelings with them. Just like you, your child prefers some ways to respond to sadness more than others. By working with your therapist, you will come to recognize what seems to work best for your child.

Coping Skills and Problem Solving for Depression

This last phase of CERT has two parts. One part involves continuing to practice the mood repair skills that helped your child to recover from sadness. The other part deals with ways to handle better those stressful situations that can make your child sad or upset. By learning so-called coping skills, your child can handle such situations more effectively when they arise in the future and thereby avoid depression. During coping skills training, you and your child may learn about additional emotion regulation tools as well as problem-solving skills.

To help remember the key problem-solving steps, the phrase WWW.Solve is used in CERT. Here are the steps:

The first **W** stands for **what** is the problem?

The second **W** stands for **who** can help to solve this problem?

The third **W** stands for **ways** to solve the problem. What are the positives and negatives of each way to solve the problem?

Following these steps can make it easier to decide if a particular problem or issue may be solved and what the best approach likely is.

How do you help your child learn to manage feelings of sadness, crankiness, and unhappiness so that those emotions do not take over? How do you also help her develop improved coping skills? The next section explains this process.

Your Role as Parents in CERT

Being the Assistant Coach

In CERT, your therapist, you as parents, and your child have to work together as a **team**. As coaches, the therapist and you will teach and guide the player, your child. Being a good coach is not easy! You will have to keep in mind and follow some rules that have been shown to help players learn. Here is a list of six important things that you, the parent, will be asked to remember when you put on your assistant coach hat.

The Rules of Coaching

A good coach:

1. **Focuses** on the player's abilities and strengths.
2. **Works** with the player on new ways to do things.
3. **Helps** the player to use different abilities to reach goals.
4. **Praises and encourages** the player to keep going!
5. **Hangs in there** and works with the player even if the coach had a bad day!
6. **Learns and practices** because coaches are made, not born.

Between-Session Assignments

At the end of each session, the therapist, you, and your child will decide on an assignment to carry out between sessions. You will be asked to coach your child in completing these assignments. Try to keep notes of your child's progress; this can help to decide what works best. Your therapist may ask you and your child to keep a list of some things that happen in a typical day. Or, you may be asked to maintain a record of when your child gets sad or upset. Depending on your child's age, he also may be asked to keep a list or to work with you on creating one. Such information can give the team a better idea of the problems that can come up. Understanding the *context* in which particular problems surface helps your therapist to identify what makes your child's sadness and crankiness worse, and what can help him feel better.

As the assistant coach, you will help your child to use mood repair tools from the three rooms in The House of ER. The tools your therapist recommends will depend on your child's age, what your child feels comfortable with, and what may have helped him in the past. Each tool should help to prevent sad and upsetting feelings from becoming stronger or taking over.

As the assistant coach, you will be asked to help your child practice using the recommended tools, keep track of the results, and report to the therapist about how the tools did or didn't work. For the tools that work, you will be asked to help your child *practice!* Repeated practice with the tools that help overcome sad feelings is very important. Remember, just like coaching players in a team; if the players don't practice, they lose their skills. *Remember, you as the parent and assistant coach are an important part of your child's recovery.*

In CERT, there is also a set of rules to help your child be a good team player. The therapist will review these rules with you and your child. Part of your role as assistant coach is to help your child follow these rules:

The Rules of Being a Good Team Player

A good team player:

1. **Will try** new ways to do things.
2. **Works with the coaches** to come up with game plans and goals.
3. **Uses words** to tell the coaches how they feel.
4. **Asks for help** when things get tough.
5. **Does *not* give up** even if a game plan doesn't work right away.
6. **Practices, practices, practices** because that's what it takes to reach the goal.

Children Who Are Sad May Act "Bad"

Children with depression often see themselves in negative ways. They have thoughts like "I'm no good." Sometimes, out of frustration, or because they feel miserable, depressed children can come across as disobedient or uncooperative. They may not follow the rules. This often leads to family members and other adults reacting negatively, which can make the child's depression worse.

When you act as the assistant coach, keep in mind that many of your child's negative behaviors are due to the depression. Depression makes children lose their motivation and interest in things, and not want to be with people. Don't forget that depressed children may come across as "bad" and may push away others, including family and friends. Remembering this will help you to not become frustrated when coaching your child.

The Phases of CERT

As the assistant coach, you will help your child use various emotion regulation tools through all stages of CERT. For some children, the tools also may help to manage other symptoms of depression, such as problems with sleep or having low self-esteem.

As your child begins to feel better and is no longer depressed, your therapist will remind you that you are nearing the last phase of CERT, coping skills training, which includes problem solving, as already mentioned. You will be asked to have your child continue to practice the emotion regulation skills, which were learned, as well as new coping strategies and problem-solving approaches that were identified.

To summarize, there are many ways children can feel better when they are sad: get a hug from a parent, jump rope, jog, be with friends, focus on specific mental pictures, be engaged in some project. Via CERT, you and your child learn when and how to use such tools to regulate sad and upsetting emotions. By practicing good mood repair, your child can recover from depression and better handle stressful events in the future.

Frequently Asked Questions

Here are some questions that parents have frequently asked and our answers. Let your therapist know if you have other questions.

Question: Do I have to be an assistant coach all the time, 24 hours a day?

Answer: No! Being the assistant coach is most important when you help your child to carry out CERT assignments, or practice new skills or ways of behaving.

Question: My child acts up mostly to get attention. Aren't some of the things in CERT just ways for my child to always be in the spotlight?

Answer: When we work as a team and make your child the key player, your child is the center of attention. However, the goal of this attention is to help your child become more effective in carrying out his everyday responsibilities and act more appropriately.

Question: My child never does what I tell her! How do I know that my child will do all these new "homework" things?

Answer: Your therapist will always review any CERT assignment with you and your child before a session is finished. The therapist will make sure that your child understands what was planned, is able to do the specific assignment, and is willing to work on it.

Question: I have read that depression is a biochemical problem in the brain. What is CERT's explanation for that?

Answer: Every human function is grounded in the biology and biochemistry of our bodies. Disturbances in feeling are therefore accompanied by some type of change in bodily systems. The use of CERT in depression is based on research that shows a link between emotions, thoughts, behavior, and inner biological processes. Thus, biochemical processes in the brain can be influenced potentially by changing a person's behavior, thinking, and social interaction.

Question: This treatment seems to require a lot of work. Can I be sure that it will cure my child's depression?

Answer: Our goal is to help your child recover from his or her current depression and have better coping skills. As of now, nobody knows for sure the exact causes of depression. Therefore, we cannot yet talk about a cure. However, the skills we teach in CERT are designed to help lessen the risk of further depression for your child, or help nip it in the bud if a depression is about to start.

Question: Now that my child is no longer depressed, can we stop doing CERT exercises, coaching sessions, and similar stuff?

Answer: Let's say that you are coaching a winning team. Do you stop coaching because the team has won? Or, let's say that you practiced good dental hygiene and got an "A" from your dentist at your last checkup. Do you then stop brushing your teeth? So, the answer is this: Whatever strategies helped your child get out of the depression will probably help her to stay free of depression. Try your best to keep up some level of practice and coaching on those strategies that were most useful!

Question: I really want to help my child—but I think that he got his moodiness and depression from his father's side of the family. So, if it's in your blood, can therapy do any good?

Answer: There is some evidence that certain people may inherit a tendency to depression. But what you may inherit from your parents is only a small part of the picture. Other parts have to do with the stresses your child faces and the ways in which she copes with emotions and problems. Even when depression runs in the family, a treatment like CERT can help.

Conclusion

Keeping a hopeful attitude and not giving up are important in CERT. If an assigned mood repair tool does not work out, the team still learns from this—it is not a failure. If your child improves but then feels sad and upset again, do not give up or blame yourself. Remember, it took some time for your child to become depressed, and the depression has lasted for a while. Therefore, it will take some time to find the best road to recovery and to stay on that road.

In CERT, the treatment team works together to help the child overcome depression. Remember, you are the expert on your child. Your child is the star player and, with practice, you can be an expert assistant coach.

References

aan het Rot, M., Mathew, S. J., & Charney, D. S. (2009). Neurobiological mechanisms in major depressive disorder. *Canadian Medical Association Journal, 180*(3), 305–313.

Achenbach, T. M. (2001). *Manual for the Child Behavior Checklist.* Burlington, VT: ASEBA.

Adolphs, R. (2002). Neural systems for recognizing emotion. *Current Opinion in Neurobiology, 12,* 169–177.

Aldao, A. (2013). The future of emotion regulation research: Capturing context. *Perspectives on Psychological Science, 8*(2), 155–172.

Aldao, A., Nolen-Hoeksema, S., & Schweizer, S. (2010). Emotion-regulation strategies across psychopathology: A meta-analytic review. *Clinical Psychology Review, 30,* 217–237.

Alderson-Day, B., & Fernyhough, C. (2015). Inner speech: Development, cognitive functions, phenomenology, and neurobiology. *Psychological Bulletin, 141*(5), 931–965.

Alexander, R., Aragón, O. R., Bookwala, J., Cherbuin, N., Gatt, J. M., Kahrilas, I. J., . . . Styliadis, C. (2021). The neuroscience of positive emotions and affect: Implications for cultivating happiness and wellbeing. *Neuroscience and Biobehavioral Reviews, 121,* 220–249.

American Academy of Child and Adolescent Psychiatry (AACAP). (2001). Practice parameter for the assessment and treatment of children and adolescents with suicidal behavior. *Journal of the American Academy of Child and Adolescent Psychiatry, 40,* 24S–51S.

American Psychiatric Association. (1980). *Diagnostic and statistical manual of mental disorders* (3rd ed.). Washington, DC: Author.

American Psychiatric Association. (1994). *Diagnostic and statistical manual of mental disorders* (4th ed.). Washington, DC: Author.

American Psychiatric Association. (2013). *Diagnostic and statistical manual of mental disorders* (5th ed.). Arlington, VA: Author.

American Psychiatric Association. (2022). *Diagnostic and statistical manual of mental disorders* (5th ed., text rev.). Arlington, VA: Author.

Amso, D., & Scerif, G. (2015). The attentive brain: Insights from developmental cognitive neuroscience. *Nature Reviews Neuroscience, 16*(10), 606–619.

Anderson, K. M., Collins, M. A., Kong, R., Fang, K., Li, J., He, T., . . . Holmes, A. J. (2020). Convergent molecular, cellular, and cortical neuroimaging signatures of major depressive disorder. *Proceedings of the National Academy of Sciences of the USA, 117*(40), 25138–25149.

Andreasen, N. C., & Wasek, P. (1980). Adjustment disorders in adolescents and adults. *Archives of General Psychiatry, 37,* 1166–1170.

Andrés, M. L., Richaud de Minzi, M. C., Castañeiras, C., Canet-Juric, L., & Rodríguez-Carvajal, R. (2016). Neuroticism and depression in children: The role of cognitive emotion regulation strategies. *Journal of Genetic Psychology, 177*(2), 55–71.

Angold, A., & Worthman, C. W. (1993). Puberty onset of gender differences in rates of depression: A developmental, epidemiologic and neuroendocrine perspective. *Journal of Affective Disorders, 29,* 145–158.

Anuar, N., Cumming, J., & Williams, S. (2016). Emotion regulation predicts imagery ability. *Imagination, Cognition, and Personality, 36*(3), 254–269.

Arnberg, A., & Öst, L. G. (2014). CBT for children with depressive symptoms: A meta-analysis. *Cognitive Behaviour Therapy, 43*(4), 275–288.

Augustine, A. A., & Hemenover, S. H. (2009). On the relative effectiveness of affect regulation strategies: A meta-analysis. *Cognition and Emotion, 23,* 1181–1220.

Avenevoli, S., & Merikangas, K. R. (2006). Implications of high-risk family studies for prevention of depression. *American Journal of Preventive Medicine, 31*(6S1), S126–S135.

Avenevoli, S., Stolar, M., Li, J., Dierker, L., & Merikangas, K. R. (2001). Comorbidity of depression in children and adolescents: Models and evidence from a prospective high-risk family study. *Biological Psychiatry, 49,* 1071–1081.

Averill, L. A., Averill, C. L., Kelmendi, B., Abdallah, C. G., & Southwick, S. M. (2018). Stress response modulation underlying the psychobiology of resilience. *Current Psychiatry Reports, 20,* 26–39.

Bahmani, Z., Clark, K., Merrikhi, Y., Mueller, A., Pettine, W., Vanegas, M. I., . . . Noudoost, B. (2019). Prefrontal contributions to attention and working memory. *Current Topics in Behavioral Neuroscience, 41,* 129–153.

Baji, I., Lopez-Duran, N. L., Kovacs, M., George, C. J., Mayer, L., Kapornai, K., . . . Vetró, Á. (2009). Age and sex analyses of somatic complaints and symptom presentation of childhood depression in a Hungarian clinical sample. *The Journal of Clinical Psychiatry, 70,* 1467–1472.

Bargh, J. A., & Chartrand, T. L. (1999). The unbearable automaticity of being. *American Psychologist, 54,* 462–479.

Bariola, E., Gullone, E., & Hughes, E. K. (2011). Child and adolescent emotion regulation: The role of parental emotion regulation and expression. *Clinical Child and Family Psychology Review, 14*(2), 198–212.

Barrett, L. F., Gross, J., Christensen, T. C., & Benvenuto, M. (2001). Knowing what you're feeling and knowing what to do about it: Mapping the relation between emotion differentiation and emotion regulation. *Cognition and Emotion, 15,* 713–724.

Barthel, A. L., Hay, A., Doan, S. N., & Hofmann, S. G. (2018). Interpersonal emotion regulation: A review of social and developmental components. *Behaviour Change, 35*(4), 203–216.

Bebko, G. M., Franconeri, S. L., Ochsner, K. N., & Chiao, J. Y. (2011). Look before you regulate: Differential perceptual strategies underlying expressive suppression and cognitive reappraisal. *Emotion, 11*(4), 732–742.

Beck, A. T. (1967). *Depression: Clinical, experimental and theoretical aspects.* New York: Harper & Row.

Beck, A. T., Rush, A. J., Shaw, B. F., & Emery, G. (1979). *Cognitive therapy of depression.* New York: Guilford Press.

Beck, A. T., Steer, R. A., & Brown, G. K. (1996). *Beck Depression Inventory–second edition (BDI-II).* San Antonio, TX: Pearson.

Beebe, D. W. (2011). Cognitive, behavioral, and functional consequences of inadequate sleep in children and adolescents. *Pediatric Clinics of North America, 58*(3), 649–665.

Belden, A. C., Luby, J. L., Pagliaccio, D., & Barch, D. M. (2014). Neural activation is associated with the cognitive emotion regulation of sadness in healthy children. *Developmental Cognitive Neuroscience, 9,* 136–147.

Berkowitz, L., & Harmon-Jones, E. (2004). Toward an understanding of the determinants of anger. *Emotion, 4,* 107–130.

Best, J. R., & Miller, P. H. (2010). A developmental perspective on executive function. *Child Development, 81*(6), 1641–1660.

Best, J. R., Miller, P. H., & Jones, L. L. (2009). Executive functions after age 5: Changes and correlates. *Developmental Review, 29*(3), 180–200.

Bettis, A. H., Siciliano, R. E., Rogers, B. P., Ichinose, M., & Compas, B. E. (2021). Neural correlates of distraction and reappraisal in the family context: Associations with symptoms of anxiety and depression in youth. *Child Neuropsychology, 27*(5), 573–586.

Betts, J., Gullone, E., & Allen, J. S. (2009). An examination of emotion regulation, temperament, and parenting style as potential predictors of adolescent depression risk status: A correlational study. *British Journal of Developmental Psychology, 27,* 473–485.

Birmaher, B., Ryan, N. D., Williamson, D. E., Brent, D. A., Kaufman, J., Dahl, R., . . . Nelson, B. (1996). Childhood and adolescent depression: A review of the past 10 years. Part I. *Journal of the American Academy of Child and Adolescent Psychiatry, 35,* 1427–1439.

Birmaher, B., Williamson, D. E., Dahl, R. E., Axelson, D. A., Kaufman, J., Dorn, L. D., & Ryan, N. D. (2004). Clinical presentation and course of depression in youth: Does onset in childhood differ from onset in adolescence? *Journal of the American Academy of Child and Adolescent Psychiatry, 43,* 63–70.

Björnsdotter, M., Gordon, I., Pelphrey, K. A., Olausson, H., & Kaiser, M. D. (2014). Development of brain mechanisms for processing affective touch. *Frontiers in Behavioral Neuroscience, 8*(24).

Boldt, L. J., Goffin, K. C., & Kochanska, G. (2020). The significance of early parent-child attachment for emerging regulation: A longitudinal investigation of processes and mechanisms from toddler age to preadolescence. *Developmental Psychology, 56*(3), 431–443.

Bonanno, G. A. (2001). Emotion self-regulation. In T. J. Mayne & G. A. Bonanno (Eds.), *Emotions: Current issues and future directions* (pp. 251–285). New York: Guilford Press.

Bonanno, G. A., & Burton, C. L. (2013). Regulatory flexibility: An individual differences perspective on coping and emotion regulation. *Perspectives on Psychological Science, 8*(6), 591–612.

Booth, J. R., Burman, D. D., Meyer, J. R., Lei, Z., Choy, J., Gitelman, D. R., . . . Mesulam, M. M. (2003). Modality-specific and -independent developmental differences in the neural substrate for lexical processing. *Journal of Neurolinguistics, 16*(4–5), 383–405.

Braungart, J. M., & Stifter, C. A. (1991). Regulation of negative reactivity during the strange situation: Temperament and attachment in 12-month-old infants. *Infant Behavior and Development, 14,* 349–364.

Braunstein, L. M., Gross, J. J., & Ochsner, K. N. (2017). Explicit and implicit emotion regulation: A multi-level framework. *Social Cognitive and Affective Neuroscience, 12*(10), 1545–1557.

Brent, D. A., Kolko, D. J., Birmaher, B., Baugher, M., Bridge, J., Roth, C., & Holder, D. (1998). Predictors of treatment efficacy in a clinical trial of three psychosocial treatments for adolescent depression. *Journal of the American Academy of Child and Adolescent Psychiatry, 37,* 906–914.

Brent, D. A., & Maalouf, F. T. (2009). Pediatric depression: Is there evidence to improve evidence-based treatments? *Journal of Child Psychology and Psychiatry, 50,* 143–152.

Brent, D. A., Perper, J. A., Moritz, G., Allman, C., Friend, A., Roth, C., . . . Baugher, M. (1993). Psychiatric risk factors for adolescent suicide: A case-control study. *Journal of the American Academy of Child and Adolescent Psychiatry, 32,* 521–529.

Bretherton, I. (1985). Attachment theory: Retrospect and prospect. *Monographs of the Society for Research in Child Development, 50* (1–2, Serial No. 209), 3–35.

Brown, G. W., Harris, T. O., & Hepworth, C. (1994). Life events and endogenous depression: A puzzle reexamined. *Archives of General Psychiatry, 51,* 525–534.

Buhle, J. T., Silvers, J. A., Wager, T. D., Lopez, R., Onyemekwu, C., Kober, H., . . . Ochsner, K. N. (2014). Cognitive reappraisal of emotion: A meta-analysis of human neuroimaging studies. *Cerebral Cortex, 24*(11), 2981–2990.

Burke, J., & Loeber, R. (2010). Oppositional defiant disorder and the explanation of the comorbidity between behavioral disorders and depression. *Clinical Psychology: Science and Practice, 17*(4), 319–326.

Burleson, M. H., & Quigley, K. S. (2021). Social interoception and social allostasis through touch: Legacy of the somatovisceral afference model of emotion. *Social Neuroscience, 16*(1), 92–102.

Bylsma, L. M., Yaroslavsky, I., Rottenberg, J.,

Kiss, E., Kapornai, K., Halas, K., . . . Kovacs, M. (2016). Familiality of mood repair responses among youth with and without histories of depression. *Cognition and Emotion, 30*(4), 807–816.

Calkins, S. D. (1994). Origins and outcomes of individual differences in emotion regulation. *Monographs of the Society for Research in Child Development, 59*(2/3), 53–72.

Calkins, S. D., Dollar, J. M., & Wideman, L. (2019). Temperamental vulnerability to emotion dysregulation and risk for mental and physical health challenges. *Development and Psychopathology, 31*(3), 957–970.

Calkins, S. D., Gill, K. L., Johnson, M. C., & Smith, C. L. (1999). Emotional reactivity and emotional regulation strategies as predictors of social behavior with peers during toddlerhood. *Social Development, 8,* 310–334.

Calkins, S. D., & Johnson, M. C. (1998). Toddler regulation of distress to frustrating events: Temperamental and maternal correlates. *Infant Behavior and Development, 21,* 379–395.

Campos, J. J., Mumme, D., Kermoian, R., & Campos, R. G. (1994). A functionalist perspective on the nature of emotion. *Monographs of the Society for Research in Child Development, 59,* 284–303.

Carolson, J. E., Geisinger, K. E., & Jonson, J. L. (Eds.). (2021). *The twenty-first mental measurements yearbook.* Lincoln: University of Nebraska Press.

Carroll, K. M., & Rounsaville, B. J. (2008). Efficacy and effectiveness in developing treatment manuals. In A. M. Nezu & C. M. Nezu (Eds.), *Evidence-based outcome research: A practical guide to conducting randomized controlled trials for psychosocial interventions* (pp. 219–244). New York: Oxford University Press.

Carver, C. S., & Scheier, M. F. (1990). Origins and functions of positive and negative affect: A control-process view. *Psychological Review, 97,* 19–35.

Chan, J. S. Y., Liu, G., Liang, D., Deng, K., Wu, J., & Yan, J. H. (2019). Therapeutic benefits of physical activity for mood: A systemic review on the effects of exercise intensity, duration, and modality [Special issue]. *The Journal of Psychology, 153*(1), 102–125.

Cheung, E. O., Gardner, W. L., & Anderson, J. F. (2015). Emotionships: Examining people's emotion-regulation relationships and their consequences for well-being. *Social Psychological and Personality Science, 6*(4), 407–414.

Cicchetti, D., Ackerman, B. P., & Izard, C. E. (1995). Emotions and emotion regulation in developmental psychopathology. *Development and Psychopathology, 7,* 1–10.

Cicchetti, D., & Toth, S. L. (1998). The development of depression in children and adolescents. *American Psychologist, 53,* 221–241.

Clark, R. A., MacGeorge, E. L., & Robinson, L. (2008). Evaluation of peer comforting strategies by children and adolescents. *Human Communication Research, 34*(2), 319–345.

Coddington, R. D. (1972). The significance of life events as etiologic factors in the diseases of children—I. A survey of professional workers. *Journal of Psychosomatic Research, 16,* 7–18.

Cole, P. M., Martin, S. E., & Dennis, T. A. (2004). Emotion regulation as a scientific construct: Methodological challenges and directions for child development research. *Child Development, 75,* 317–333.

Cole, P. M., Ram, N., & English, M. S. (2019). Toward a unifying model of self-regulation: A developmental approach. *Child Development Perspectives, 13*(2), 91–96.

Collins, N. L., & Read, S. J. (1990). Adult attachment, working models, and relationship quality in dating couples. *Journal of Personality and Social Psychology, 58,* 644–663.

Compas, B. E. (1987). Coping with stress during childhood and adolescence. *Psychological Bulletin, 101,* 393–403.

Compas, B. E., Connor-Smith, J., & Jaser, S. S. (2004). Temperament, stress reactivity, and coping: Implications for depression in childhood and adolescence. *Journal of Clinical Child and Adolescent Psychology, 33,* 21–31.

Compas, B. E., Jaser, S. S., Bettis, A. H., Watson, K. H., Gruhn, M. A., Dunbar, J, P., . . . Thigpen, J. C. (2017). Coping, emotion regulation, and psychopathology in childhood and adolescence: A meta-analysis and narrative review. *Psychological Bulletin, 143*(9), 939–991.

Compas, B. E., Orosan, P. G., & Grant, K. E.

(1993). Adolescent stress and coping: Implications for psychopathology during adolescence. *Journal of Adolescence, 16*, 331–349.

Cooke, J. E., Kochendorfer, L. B., Stuart-Parrigon, K. L., Koehn, A. J., & Kerns, K. A. (2019). Parent-child attachment and children's experience and regulations of emotion: A meta-analytic review. *Emotion, 19*(6), 1103–1126.

Cooney, R. E., Joormann, J., Atlas, L. Y., Eugène, F., & Gotlib, I. H. (2007). Remembering the good times: Neural correlates of affect regulation. *Neuroreport, 18*, 1771–1774.

Cooper, M. L., Frone, M. R., Russell, M., & Mudar, P. (1995). Drinking to regulate positive and negative emotions: A motivational model of alcohol use. *Journal of Personality and Social Psychology, 69*, 990–1005.

Copeland, W. E., Alaie, I., Jonsson, U., & Shanahan, L. (2021). Associations of childhood and adolescent depression with adult psychiatric and functional outcomes. *Journal of the American Academy of Child and Adolescent Psychiatry, 60*(5), 604–611.

Costello, E. J., Erkanli, A., & Angold A. (2006). Is there an epidemic of child or adolescent depression? *Journal of Child Psychology and Psychiatry, 47*, 1263–1271.

Courage, M. L., & Howe, M. L. (2002). From infant to child: The dynamics of cognitive change in the second year of life. *Psychological Bulletin, 128*, 250–277.

Coyne, J. C., Downey, G., & Boergers, J. (1992). Depression in families: A systems perspective. In D. Cicchetti & S. L. Toth (Eds.), *Rochester Symposium on Developmental Psychopathology: Vol 4. Developmental Perspectives on Depression* (pp. 211–249). Rochester, NY: University of Rochester Press.

Cracco, E., Goossens, L., & Braet, C. (2017). Emotion regulation across childhood and adolescence: Evidence for a maladaptive shift in adolescence. *European Child and Adolescent Psychiatry, 26*(8), 909–921.

Criss, M. M., Morris, A. S., Ponce-Garcia, E., Cui, L., & Silk, J. S. (2016). Pathways to adaptive emotion regulation among adolescence from low-income families. *Family Relations, 65*(3), 517–529.

Crucianelli, L., & Filippetti, M. L. (2020). Developmental perspectives on interpersonal affective touch. *Topoi, 39*(3), 575–586.

Crugnola, C. R., Tambelli, R., Spinelli, M., Gazzotti, S., Caprin, C., & Albizzati, A. (2011). Attachment patterns and emotion regulation strategies in the second year. *Infant Behavior and Development, 34*(1), 136–151.

Cumming, J., & Williams, S. E. (2013). Introducing the revised applied model of deliberate imagery use for sport, dance, exercise, and rehabilitation. *Movement and Sports Science-Science and Motricité, 82*, 69–81.

Cummings, C. M., Caporino, N. E., & Kendall, P. C. (2014). Comorbidity of anxiety and depression in children and adolescents: 20 years after. *Psychological Bulletin, 140*(3), 816–845.

Curry, J., Silva, S., Rohde, P., Ginsburg, G., Kratochvil, C., Simons, A., . . . March, J. (2011). Recovery and recurrence following treatment for adolescent major depression. *Archives of General Psychiatry, 68*(3), 263–269.

Cyranowski, J. M., Frank, E., Young, E., & Shear, M. K. (2000). Adolescent onset of the gender difference in lifetime rates of major depression. A theoretical model. *Archives of General Psychiatry, 57*, 21–27.

Czaja, J., Rief, W., & Hilbert, A. (2009). Emotion regulation and binge eating in children. *International Journal of Eating Disorders, 42*(4), 356–362.

Daches, S., Yaroslavsky, I., & Kovacs, M. (2019). The persistence of hedonically-based mood repair among young offspring at high- and low-risk for depression. *Cognition and Emotion, 34*(3), 568–580.

Dahl, R. E. (1996). The regulation of sleep and arousal: Development and psychopathology. *Development and Psychopathology, 8*, 3–27.

Daniel, S. S., & Goldston, D. B. (2012). Hopelessness and lack of connectedness to others as risk factors for suicidal behavior across the lifespan: Implications for cognitive-behavioral treatment. *Cognitive and Behavioral Practice, 19*(2), 288–300.

Davidson, R. J., Jackson, D. C., & Kalin, N. H. (2000). Emotion, plasticity, context, and regulation: Perspectives from affective neuroscience. *Psychological Bulletin, 126*, 890–909.

Davis, E. L., Levine, L. J., Lench, H. C., & Quas, J. A. (2010). Metacognitive emotion regulation: Children's awareness that changing thoughts and goals can alleviate negative emotions. *Emotion, 10,* 498–510.

de Greeff, J. W., Bosker, R. J., Oosterlaan, J., Visscher, C., & Hartman, E. (2017). Effects of physical activity on executive functions, attention, and academic performance in preadolescent children: A meta-analysis. *Journal of Science and Medicine in Sport, 21*(5), 501–507.

DeCou, C. R., Comtois, K. A., & Landes, S. J. (2019). Dialectical behavior therapy is effective for the treatment of suicidal behavior: A meta-analysis. *Behavior Therapy, 50*(1), 60–72.

Dempster, E. L., Burcescu, I., Wigg, K., Kiss, E., Baji, I., Gadoros, J., . . . Barr, C. L. (2007). Evidence of an association between the vasopressin V1b receptor gene (AVPR1B) and childhood-onset mood disorders. *Archives of General Psychiatry, 64,* 1189–1195.

Dennis, T. A., & Kelemen, D. A. (2009). Preschool children's views on emotion regulation: Functional associations and implications for social-emotional adjustment. *International Journal of Behavioral Development, 33,* 243–252.

Derogatis, L. R., & Unger, R. (2010). Symptom Checklist-90—revised. In I. B. Weiner & W. E. Craighead (Eds.), *The Corsini encyclopedia of psychology* (Vol. 4, pp. 1743–1744). Hoboken, NJ: Wiley.

DeWall, C. N., Twenge, J. M., Koole, S. L., Baumeister, R. F., Marquez, A., & Reid, M. W. (2011). Automatic emotion regulation after social exclusion: Tuning to positivity. *Emotion, 11,* 623–636.

Diamond, A. (2013). Executive functions. *Annual Review of Psychology, 64,* 135–168.

Diener, M. L., & Mangelsdorf, S. C. (1999). Behavioral strategies for emotion regulation in toddlers: Associations with maternal involvement and emotional expressions. *Infant Behavior and Development, 22,* 569–583.

Dietz, L. J., Birmaher, B., Williamson, D. E., Silk, J. S., Dahl, R. E., Axelson, D. A., . . . Ryan, N. D. (2008). Mother-child interactions in depressed children and children at high risk and low risk for future depression. *Journal of the American Academy of Child and Adolescent Psychiatry, 47*(5), 574–582.

Dietz, L. J., Mufson, L., Irvine, H., & Brent, D. A. (2008). Family-based interpersonal psychotherapy for depressed preadolescents: An open-treatment trial. *Early Intervention in Psychiatry, 2,* 154–161.

Dietz, L. J., Weinberg, R. J., Brent, D. A., & Mufson, L. (2015). Family-based interpersonal psychotherapy for depressed preadolescents: Examining efficacy and potential treatment mechanisms. *Journal of the American Academy of Child and Adolescent Psychiatry, 54*(3), 191–199.

DiGiuseppe, R., Linscott, J., & Jilton, R. (1996). Developing the therapeutic alliance in child-adolescent psychotherapy. *Applied and Preventive Psychology, 5*(2), 85–100.

DiMaggio, R., Zappulla, C., & Pace, U. (2016). The relationship between emotion knowledge, emotion regulation and adjustment in preschoolers: A mediation model. *Journal of Child and Family Studies, 25*(8), 2626–2635.

Dougherty, L. R., Blankenship, S. L., Spechler, P. A., Padmala, S., & Pessoa, L. (2015). An fMRI pilot study of cognitive reappraisal in children: Divergent effects on brain and behavior. *Journal of Psychopathology and Behavioral Assessment, 37*(4), 634–644.

Dowell, K. A., & Ogles, B. M. (2010). The effects of parent participation on child psychotherapy outcome: A meta-analytic review. *Journal of Clinical Child and Adolescent Psychology, 39*(2), 151–162.

Drake, J. E., & Winner, E. (2013). How children use drawing to regulate their emotions. *Cognition and Emotion, 27*(3), 512–520.

Duggal, S., Carlson, E. A., Sroufe, L. A., & Egeland, B. (2001). Depressive symptomatology in childhood and adolescence. *Development and Psychopathology, 13,* 143–164.

Dunn, V., & Goodyer, I. M. (2006). Longitudinal investigation into childhood- and adolescence-onset depression: Psychiatric outcome in early adulthood. *British Journal of Psychiatry, 188,* 216–222.

Eckshtain, D., Kuppens, S., Ugueto, A., Ng, M. Y., Vaughn-Coaxum, R., Corteselli, K., & Weisz, J. R. (2020). Meta-analysis: 13-year follow-up of psychotherapy effects on youth depression. *Journal of the American Academy of Child and Adolescent Psychiatry, 59*(1), 45–63.

Eid, R. S., Gobinath, A. R., & Galea, L. A. M. (2019). Sex differences in depression: Insights from clinical and preclinical studies. *Progress in Neurobiology, 176*, 86–102.

Eisenberg, N., Fabes, R. A., Guthrie, I. K., & Reiser, M. (2000). Dispositional emotionality and regulation: Their role in predicting quality of social functioning. *Journal of Personality and Social Psychology, 78*, 136–157.

Eisenberg, N., Fabes, R. A., Murphy, B., Maszk, P., Smith, M., & Karbon, M. (1995). The role of emotionality and regulation in children's social functioning: A longitudinal study. *Child Development, 66*, 1360–1384.

Eisenberg, N., & Morris, A. S. (2002). Children's emotion-related regulation. In R. V. Kail (Ed.), *Advances in child development and behavior* (Vol. 30, pp. 189–229). Amsterdam: Academic Press.

Ekas, N. V., Lickenbrock, D. M., & Braungart-Rieker, J. M. (2013). Developmental trajectories of emotion regulation across infancy: Do age and the social partner influence temporal patterns? *Infancy, 18*(5), 729–754.

Ekman, P. (1992). An argument for basic emotions. *Cognition and Emotion, 6*, 169–200.

Endler, N. S., & Parker, J. D. A. (1990a). *Coping Inventory for Stressful Situations (CISS): Manual.* New York: Multi-Health Systems.

Endler, N. S., & Parker, J. D. A. (1990b). Multidimensional assessment of coping: A critical evaluation. *Journal of Personality and Social Psychology, 58*, 844–854.

Erber, R., & Erber, M. W. (2000). The self-regulation of moods: Second thoughts on the importance of happiness in everyday life. *Psychological Inquiry, 11*, 142–148.

Erber, R., & Tesser, A. (1992). Task effort and the regulation of mood: The absorption hypothesis. *Journal of Experimental Social Psychology, 28*, 339–359.

Evans, A. M., Athenstaedt, U., & Krueger, J. I. (2013). The development of trust and altruism during childhood. *Journal of Economic Psychology, 36*, 82–95.

Farver, J. M., & Branstetter, W. H. (1994). Preschoolers' prosocial responses to their peers' distress. *Developmental Psychology, 30*(3), 334–341.

Feighner, J. P., Robins, E., Guze, S. B., Woodruff, R. A., Winokur, G., & Munoz, R. (1972). Diagnostic criteria for use in psychiatric research. *Archives of General Psychiatry, 26*, 57–63.

Feinstein, B. A., Hershenberg, R., Bhatia, V., Latack, J. A., Meuwly, N., & Davila, J. (2013). Negative social comparison on Facebook and depressive symptoms: Rumination as a mechanism. *Psychology of Popular Media Culture, 2*(3), 161–170.

Feng, X., Keenan, K., Hipwell, A. E., Henneberger, A. K., Rischall, M. S., Butch, J., . . . Babinski, D. E. (2009). Longitudinal associations between emotion regulation and depression in preadolescent girls: Moderation by the caregiving environment. *Developmental Psychology, 45*, 798–808.

Ferguson, M. J., & Zayas, V. (2009). Automatic evaluation. *Current Directions in Psychological Science, 18*, 362–366.

Ferro, T., Verdeli, H., Pierre, F., & Weissman, M. M. (2000) Screening for depression in mothers bringing their offspring for evaluation or treatment of depression. *American Journal of Psychiatry, 157*(3), 375–379.

Field, T., Martinez, A., Nawrocki, T., Pickens, J., Fox, N. A., & Schanberg, S. (1998). Music shifts frontal EEG in depressed adolescents. *Adolescence, 33*, 109–116.

Figueira, J. S. B., Pacheco, L. B., Lobo, I., Volchan, E., Pereira, M. G., de Oliveira, L., & David, I. A. (2018). "Keep that in mind!" The role of positive affect in working memory for maintaining goal-relevant information. *Frontiers in Psychology, 9*, 1228.

Fox, N. A., & Calkins, S. D. (2003). The development of self-control of emotion: Intrinsic and extrinsic influences. *Motivation and Emotion, 27*, 7–26.

Frances, A., Widiger, T., & Fyer, M. R. (1990). The influence of classification methods on comorbidity. In J. D. Maser & C. R. Cloninger (Eds.), *Comorbidity of mood and anxiety disorders* (pp. 41–59). Washington, DC: American Psychiatric Press.

Franzen, P. L., & Buysse, D. J. (2008). Sleep disturbances and depression: Risk relationships for subsequent depression and therapeutic implications. *Dialogues in Clinical Neuroscience, 10*(4), 473–481.

Frauenglass, M. H., & Diaz, R. M. (1985).

Self-regulatory functions of children's private speech: A critical analysis of recent challenges to Vygotsky's theory. *Developmental Psychology, 21,* 357–364.

Frey, M., Obermeier, V., von Kries, R., & Schulte-Körme, G. (2020). Age and sex specific incidence for depression from early childhood to adolescence: A 13-year long longitudinal analysis of German health insurance data. *Journal of Psychiatric Research, 129,* 17–23.

Fuhrman, P., Equit, M., Schmidt, K., & von Gontard, A. (2014). Prevalence of depression symptoms and associated developmental disorders in preschool children: A population-based study. *European Child & Adolescent Psychiatry, 23,* 219–224.

Fujiki, M., Brinton, B., & Clarke, D. (2002). Emotion regulation in children with specific language impairment. *Language, Speech, and Hearing Services in Schools, 33,* 102–111.

Garber, J., Braafladt, N., & Weiss, B. (1995). Affect regulation in depressed and nondepressed children and young adolescents. *Development and Psychopathology, 7,* 93–115.

Garber, J., Ciesla, J. A., McCauley, E., Diamond, G., & Schloredt, K. A. (2011). Remission of depression in parents: Links to healthy functioning in their children. *Child Development, 82,* 226–243.

Garnefski, N., & Kraaij, V. (2006). Relationships between cognitive emotion regulation strategies and depressive symptoms: A comparative study of five specific samples. *Personality and Individual Differences, 40*(8), 1659–1669.

Garnefski, N., & Kraaij, V. (2018). Specificity of relations between adolescents' cognitive emotion regulation strategies and symptoms of depression and anxiety. *Cognition and Emotion, 32*(7), 1401–1408.

Garnefski, N., Rieffe, C., Jellesma, F., Terwogt, M. M., & Kraaij, V. (2007). Cognitive emotion regulation strategies and emotional problems in 9–11-year-old children: The development of an instrument. *European Child and Adolescent Psychiatry, 16,* 1–9.

Garrison, K. E., & Schmeichel, B. J. (2022). Getting over it: Working memory capacity and affective responses to stressful events in daily life. *Emotion, 22*(3), 418–429.

Garvey, K. A., Penn, J. V., Campbell, A. L., Esposito-Smythers, C., & Spirito, A. (2009). Contracting for safety with patients: Clinical practice and forensic implications. *Journal of the American Academy of Psychiatry Law, 37*(3), 363–370.

Geller, B., Fox, L. W., & Clark, K. A. (1994). Rate and predictors of prepubertal bipolarity during follow-up of 6- to 12-year-old depressed children. *Journal of the American Academy of Child and Adolescent Psychiatry, 33,* 461–468.

Genuth, A., & Drake, J. E. (2021). The benefits of drawing to regulate sadness and anger: Distraction versus expression. *Psychology of Aesthetics, Creativity, and the Arts, 15*(1), 91–99.

Gili, M., Castellvi, P., Vives, M., de la Torre-Luque, A., Almenara, J., Blasco, M. J., . . . Roca, M. (2019). Mental disorders as risk factors for suicidal behavior in young people: A meta-analysis and systematic review of longitudinal studies. *Journal of Affective Disorders, 245,* 152–162.

Gladstone, T. R. G., Diehl, A., Thomann, L. O., & Beardslee, W. R. (2019). The association between parental depression and child psychosocial intervention outcomes: Directions for future research. *Harvard Review of Psychiatry, 27*(4), 241–253.

Goodman, S. H. (2020). Intergenerational transmission of depression. *Annual Review of Clinical Psychology, 16,* 213–238.

Goodman, S. H., Simon, H. F. M., Shamblaw, A. L., & Kim, C. Y. (2020). Parenting as a mediator of associations between depression in mothers and children's functioning: A systematic review and meta-analysis. *Clinical Child and Family Psychology Review, 23,* 427–460.

Goodyer, I. M., Herbert, J., Secher, S. M., & Pearson, J. (1997). Short-term outcome of major depression: I. Comorbidity and severity at presentation as predictors of persistent disorder. *Journal of the American Academy of Child and Adolescent Psychiatry, 36,* 179–187.

Grant, K. E., Compass, B. E., Thurm, A. E., McMahon, S. D., & Gipson, P. Y. (2004). Stressors and child and adolescent psychopathology: Measurement issues and prospective effects. *Journal of Clinical*

Child and Adolescent Psychology, 33(2), 412–425.

Graziano, P. A., Reavis, R. D., Keane, S. P., & Calkins, S. D. (2007). The role of emotion regulation in children's early academic success. *Journal of School Psychology, 45,* 3–19.

Grenell, A., Prager, E. O., Schaefer, C., Kross, E., Duckworth, A. L., & Carlson, S. M. (2019). Individual differences in the effectiveness of self-distancing for young children's emotion regulation. *British Journal of Developmental Psychology, 37*(1), 84–100.

Grolnick, W. S., Bridges, L. J., & Connell, J. P. (1996). Emotion regulation in two-year-olds: Strategies and emotional expression in four contexts. *Child Development, 67,* 928–941.

Gross, J. J. (1998). The emerging field of emotion regulation: An integrative review. *Review of General Psychology, 2,* 271–299.

Gross, J. J. (1999). Emotion regulation: Past, present, future. *Cognition and Emotion, 13,* 551–573.

Gross, J. J. (2014). Emotion regulation: Conceptual and empirical foundations. In J. J. Gross (Ed.), *Handbook of emotion regulation* (2nd ed., pp. 3–20). New York: Guilford Press.

Gullone, E., Hughes, E. K., King, N. J., & Tonge, B. (2010). The normative development of emotion regulation strategy use in children and adolescents: A 2-year follow-up study. *The Journal of Child Psychology and Psychiatry, 51,* 567–574.

Gummerum, M., & López-Pérez, B. (2020). "You shouldn't feel this way!": Children's and adolescents' interpersonal emotion regulation of victims' and violators' feelings after social exclusion. *Cognitive Development, 54,* Article 100874.

Hammen, C. (2005). Stress and depression. *Annual Review of Clinical Psychology, 1,* 293–319.

Hammen, C. L. (2015). Stress and depression: Old questions, new approaches. *Current Opinion in Psychology, 4,* 80–85.

Hammen, C., Rudolph, K., Weisz, J., Rao, U., & Burge, D. (1999). The context of depression in clinic-referred youth: Neglected areas in treatment. *Journal of the American Academy of Child and Adolescent Psychiatry, 38,* 64–71.

Harman, C., Rothbart, M. K., & Posner, M. I. (1997). Distress and attention interactions in early infancy. *Motivation and Emotion, 21,* 27–43.

Harrington, E. M., Trevino, S. D., Lopez, S., & Giuliani, N. R. (2020). Emotion regulation in early childhood: Implications for socioemotional and academic components of school readiness. *Emotion 20*(1), 48–53.

Harter, S. (2006). The self. In N. Eisenberg, W. Damon, & R. M. Lerner (Eds.), *Handbook of psychology: Social, emotional, and personality development* (pp. 505–570). Hoboken, NJ: Wiley.

Harter, S. (2012). *The construction of the self: Developmental and sociocultural foundations* (2nd ed). New York: Guilford Press.

Harvey, A. G., Murray, G., Chandler, R. A., & Soehner, A. (2011). Sleep disturbance as transdiagnostic: Consideration of neurobiological mechanisms. *Clinical Psychology Review, 31*(2), 225–235.

Hatkevich, C., Penner, F., & Sharp, C. (2019). Difficulties in emotion regulation and suicide ideation and attempt in adolescent inpatients. *Psychiatry Research, 271,* 230–238.

Heim, C., & Binder, E. B. (2012). Current research trends in early life stress and depression: Review of human studies on sensitive periods, gene-environment interactions, and epigenetics. *Experimental Neurology, 233,* 102–111.

Heimpel, S. A., Wood, J. V., Marshall, M. A., & Brown, J. D. (2002). Do people with low self-esteem really want to feel better? Self-esteem differences in motivation to repair negative moods. *Journal of Personality and Social Psychology, 82,* 128–147.

Heiy, J. E., & Cheavens J. S. (2014). Back to basics: A naturalistic assessment of the experience and regulation of emotion. *Emotion, 14*(5), 878–891.

Hemenover, S. H., Augustine, A. A., Shulman, T., Tran, T. Q., & Barlett, C. P. (2008). Individual differences in negative affect repair. *Emotion, 8,* 468–478.

Hendry, A. Johnson, M. H., & Holmboe, K. (2019). Early development of visual attention: Change, stability, and longitudinal associations. *Annual Review of Developmental Psychology, 1*(1), 251–275.

Herd, T., King-Casas, B., & Kim-Spoon, J. (2020). Developmental changes in emotion regulation during adolescence: Associations with socioeconomic risk and family emotional context. *Journal of Youth and Adolescence, 49,* 1545–1557.

Hermes, J., Behne, T., & Rakoczy, H. (2018). The development of selective trust: Prospects for a dual-process account. *Child Development Perspectives, 12*(2), 134–138.

Hertenstein, M. J., & Campos, J. J. (2001). Emotion regulation via maternal touch. *Infancy, 2*(4), 549–566.

Hertenstein, M. J., Keltner, D., App, B., Bulleit, B. A., & Jaskolka, A. R. (2006). Touch communicates distinct emotions. *Emotion, 6,* 528–533.

Heyes, S. B., Pictet, A., Mitchell, H., Raeder, S. M., Lau, J. Y. F., Holmes, E. A., & Blackwell, S. E. (2017). Mental imagery-based training to modify mood and cognitive bias in adolescents: Effects of valence and perspective. *Cognitive Therapy and Research, 41*(1), 73–88.

Hiekkaranta, A. P., Kirtley, O. J., Lafit, G., Decoster, J., Derom, C., de Hert, M., . . . Myin-Germeys, I. (2021). Emotion regulation in response to daily negative and positive events in youth: The role of event intensity and psychopathology. *Behaviour Research and Therapy, 144,* Article 103916.

Hobson, C. J., Kamen, J., Szostek, J., Nethercut, C. M., Tiedmann, J. W., & Wojnarowicz, S. (1998). Stressful life events: A revision and update of the social readjustment rating scale. *International Journal of Stress Management, 5,* 1–23.

Hofer, M. A. (1994). Hidden regulators in attachment, separation, and loss. *Monographs of the Society for Research in Child Development, 59* (2/3), 192–207.

Holmes, T. H., & Rahe, R. H. (1967). The social readjustment rating scale. *Journal of Psychosomatic Research, 11*(2), 213–218.

Howard, K. I., Kopta, S. M., Krause, M. S., & Orlinsky, D. E. (1986). The dose-effect relationship in psychotherapy. *American Psychologist, 41,* 159–164.

Hsu, N. S., Novick, J. M., & Jaeggi, S. M. (2014). The development and malleability of executive control abilities. *Frontiers in Behavioral Neuroscience, 8,* 221.

Imeri, L., & Opp, M. R. (2009). How (and why) the immune system makes us sleep. *Nature Reviews Neuroscience, 10*(3), 199–210.

Isen, A. M. (1985). Asymmetry of happiness and sadness in effects on memory in normal college students: Comment on Hasher, Rose, Zacks, Sanft, and Doren. *Journal of Experimental Psychology: General, 114,* 388–391.

Iwanski, A., Lichtenstein, L., Muhling, L. E., & Zimmermann, P. (2021). Effects of father and mother attachment on depressive symptoms in middle childhood and adolescence: The mediating role of emotion regulation. *Brain Sciences, 11*(9), 1153.

Izard, C. E., & Ackerman, B. P. (2000). Motivational, organizational, and regulatory functions of discrete emotions. In M. Lewis & J. M. Haviland-Jones (Eds.), *Handbook of emotions* (2nd ed., pp. 253–264). New York: Guilford Press.

Jean, A. D. L., Stack, D. M., & Arnold, S. (2014). Investigating maternal touch and infants' self-regulatory behaviours during a modified face-to-face still-face with touch procedure. *Infant and Child Development, 23*(6), 557–574.

Joiner, T. E., Jr. & Metalsky, G. I. (1995). A prospective test of an integrative interpersonal theory of depression: A naturalistic study of college roommates. *Journal of Personality and Social Psychology, 69,* 778–788.

Jones, N. A., & Field, T. (1999). Massage and music therapies attenuate frontal EEG asymmetry in depressed adolescents. *Adolescence, 34,* 529–534.

Jones, R., Yates, W. R., & Zhou, M. H. (2002). Readmission rates for adjustment disorders: Comparison with other mood disorders. *Journal of Affective Disorders, 71,* 199–203.

Jönsson, E. H., Kotilahti, K., Heiskala, J., Wasling, H. B., Olausson, H., Croy, I., . . . Nissilä, I. (2018). Affective and non-affective touch evoke differential brain responses in 2-month-old infants. *NeuroImage, 169,* 162–171.

Joormann, J., Siemer M., & Gotlib, I. H. (2007). Mood regulation in depression: Differential effects of distraction and recall of happy memories on sad mood. *Journal of Abnormal Psychology, 116,* 484–490.

Josephson, B. R., Singer, J. A., & Salovey, P. (1996). Mood regulation and memory: Repairing sad moods with happy memories. *Cognition and Emotion, 10,* 437–444.

Joshanloo, M., & Weijers, D. (2014). Aversion to happiness across cultures: A review of where and why people are averse to happiness. *Journal of Happiness Studies, 15,* 717–735.

Karreman, A., van Tuijl, C., van Aken, M. A. G., & Deković, M. (2006). Parenting and self-regulation in preschoolers: A meta-analysis. *Infant and Child Development, 15*(6), 561–579.

Karver, M., Shirk, S., Handelsman, J. B., Fields, S., Crisp, H., Gudmundsen, G., & McMakin, D. (2008). Relationship processes in youth psychotherapy: Measuring alliance, alliance-building behaviors, and client involvement. *Journal of Emotional and Behavioral Disorders, 16*(1), 15–28.

Kaslow, N. J., Deering, C. G., & Racusin, G. R. (1994). Depressed children and their families. *Clinical Psychology Review, 14,* 39–59.

Kato, T. (2015). The impact of coping flexibility on the risk of depressive symptoms. *PLoS One, 10*(5), e0128307.

Katz, L. Y., Cox, B. J., Gunasekara, S., & Miller, A. L. (2004). Feasibility of dialectical behavior therapy for suicidal adolescent inpatients. *Journal of the American Academy of Child and Adolescent Psychiatry, 43*(3), 276–282.

Kaufman, J., Birmaher, B., Brent, D. A., Rao, U., Flynn, C., Moreci, P., . . . Ryan, N. (1997). Schedule for Affective Disorders and Schizophrenia for School-Age Children–Present and Lifetime version (K-SADS-PL): Initial reliability and validity data. *Journal of the American Academy of Child and Adolescent Psychiatry, 36,* 980–988.

Kemp, J. V. A., Bernier, E., Label, C., & Kopala-Sibley, D. C. (2022). Associations between parental mood and anxiety psychopathology and offspring brain structure: A scoping review. *Clinical Child and Family Psychology Review, 25*(1), 222–247.

Kendler, K. S., Thornton, L. M., & Prescott, C. A. (2001). Gender differences in the rates of exposure to stressful life events and sensitivity to their depressogenic effects. *American Journal of Psychiatry, 158,* 587–593.

Kessler, R. C. (1997). The effects of stressful life events on depression. *Annual Review of Psychology, 48,* 191–214.

Kessler, R. C., & Walters, E. E. (1998). Epidemiology of DSM-III-R major depression and minor depression among adolescents and young adults in the National Comorbidity Survey. *Depression and Anxiety, 7,* 3–14.

Kirsch, I. S., Jungeblut, A., Jenkins, L., & Kolstad, A. (2002). *Adult literacy in America: A first look at the findings of the National Adult Literacy Survey* (3rd ed.). Washington, DC: National Center for Education Statistics.

Kiss, E., Gentzler, A. M., George, C., Kapornai, K., Tamás, Z., Kovacs, M., & Vetró, Á. (2007). Factors influencing mother-child reports of depressive symptoms and agreement among clinically referred depressed youngsters in Hungary. *Journal of Affective Disorders, 100,* 143–151.

Klein, D. N., Lewinsohn, P. M., Seeley, J. R., & Rohde, P. (2001). A family study of major depressive disorder in a community sample of adolescents. *Archives of General Psychiatry, 58,* 13–20.

Klenberg, L., Korkman, M., & Lahti-Nuuttila, P. (2001). Differential development of attention and executive functions in 3- to 12-year-old Finnish children. *Developmental Neuropsychology, 20,* 407–428.

Klerman, G. L., Weissman, M. M., Rounsaville, B. J., & Chevron, E. S. (1984). *Interpersonal psychotherapy of depression.* New York: Basic Books.

Knudsen, E. I. (2018). Neural circuits that mediate selective attention: A comparative perspective. *Trends in Neurosciences, 41*(11), 789–805.

Kobak, R. R., & Sceery, A. (1988). Attachment in late adolescence: Working models, affect regulation, and representations of self and others. *Child Development, 59,* 135–146.

Kobayashi, R., Miyatani, M., & Nakao, T. (2021). High working memory capacity facilitates distraction as an emotion regulation strategy. *Current Psychology, 40,* 1159–1167.

Koole, S. L. (2009). The psychology of emotion regulation: An integrative review. *Cognition and Emotion, 23,* 4–41.

Koole, S. L., Webb, T. L., & Sheeran, P. L.

(2015). Implicit emotion regulation: Feeling better without knowing why. *Current Opinion in Psychology, 3,* 6–10.

Kopp, C. B. (1989). Regulation of distress and negative emotions: A developmental view. *Developmental Psychology, 25,* 343–354.

Korkman, M. (2001). Introduction to the special issue on normal neuropsychological development in the school-age years. *Developmental Neuropsychology, 20*(1), 325–330.

Korkman, M., Kemp, S. L., & Kirk, U. (2001). Effects of age on neurocognitive measures of children ages 5 to 12: A cross-sectional study on 800 children from the United States. *Developmental Neuropsychology, 20*(1), 331–354.

Korkman, M., Lahti-Nuuttila, P., Laasonen, M., Kemp, S. L., & Holdnack, J. (2013). Neurocognitive development in 5- to 16-year-old North American children: A cross-sectional study. *Child Neuropsychology, 19*(5), 516–539.

Kovacs, M. (1986). A developmental perspective on methods and measures in the assessment of depressive disorders: The clinical interview. In M. Rutter, C. Izard, & P. Read (Eds.), *Depression in young people: Developmental and clinical perspectives* (pp. 435–465). New York: Guilford Press.

Kovacs, M. (1996). Presentation and course of major depressive disorder during childhood and later years of the life span. *Journal of the American Academy of Child and Adolescent Psychiatry, 35,* 705–715.

Kovacs, M. (2009). *Manual of contextual emotion regulation therapy for depression in childhood—revised (CERT-CR)* [Self-published]. Pittsburgh, PA: University of Pittsburgh School of Medicine, Department of Psychiatry.

Kovacs, M., Akiskal, H. S., Gatsonis, C., & Parrone, P. L. (1994). Childhood-onset dysthymic disorder: Clinical features and prospective naturalistic outcome. *Archives of General Psychiatry, 51,* 365–374.

Kovacs, M., & Bastiaens, L. J. (1995). The psychotherapeutic management of major depressive and dysthymic disorders in childhood and adolescence: Issues and prospects. In I. M. Goodyer (Ed.), *The depressed child and adolescent: Developmental and clinical perspectives* (pp. 281–310). New York: Cambridge University Press.

Kovacs, M., Devlin, B., Pollock, M., Richards, C., & Mukerji, P. (1997). A controlled family history study of childhood-onset depressive disorder. *Archives of General Psychiatry, 54,* 613–623.

Kovacs, M., Feinberg, T. L., Crouse-Novak, M. A., Paulauskas, S. L., & Finkelstein, R. (1984a). Depressive disorders in childhood: I. A longitudinal prospective study of characteristics and recovery. *Archives of General Psychiatry, 41,* 229–237.

Kovacs, M., Feinberg, T. L., Crouse-Novak, M. A., Paulauskas, S. L., Pollock, M., & Finkelstein, R. (1984b). Depressive disorders in childhood: II. A longitudinal study of the risk for a subsequent major depression. *Archives of General Psychiatry, 41,* 643–649.

Kovacs, M., Gatsonis, C., Paulauskas, S. L., & Richards, C. (1989). Depressive disorders in childhood: IV. A longitudinal study of comorbidity with and risk factors for anxiety disorders. *Archives of General Psychiatry, 46,* 776–782.

Kovacs, M., Gatsonis, C., Pollock, M., & Parrone, P. L. (1994). A controlled prospective study of DSM-III adjustment disorder in childhood. *Archives of General Psychiatry, 51,* 535–541.

Kovacs, M., & George, C. J. (2020). Maladaptive mood repair predicts suicidal behaviors among young adults with depression histories. *Journal of Affective Disorders, 265,* 558–566.

Kovacs, M., Goldston, D., & Gatsonis, C. (1993). Suicidal behaviors and childhood-onset depressive disorders: A longitudinal investigation. *Journal of the American Academy of Child and Adolescent Psychiatry, 32,* 8–20.

Kovacs, M., Joormann, J., & Gotlib, I. H. (2008). Emotion (dys)regulation and links to depressive disorders. *Child Development Perspectives, 2,* 149–155.

Kovacs, M., Lopez-Duran, N. L., Mayer, L., George, C., Baji, L., Kiss, E., . . . Kapornai, K. (2019). The development of mood repair response repertories: I. Age-related changes among 7- to 14-year-old depressed and control children and adolescents. *Journal of Clinical Child and Adolescent Psychology, 48*(1), 143–152.

Kovacs, M., & Multi-Health Systems (MHS)

Staff (2011). *Children's Depression Inventory—second edition.* North Tonawanda, NY: MHS.

Kovacs, M., Obrosky, D. S., Gatsonis, C., & Richards, C. (1997). First-episode major depressive and dysthymic disorder in childhood: Clinical and sociodemographic factors in recovery. *Journal of the American Academy of Child and Adolescent Psychiatry, 36,* 777–784.

Kovacs, M., Obrosky, S., & George, C. (2016). The course of major depressive disorder from childhood to young adulthood: Recovery and recurrence in a longitudinal observational study. *Journal of Affective Disorders, 203,* 374–381.

Kovacs, M., & Paulauskas, S. L. (1984). Developmental stage and the expression of depressive disorders in children: An empirical analysis. In D. Cicchetti, & K. Schneider-Rosen (Eds.), *Childhood depression* (New Directions for Child Development, Issue 26, pp. 59–80). San Francisco: Jossey-Bass.

Kovacs, M., Paulauskas, S., Gatsonis, C., & Richards, C. (1988). Depressive disorders in childhood. III. A longitudinal study of comorbidity with and risk for conduct disorders. *Journal of Affective Disorders, 15,* 205–217.

Kovacs, M., Rottenberg, J., & George, C. (2009). Maladaptive mood repair responses distinguish young adults with early-onset depressive disorders and predict future depression outcomes. *Psychological Medicine, 39,* 1841–1854.

Kovacs, M., & Sherrill, J. T. (2001). The psychotherapeutic management of major depressive and dysthymic disorders in childhood and adolescence: Issues and prospects. In I. M. Goodyer (Ed.), *The depressed child and adolescent* (2nd ed., pp. 325–352). New York: Cambridge University Press.

Kovacs, M., Sherrill, J., George, C. J., Pollock, M., Tumuluru, R. V., & Ho, V. (2006). Contextual emotion-regulation therapy for childhood depression: Description and pilot testing of a new intervention. *Journal of the American Academy of Child and Adolescent Psychiatry, 45,* 892–903.

Kovacs, M., Yaroslavsky, I., Rottenberg, J., George, C. J., Baji, I., Benák, I., . . . Kapornai, K. (2015). Mood repair via attention refocusing or recall of positive autobiographical memories by adolescents with pediatric-onset major depression. *Journal of Child Psychology and Psychiatry, 56*(10), 1108–1117.

Kraaij, V., & Garnefski, N. (2019). The behavioral emotion regulation questionnaire: Development, psychometric properties and relationships with emotional problems and the cognitive emotion regulation questionnaire. *Personality and Individual Differences, 137,* 56–61.

Kramer, A. F., Gonzalez de Sather, J. C. M., & Cassavaugh, N. D. (2005). Development of attentional and oculomotor control. *Developmental Psychology, 41,* 760–772.

Kramer, L. (2014). Learning emotional understanding and emotion regulation through sibling interaction. *Early Education and Development, 25*(2), 160–184.

Kronk, C. M. (1994). Private speech in adolescents. *Adolescence, 29,* 781–804.

Kudinova, A. Y., James, K., & Gibb, B. E. (2018). Cognitive reappraisal and depression in children with a parent history of depression. *Journal of Abnormal Child Psychology, 46,* 849–856.

Kuhl, P. K. (2000). A new view of language acquisition. *Proceedings of the National Academy of Sciences of the United States of America, 97*(22), 11850–11857.

Kuhn, D. (2000). Metacognitive development. *Current Directions in Psychological Science, 9,* 178–181.

Lacey, M. F., Wilhelm, R. A., & Gable, P. A. (2021). What is it about positive affect that alters attentional scope? *Current Opinion in Behavioral Sciences, 39,* 185–189.

Larsen, R. J. (2000). Toward a science of mood regulation. *Psychological Inquiry, 11,* 129–141.

Larsen, R. J., & Diener, E. (1987). Affect intensity as an individual difference characteristic: A review. *Journal of Research in Personality, 21,* 1–39.

Lavelli, M., Carra, C., Rossi, G., & Keller, H. (2019). Culture-specific development of early mother-infant emotional co-regulation: Italian, Cameroonian, and West African immigrant dyads. *Developmental Psychology, 55*(9), 1850–1867.

Lawrence, H. R., Burke, T. A., Sheehan, A. E.,

Pastro, B., Levin, R. Y., Walsh, R. F. L., . . . Liu, R. T. (2021). Prevalence and correlates of suicidal ideation and suicide attempts in preadolescent children: A US population-based study. *Translational Psychiatry, 11*(1), 489.

Lazarus, R. S., & Folkman, S. (1984). *Stress, appraisal, and coping.* New York: Springer.

Lazarus, R. S., & Folkman, S. (1991). The concept of coping. In A. Monat & R. S. Lazarus (Eds.), *Stress and coping. An anthology* (pp. 189–206). New York: Columbia University Press.

LeBourgeois, M. K., Giannotti, F., Cortesi, F., Wolfson, A. R., & Harsh, J. (2005). The relationship between reported sleep quality and sleep hygiene in Italian and American adolescents. *Pediatrics, 115*(1), 257–265.

Lee, T.-W., & Xue, S.-W. (2018). Does emotion regulation engage the same neural circuit as working memory? A meta-analytical comparison between cognitive reappraisal of negative emotion and 2-back working memory task. *PLOS ONE, 13*(9), Article e0203753.

Leehr, E. J., Krohmer, K., Schag, K., Dresler, T., Zipfel, S., & Giel, K. E. (2015). Emotion regulation model in binge eating disorder and obesity—a systematic review. *Neuroscience and Biobehavioral Reviews, 49,* 125–134.

LeMoult, J. (2020). From stress to depression: Bringing together cognitive and biological science. *Current Directions in Psychological Science, 29*(6), 592–598.

LeMoult, J., Humphreys, K. L., Tracy, A., Hoffmeister, J.-A., Ip, E., & Gotlib, I. H. (2020). Meta-analysis: Exposure to early life stress and risk for depression in childhood and adolescence. *Journal of the American Academy of Child and Adolescent Psychiatry, 59*(7), 842–855.

Lennarz, H. K., Hollenstein, T., Lichtwarck-Aschoff, A., Kuntsche, E., & Granic, I. (2019). Emotion regulation in action: Use, selection, and success of emotion regulation in adolescents' daily lives. *International Journal of Behavioral Development, 43*(1), 1–11.

Lepore, S. J. (1997). Expressive writing moderates the relation between intrusive thoughts and depressive symptoms. *Journal of Personality and Social Psychology, 5,* 1030–1037.

Levy, K. N., Ellison, W. D., Scott, L. N., & Bernecker, S. L. (2011). Attachment style. *Journal of Clinical Psychology: In Session, 67*(2), 193–203.

LeWinn, K. Z., Strigo, I. A., Connolly, C. G., Ho, T. C., Tymofiyeva, O., Sacchet, M. D., . . . Yang, T. T. (2018). An exploratory examination of reappraisal success in depressed adolescents: Preliminary evidence of functional differences in cognitive control brain regions. *Journal of Affective Disorders, 240,* 155–164.

Lewinsohn, P. M., & Graf, M. (1973). Pleasant activities and depression. *Journal of Consulting and Clinical Psychology, 41,* 261–268.

Lewinsohn, P. M., Hops, H., Roberts, R. E., Seeley, J. R., & Andrews, J. A. (1993). Adolescent psychopathology: I. Prevalence and incidence of depression and other DSM-III-R disorders in high school students. *Journal of the Abnormal Psychology, 102,* 133–144.

Lewinsohn, P. M., Rohde, P., & Seeley, J. R. (1998). Major depressive disorder in older adolescents: Prevalence, risk factors, and clinical implications. *Clinical Psychology Review, 18,* 765–794.

Lewinsohn, P. M., Sullivan, J. M., & Grosscup, S. J. (1980). Changing reinforcing events: An approach to the treatment of depression. *Psychotherapy: Theory, Research, and Practice, 17,* 322–334.

Lewis, F. C., Reeve, R. A., & Johnson, K. A. (2018). A longitudinal analysis of the attention networks in 6- to 11-year-old children. *Child Neuropsychology, 24*(2), 145–165.

Liu, X., Buysse, D. J., Gentzler, A. L., Kiss, E., Mayer, L., Kapornai, K., . . . Kovacs, M. (2007). Insomnia and hypersomnia associated with depressive phenomenology and comorbidity in childhood depression. *Sleep, 30*(1), 83–90.

Liu, X., Gentzler, A. L., Tepper, P., Kiss, E., Kothencné, V. O., Tamás, Z., . . . Kovacs, M. (2006). Clinical features of depressed children and adolescents with various forms of suicidality. *Journal of Clinical Psychiatry, 67,* 1442–1450.

Loevaas, M. E. S., Sund, A. M., Patras, J., Martinsen, K., Hjemdal, O., Neumer, S.-P., . . . Reinfjell, T. (2018). Emotion regulation and its relation to symptoms of anxiety and depression in children aged 8–12 years:

Does parental gender play a differentiating role? *BMC Psychology, 6*(42).

López-Pérez, B., & Pacella D. (2021). Interpersonal emotion regulation in children: Age, gender, and cross-cultural differences using a serious game. *Emotion, 21*(1), 17–27.

López-Pérez, B., Wilson, E. L., Dellaria, G., & Gummerum, M. (2016). Developmental differences in children's interpersonal emotion regulation. *Motivation and Emotion, 40*(5), 767–780.

Luby, J. L., Barch, D. M., Whalen, D., Tillman, R., & Freedland, K. E. (2018). A randomized controlled trial of parent-child psychotherapy targeting emotion development for early childhood depression. *American Journal of Psychiatry, 175*(11), 1102–1110.

Luby, J. L., Belden, A. C., & Spitznagel, E. (2006). Risk factors for preschool depression: The mediating role of early stressful life events. *Journal of Child Psychology and Psychiatry, 47,* 1292–1298.

Luby, J. L., Heffelfinger, A. K., Mrakotsky, C., Brown, K. M., Hessler, M. J., Wallis, J. M., & Spitznagel, E. L. (2003). The clinical picture of depression in preschool children. *Journal of the American Academy Child and Adolescent Psychiatry, 42*(3), 340–348.

Luby, J. L., Heffelfinger, A. K., Mrakotsky, C., Hessler, M. J., Brown, K. M., & Hildebrand, T. (2002). Preschool major depressive disorder: Preliminary validation for developmentally modified DSM-IV criteria. *Journal of the American Academy of Child and Adolescent Psychiatry, 41*(8), 928–937.

Luby, J. L., Whalen, D., Tillman, R., & Barch, D. M. (2019). Clinical and psychosocial characteristics of young children with suicidal ideation, behaviors, and nonsuicidal self-injurious behaviors. *Journal of the American Academy of Child and Adolescent Psychiatry, 58*(1), 117–127.

Lucas-Molina, B., Quintanilla, L., Sarmento-Henrique, R., Babarro, J. M., & Giménez-Dasí, M. (2020). The relationship between emotion regulation and emotion knowledge in preschoolers: A longitudinal study. *International Journal of Environmental Research and Public Health, 17*(16), 5726.

Luinge, M. R., Post, W. J., Wit, H. P., & Goorhuis-Brouwer, S. M. (2006). The ordering of milestones in language development for children from 1 to 6 years of age. *Journal of Speech, Language, and Hearing Research, 49*(5), 923–940.

Luminet, O., Bouts, P., Delie, F., Manstead, A. S. R., & Rimé, B. (2000). Social sharing of emotion following exposure to a negatively valenced situation. *Cognition and Emotion, 14,* 661–688.

Lyubomirsky, S., Kasri, F., & Zehm, K. (2003). Dysphoric rumination impairs concentration on academic tasks. *Cognitive Therapy and Research, 27,* 309–330.

Lyubomirsky, S., & Nolen-Hoeksema, S. (1993). Self-perpetuating properties of dysphoric rumination. *Journal of Personality and Social Psychology, 65,* 339–349.

Ma, X., Tamir, M., & Miyamoto, Y. (2018). A socio-cultural instrumental approach to emotion regulation: Culture and the regulation of positive emotions. *Emotion, 18*(1), 138–152.

Maalouf, F. T., & Brent, D. A. (2012). Child and adolescent depression intervention overview: What works, for whom and how well? *Child and Adolescent Psychiatric Clinics of North America, 21*(2), 299–312.

Mangelsdorf, S. C., Shapiro, J. R., & Marzolf, D. (1995). Developmental and temperamental differences in emotion regulation in infancy. *Child Development, 66,* 1817–1828.

Manian, N., & Bornstein, M. H. (2009). Dynamics of emotion regulation in infants of clinically depressed and nondepressed mothers. *Journal of Child Psychology and Psychiatry, 50,* 1410–1418.

Manly, T., Anderson, V., Nimmo-Smith, I., Turner, A., Watson, P., & Robertson, I. H. (2001). The differential assessment of children's attention: The test of everyday attention for children (TEA-Ch), normative sample and ADHD performance. *The Journal of Child Psychology and Psychiatry, 42*(8), 1065–1081.

Maria, A., Hirvi, P., Kotilahti, K., Heiskala, J., Tuulari, J. J., Karlsson, L., . . . Nissilä, I. (2022). Imaging affective and non-affective touch processing in two-year-old children. *NeuroImage, 251,* Article 118983.

Maser, J. D., & Cloninger, C. R. (Eds.). (1990). *Comorbidity of mood and anxiety disorders.*

Washington, DC: American Psychiatric Press.

Masi, G., Millepiedi, S., Mucci, M., Pascale, R. R., Perugi, G., & Akiskal, H. S. (2003). Phenomenology and comorbidity of dysthymic disorder in 100 consecutively referred children and adolescents: Beyond DSM-IV. *Canadian Journal of Psychiatry, 48*(2), 99–105.

Maswood, R., Rasmussen, A. S., & Rajaram, S. (2019). Collaborative remembering of emotional autobiographical memories: Implications for emotion regulation and collective memory. *Journal of Experimental Psychology: General, 148*(1), 65–79.

Matsumoto, D., Yoo, S. H., Nakagawa, S., & 37 members of the Multinational Study of Cultural Display Rules. (2008). Culture, emotion regulation, and adjustment. *Journal of Personality and Social Psychology, 94*(6), 925–937.

Mauss, I. B., Bunge, S. A., & Gross, J. J. (2007). Automatic emotion regulation. *Social and Personality Psychology Compass, 1/1,* 146–167.

Mayer, L., Lopez-Duran, N. L., Kovacs, M., George, C. J., Baji, I., Kapornai, K., . . . Vetró, Á. (2009). Stressful life events in a clinical sample of depressed children in Hungary. *Journal of Affective Disorders, 115,* 207–214.

McCauley, E., Myers, K., Mitchell, J., Calderon, R., Schloredt, K., & Treder, R. (1993). Depression in young people: Initial presentation and clinical course. *Journal of the American Academy of Child and Adolescent Psychiatry, 32,* 714–722.

McDermott, J. F., & Char, W. F. (1984). Stage-related models of psychotherapy with children. *Journal of the American Academy of Child Psychiatry, 23,* 537–543.

McDonough-Caplan, H., Klein, D. N., & Beauchaine, T. P. (2018). Comorbidity and continuity of depression and conduct problems from elementary school to adolescence. *Journal of Abnormal Psychology, 127*(3), 326–337.

McIntosh, A. M., Sullivan, P. F., & Lewis, C. M. (2019). Uncovering the genetic architecture of major depression. *Neuron, 102,* 91–103.

McLeod, B. D., Wood, J. J., & Weisz, J. R. (2007). Examining the association between parenting and childhood anxiety: A meta-analysis. *Clinical Psychology Review, 27,* 155–172.

McRae, K., Gross, J. J., Weber, J., Robertson, E. R., Sokol-Hessner, P., Ray, R. D., . . . Ochsner, K. N. (2012). The development of emotion regulation: An fMRI study of cognitive reappraisal in children, adolescents and young adults. *Social Cognitive and Affective Neuroscience, 7*(1), 11–22.

Melero, S., Orgilés, M., Espada, J. P., & Morales, A. (2021). How does depression facilitate psychological difficulties in children? The mediating role of cognitive emotion regulation strategies. *Clinical Psychology and Psychotherapy, 28*(2), 384–393.

Melvin, G. A., Dudley, A. L., Gordon, M. S., Ford, S., Taffe, J., & Tonge, B. J. (2013). What happens to depressed adolescents? A follow-up study into early adulthood. *Journal of Affective Disorders, 151*(1), 298–305.

Messer, S. C., & Gross, A. M. (1995). Childhood depression and family interaction: A naturalistic observation study. *Journal of Clinical Child Psychology, 24,* 77–88.

Miguel, H. O., Gonçalves, Ó. F., Cruz, S., & Sampaio, A. (2019a). Infant brain response to affective and discriminative touch: A longitudinal study using fNIRS. *Social Neuroscience, 14*(5), 571–582.

Miguel, H. O., Gonçalves, Ó. F., & Sampaio, A. (2019b). Behavioral response to tactile stimuli relates to brain response to affective touch in 12-month-old infants. *Developmental Psychobiology, 62*(1), 107–115.

Miguel, H. O., Lisboa, I. C., Gonçalves, Ó., & Sampaio, A. (2019c). Brain mechanisms for processing discriminative and affective touch in 7-month-old infants. *Developmental Cognitive Neuroscience, 35,* 20–27.

Mikolajczak, M., Petrides, K. V., & Hurry, J. (2009). Adolescents choosing self-harm as an emotion regulation strategy: The protective role of trait emotional intelligence. *British Journal of Clinical Psychology, 48*(2), 181–193.

Mikulincer, M., Shaver, P. R., & Pereg, D. (2003). Attachment theory and affect regulation: The dynamics, development, and cognitive consequences of attachment-related strategies. *Motivation and Emotion, 27,* 77–102.

Miller, E. K., & Buschman, T. J. (2013). Cortical circuits for the control of attention. *Current Opinion in Neurobiology, 23*(2), 216–222.

Moreau, D., Mufson, L., Weissman, M. M., & Klerman, G. L. (1991). Interpersonal psychotherapy for adolescent depression: Description of modification and preliminary application. *Journal of the American Academy of Child and Adolescent Psychiatry, 30*, 642–651.

Morris. A. S., Criss, M. M., Silk, J. S., & Houltberg, B. J. (2017). The impact of parenting on emotion regulation during childhood and adolescence. *Child Development Perspectives, 11*(4), 233–238.

Morris, A. S., Silk, J. S., Morris, M. D. S., Steinberg, L., Aucoin, K. J., & Keyes, A. W. (2011). The influence of mother–child emotion regulation strategies on children's expression of anger and sadness. *Developmental Psychology, 47*(1), 213–225.

Morris, A. S., Silk, J. S., Steinberg, L., Myers, S. S., & Robinson, L. R. (2007). The role of the family context in the development of emotion regulation. *Social Development, 16*, 361–388.

Morris, W. N. (2000). Some thoughts about mood and its regulation. *Psychological Inquiry, 11*, 200–202.

Morris, W. N., & Reilly, N. P. (1987). Toward the self-regulation of mood: Theory and research. *Motivation and Emotion, 11*, 215–249.

Morrow, J., & Nolen-Hoeksema, S. (1990). Effects of responses to depression on the remediation of depressive affect. *Journal of Personality and Social Psychology, 58*, 519–527.

Mufson, L., Moreau, D., Weissman, M. M., Wickramaratne, P., Martin, J., & Samoilov, A. (1994). Modification of interpersonal psychotherapy with depressed adolescents (IPT-A): Phase I and II studies. *Journal of the American Academy of Child and Adolescent Psychiatry, 33*, 695–705.

Muijs, D., & Bokhove, C. (2020). *Metacognition and self-regulation: Evidence review.* London: Education Endowment Foundation.

Murray, E. A. (2007). The amygdala, reward and emotion. *Trends in Cognitive Sciences, 11*, 489–497.

Neacsiu, A. D., Fang, C. M., Rodriguez, M., & Rosenthal, M. Z. (2018). Suicidal behavior and problems with emotion regulation. *Suicide and Life-Threatening Behavior, 48*(1), 52–74.

Nestler, E. J., & Carlezon, W. A., Jr. (2006). The mesolimbic dopamine reward circuit in depression. *Biological Psychiatry, 59*, 1151–1159.

Neuman, R. J., Geller, B., Rice, J. P., & Todd, R. D. (1997). Increased prevalence and earlier onset of mood disorders among relatives of prepubertal versus adult probands. *Journal of the American Academy of Child and Adolescent Psychiatry, 36*, 466–473.

Newcorn, J. H., & Strain, J. (1992). Adjustment disorder in children and adolescents. *Journal of the American Academy of Child and Adolescent Psychiatry, 31*, 318–327.

Niven, K., Totterdell, P., & Holman, D. (2009). A classification of controlled interpersonal affect regulation strategies. *Emotion, 9*, 498–509.

Nock, M. K., Borges, G., Bromet, E. J., Cha, C. B., Kessler, R. C., & Lee, S. (2008) Suicide and suicidal behavior. *Epidemiologic Reviews, 30*(1), 133–154.

Nolen-Hoeksema, S., & Girgus, J. S. (1994). The emergence of gender differences in depression during adolescence. *Psychological Bulletin, 115*, 424–443.

Nook, E. C., Bustamante, C. M. V., Cho, H. Y., & Somerville, L. H. (2020). Use of linguistic distancing and cognitive reappraisal strategies during emotion regulation in children, adolescents, and young adults. *Emotion, 20*(4), 525–540.

Ogren, M., & Johnson, S. P. (2020). Factors facilitating early emotion understanding development: Contributions to individual differences. *Human Development, 64*(3), 108–118.

Olausson, H., Lamarre, Y., Backlund, H., Morin, C., Wallin, B. G., Starck, G., . . . Bushnell, M. C. (2002). Unmyelinated tactile afferents signal touch and project to insular cortex. *Nature Neuroscience, 5*, 900–904.

Olulade, O. A., Seydell-Greenwald, A., Chambers, C. E., Turkeltaub, P. E., Dromerick, A. W., Berl, M. M., . . . Newport, E. L. (2020). The neural basis of language development: Changes in lateralization over age. *Proceedings of the National Academy of Sciences of the United States of America, 117*(38), 23477–23483.

Orvell, A., Ayduk, Ö., Moser, J. S., Gelman, S. A., & Kross, E. (2019). Linguistic shifts: A relatively effortless route to emotion regulation? *Current Directions in Psychological Science, 28*(6), 567–573.

Palagini, L., Gemignani, A., & Guazzelli, M. (2012). Significance of REM sleep in depression: Effects on neurogenesis. *Journal of Sleep Disorders and Therapy, 1*(3), e109.

Pagliaccio, D., Alqueza, K. L., Marsh, R., & Auerbach, R. P. (2020). Brain volume abnormalities in youth at high risk for depression: Adolescent brain and cognitive development study. *Journal of the American Academy of Child and Adolescent Psychiatry, 59*(10), 1178–1188.

Park, C., Rosenblat, J. D., Brietzke, E., Pan, Z., Lee, Y., Cao, B., . . . McIntyre, R. S. (2019). Stress, epigenetics and depression: A systematic review. *Neuroscience and Biobehavioral Reviews, 102*, 139–152.

Parkinson, B., & Totterdell, P. (1999). Classifying affect-regulation strategies. *Cognition and Emotion, 13*, 277–303.

Parrott, W. G. (1993). Beyond hedonism: Motives for inhibiting good moods and for maintaining bad moods. In D. M. Wegner & J. W. Pennebaker (Eds.), *Handbook of mental control* (pp. 278–305). Englewood Cliffs, NJ: Prentice Hall.

Parsafar, P., Fontanilla, F. L., & Davis, E. L. (2019). Emotion regulation strategy flexibility in childhood: When do children switch between different strategies? *Journal of Experimental Child Psychology, 183*, 1–18.

Paul, K., Pourtois, G., van Steenbergen, H., Gable, P., & Dreisbach, G. (2021). Finding a balance: Modulatory effects of positive affect on attentional and cognitive control. *Current Opinion in Behavioral Sciences, 39*, 136–141.

Peña-Sarrionandia, A., Mikolajczak, M., & Gross, J. J. (2015). Integrating emotion regulation and emotional intelligence traditions: A meta-analysis. *Frontiers in Psychology, 6*, Article 160.

Perone, S., Simmering, V. R., & Buss, A. T. (2021). A dynamical reconceptualization of executive-function development. *Perspectives on Psychological Science, 16*(6), 1198–1208.

Petersen, S. E., & Posner, M. I. (2012). The attention system of the human brain: 20 years after. *Annual Review of Neuroscience, 35*, 73–89.

Pomerantz, E. M., & Rudolph, K. D. (2003). What ensues from emotional distress? Implications for competence estimation. *Child Development, 74*, 329–345.

Pons, F., Harris, P. L., & de Rosnay, M. (2004). Emotion comprehension between 3 and 11 years: Developmental periods and hierarchical organization. *European Journal of Developmental Psychology, 1*, 127–152.

Pons, F., Lawson, J., Harris, P. L., & de Rosnay, M. (2003). Individual differences in children's emotion understanding: Effects of age and language. *Scandinavian Journal of Psychology, 44*, 347–353.

Portugal, E. M. M., Cevada, T., Monteiro-Junior, R. S., Guimarães, T. T., da Cruz Rubini, E., Lattari, E., . . . Deslandes, A. C. (2013). Neuroscience of exercise: From neurobiology mechanisms to mental health. *Neuropsychobiology, 68*(1), 1–14.

Posner, M. I., & Rothbart, M. K. (2000). Developing mechanisms of self-regulation. *Development and Psychopathology, 12*(3), 427–441.

Post, R. M. (1992). Transduction of psychosocial stress into the neurobiology of recurrent affective disorder. *American Journal of Psychiatry, 149*, 999–1010.

Puig-Antich, J., Dahl, R., Ryan, N., Novacenko, H., Goetz, D., Goetz, R., . . . Klepper, T. (1989). Cortisol secretion in prepubertal children with major depressive disorder. *Archives of General Psychiatry, 46*, 801–809.

Puig-Antich, J., Lukens, E., Davies, M., Goetz, D., Brennan-Quattrock, J., & Todak, G. (1985a). Psychosocial functioning in prepubertal major depressive disorders: I. Interpersonal relationships during the depressive episode. *Archives of General Psychiatry, 42*, 500–507.

Puig-Antich, J., Lukens, E., Davies, M., Goetz, D., Brennan-Quattrock, J., & Todak, G. (1985b). Psychosocial functioning in prepubertal major depressive disorders: II. Interpersonal relationships after sustained recovery from affective episode. *Archives of General Psychiatry, 42*, 511–517.

Puig-Antich, J., Perel, J. M., Lupatkin, W., Chambers, W. J., Shea, C., Tabrizi, M. A., & Stiller, R. L. (1979). Plasma levels of imipramine (IMI) and desmethylimipramine (DMI) and clinical response in prepubertal major depressive disorder: A preliminary report. *Journal of the American Academy of Child and Adolescent Psychiatry, 18,* 616–627.

Quirin, M., Bode, R. C., & Kuhl, J. (2011). Recovering from negative events by boosting implicit positive affect. *Cognition and Emotion, 25*(3), 559–570.

Rao, U., & Chen, L.-A. (2009). Characteristics, correlates, and outcomes of childhood and adolescent depressive disorders. *Dialogues in Clinical Neuroscience, 11*(1), 45–62.

Rao, U., Ryan, N. D., Birmaher, B., Dahl, R. E., Williamson, D. E., Kaufman, J., . . . Nelson, B. (1995). Unipolar depression in adolescents: Clinical outcome in adulthood. *Journal of the American Academy of Child and Adolescent Psychiatry, 34,* 566–578.

Rao, U., Weissman, M. M., Martin, J. A., & Hammond, R. W. (1993). Childhood depression and risk of suicide: A preliminary report of a longitudinal study. *Journal of the American Academy of Child and Adolescent Psychiatry, 32,* 21–27.

Ratcliff, K. A., Vazquez, L. C., Lunkenheimer, E. S., & Cole, P. M. (2021). Longitudinal changes in young children's strategy use for emotion regulation. *Developmental Psychology, 57*(9), 1471–1486.

Rathus, J. H. & Miller, A. L. (2002). Dialectical behavior therapy adapted for suicidal adolescents. *Suicide and Life-Threatening Behavior, 32*(2), 146–157.

Rathus, J. H., & Miller, A. L. (2015). *DBT skills manual for adolescents.* New York: Guilford Press.

Rehm, L. P. (1977). A self-control model of depression. *Behavior Therapy, 8,* 787–804.

Reijntjes, A., Stegge, H., Terwogt, M. M., & Hurkens, E. (2007). Children's depressive symptoms and their regulation of negative affect in response to vignette depicted emotion-eliciting events. *International Journal of Behavioral Development, 31,* 49–58.

Reijntjes, A., Stegge, H., Terwogt, M. M., Kamphuis, J. H., & Telch, M. J. (2006a). Children's coping with *in vivo* peer rejection: An experimental investigation. *Journal of Abnormal Child Psychology, 34,* 877–889.

Reijntjes, A., Stegge, H., Terwogt, M. M., Kamphuis, J. H., & Telch, M. J. (2006b). Emotion regulation and its effects on mood improvement in response to an *in vivo* peer rejection challenge. *Emotion, 6,* 543–552.

Reindl, M., Gniewosz, B., & Reinders, H. (2016). Socialization of emotion regulation strategies through friends. *Journal of Adolescence, 49,* 146–157.

Reinherz, H. Z., Giaconia, R. M., Pakiz, B., Silverman, A. B., Frost, A. K., & Lefkowitz, E. S. (1993). Psychosocial risks for major depression in late adolescence: A longitudinal community study. *Journal of the American Academy of Child and Adolescent Psychiatry, 32,* 1155–1163.

Richland, L. E., & Burchinal, M. R. (2013). Early executive function predicts reasoning development. *Psychological Science, 24*(1), 87–92.

Rippere, V. (1977). What's the thing to do when you're feeling depressed?—A pilot study. *Behaviour Research and Therapy, 15,* 185–191.

Rippere, V. (1979). Scaling the helpfulness of antidepressive activities. *Behaviour Research and Therapy, 17,* 439–449.

Robinson, K., Garisch, J. A., & Wilson, M. S. (2021). Nonsuicidal self-injury thoughts and behavioural characteristics: Associations with suicidal thoughts and behaviours among community adolescents. *Journal of Affective Disorders, 282,* 1247–1254.

Robson, D. A., Allen, M. S., & Howard, S. J. (2020). Self-regulation in childhood as a predictor of future outcomes: A meta-analytic review. *Psychological Bulletin, 146*(4), 324–354.

Rogers, C. R. (1961). *On becoming a person: A therapist's view of psychotherapy.* Boston: Houghton Mifflin.

Rogers, C. R. (1980). *A way of being.* Boston: Houghton Mifflin.

Rood, L., Roelofs, J., Bögels, S. M., Nolen-Hoeksema, S., & Schouten, E. (2009). The influence of emotion-focused rumination and distraction on depressive symptoms in non-clinical youth: A meta-analytic review. *Clinical Psychology Review, 29,* 607–616.

Rothbart, M. K., Ziaie, H., & O'Boyle, C. G.

(1992). Self-regulation and emotion in infancy. *New Directions for Child Development, 55,* 7–23.

Rottenberg, J., & Gross, J. J. (2007). Emotion and emotion regulation: A map for psychotherapy researchers. *Clinical Psychology: Science and Practice, 14,* 323–328.

Ruff, H. A., & Lawson, K. R. (1990). Development of sustained, focused attention in young children during free play. *Developmental Psychology, 26,* 85–93.

Rutter, M. (2011). Research review: Child psychiatric diagnosis and classification: Concepts, findings, challenges and potential. *Journal of Child Psychology and Psychiatry, 52,* 647–660.

Sala, M. N., Pons, F., & Molina, P. (2014). Emotion regulation strategies in preschool children. *British Journal of Developmental Psychology, 32*(4), 440–453.

Salk, R. H., Hyde, J. S., & Abramson, L. Y. (2017). Gender differences in depression in representative national samples: Meta-analyses of diagnoses and symptoms. *Psychological Bulletin, 143*(8), 783–822.

Salk, R. H., Petersen, J. L., Abramson, L. Y., & Hyde, J. S. (2016) The contemporary face of gender differences and similarities in depression throughout adolescence: Development and chronicity. *Journal of Affective Disorders, 205,* 28–35.

Salovey, P., & Grewal, D. (2005). The science of emotional intelligence. *Current Directions in Psychological Science, 14,* 281–285.

Salovey, P., Stroud, L. R., Woolery, A., & Epel, E. S. (2002). Perceived emotional intelligence, stress reactivity, and symptom reports: Further explorations using the trait meta-mood scale. *Psychology and Health, 17,* 611–627.

Samson, A. C., & Gross, J. J. (2012). Humour as emotion regulation: The differential consequences of negative versus positive humour. *Cognition and Emotion, 26*(2), 375–384.

Santucci, A. K., Silk, J. S., Shaw, D. S., Gentzler, A., Fox, N. A., & Kovacs, M. (2008). Vagal tone and temperament as predictors of emotion regulation strategies in young children. *Developmental Psychobiology, 50,* 205–216.

Schäfer, J. Ö., Naumann, E., Holmes, E. A., Tuschen-Caffier, B., & Samson, A. C. (2017). Emotion regulation strategies in depressive and anxiety symptoms in youth: A meta-analytic review. *Journal of Youth Adolescence, 46*(2), 261–276.

Schwager, S., & Rothermund, K. (2013). Counter-regulation triggered by emotions: Positive/negative affective states elicit opposite valence biases in affective processing. *Cognition and Emotion, 27*(5), 839–855.

Schweizer, S., Gotlib, I. H., & Blakemore, S.-J. (2020). The role of affective control in emotion regulation during adolescence. *Emotion, 20*(1), 80–86.

Scully, J. A., Tosi, H., & Banning, K. (2000). Life event checklists: Revisiting the social readjustment rating scale after 30 years. *Educational and Psychological Measurement, 60*(6), 864–876.

Seah, T. H. S., Matt, L. M., & Coifman, K. G. (2021). Spontaneous self-distancing mediates the association between working memory capacity and emotion regulation success. *Clinical Psychological Science, 9*(1), 79–96.

Selman, R. L., Jaquette, D., & Lavin, D. R. (1977). Interpersonal awareness in children: Toward an integration of developmental and clinical child psychology. *American Journal of Orthopsychiatry, 47,* 264–274.

Shafir, T. (2015). Movement-based strategies for emotion regulation. In M. L. Bryant (Ed.), *Handbook on Emotion regulation: Cognitive effects and social consequences* (pp. 231–249). Hauppauge, NY: Nova Science.

Shanmugan, S., & Satterthwaite, T. D. (2016). Neural markers of the development of executive function: Relevance for education. *Current Opinion in Behavioral Sciences, 10,* 7–13.

Shaw, W. S., Dimsdale, J. E., & Patterson, T. L. (2008). Stress and life events measures. In A. J. Rush, Jr., M. B. First, & D. Blacker (Eds.), *Handbook of psychiatric measures* (pp. 193–210). Washington, DC: American Psychiatric Publishing.

Sheeber, L., Hops, H., & Davis, B. (2001). Family processes in adolescent depression. *Clinical Child and Family Psychology Review, 4,* 19–35.

Shirk, S. R., & Karver, M. (2003). Prediction of treatment outcome from relationship variables in child and adolescent therapy: A meta-analytic review. *Journal of Consulting and Clinical Psychology, 71*(3), 452–464.

Siener, S., & Kerns, K. A. (2012). Emotion regulation and depressive symptoms in preadolescence. *Child Psychiatry and Human Development, 43,* 414–430.

Silk, J. S., Shaw, D. S., Skuban, E. M., Oland, A. A., & Kovacs, M. (2006). Emotion regulation strategies in offspring of childhood-onset depressed mothers. *Journal of Child Psychology and Psychiatry, 47,* 69–78.

Silk, J. S., Steinberg, L., & Morris, A. S. (2003). Adolescents' emotion regulation in daily life: Links to depressive symptoms and problem behavior. *Child Development, 74,* 1869–1880.

Silkenbeumer, J. R., Schiller, E.-M., & Kärtner, J. (2018). Co- and self-regulation of emotions in the preschool setting. *Early Childhood Research Quarterly, 44,* 72–81.

Silvers, J. A. (2020). Extinction learning and cognitive reappraisal: Windows into the neurodevelopment of emotion regulation. *Child Development Perspectives, 14*(3), 178–184.

Silvers, J. A., McRae, K., Gabrieli, J. D. E., Gross, J. J., Remy, K. A., & Ochsner, K. N. (2012). Age-related differences in emotional reactivity, regulation, and rejection sensitivity in adolescence. *Emotion, 12*(6), 1235–1247.

Sim, L., Adrian, M., Zeman, J., Cassano, M., & Friedrich, W. N. (2009). Adolescent deliberate self-harm: Linkages to emotion regulation and family emotional climate. *Journal of Research on Adolescence, 19,* 75–91.

Smith, M., & Walden, T. (2001). An exploration of African American preschool-aged children's behavioral regulation in emotionally arousing situations. *Child Study Journal, 31*(1), 13–45.

Solomon, D. A., Keller, M. B., Leon, A. C., Mueller, T. I., Shea, M. T., Warshaw, M., . . . Endicott, J. (1997). Recovery from major depression: A 10-year prospective follow-up across multiple episodes. *Archives of General Psychiatry, 54,* 1001–1006.

Spirito, A., & Esposito-Smythers, C. (2006). Addressing adolescent suicidal behavior: Cognitive-behavioral strategies. In P. C. Kendall (Ed.), *Child and adolescent therapy: Cognitive-behavioral procedures* (3rd ed., pp. 217–242). New York: Guilford Press.

Sroufe, L. A. (1995). *Emotional development: The organization of emotional life in the early years.* Cambridge, UK: Cambridge University Press.

Stansbury, K., & Sigman, M. (2000). Responses of preschoolers in two frustrating episodes: Emergence of complex strategies for emotion regulation. *Journal of Genetic Psychology, 161,* 182–202.

Stapinski, L. A., Edwards, A. C., Hickman, M., Araya, R., Teesson, M., Newton, N. C., . . . Heron, J. (2016). Drinking to cope: A latent class analysis of coping motives for alcohol use in a large cohort of adolescents. *Prevention Science, 17(5),* 584–594.

Stark, K. D., Hargrave, J., Sander, J., Custer, G., Schnoebelen, S., Simpson, J., & Mohar, J. (2006). Treatment of childhood depression: The ACTION treatment program. In P. C. Kendall (Ed.), *Child and adolescent therapy: Cognitive-behavioral procedures* (3rd ed., pp. 169–216). New York: Guilford Press.

Stark, K. D., Reynolds, W. M., & Kaslow, N. J. (1987). A comparison of the relative efficacy of self-control therapy and a behavioral problem-solving therapy for depression in children. *Journal of Abnormal Child Psychology, 15,* 91–113.

Steel, C., Wright, K., Goodwin, G., Simon, J., Morant, N., Taylor, R., . . . Holmes, E. (2020). The IBER study: Study protocol for a feasibility randomised controlled trial of imagery based emotion regulation for the treatment of anxiety in bipolar disorder. *Pilot and Feasibility Studies, 6*(1), Article 83.

Stegge, H., & Terwogt, M. M. (2007). Awareness and regulation of emotion in typical and atypical development. In J. J. Gross (Ed.), *Handbook of emotion regulation* (pp. 269–286). New York: Guilford Press.

Stein, T., & Peelen, M. V. (2021). Dissociating conscious and unconscious influences on visual detection effects. *Nature Human Behaviour, 5*(5), 612–624.

Steinberg, L. (2005). Cognitive and affective development in adolescence. *Trends in Cognitive Sciences, 9,* 69–74.

Stifter, C. A., & Braungart, J. M. (1995). The regulation of negative reactivity in infancy:

Function and development. *Developmental Psychology, 31,* 448–455.

Strauss, J., Barr, C. L., George, C. J., Devlin, B., Vetró, Á., Kiss, E., . . . Kennedy, J. L. (2005). Brain-derived neurotrophic factor variants are associated with childhood-onset mood disorder: Confirmation in a Hungarian sample. *Molecular Psychiatry, 10,* 861–867.

Strick, M., Holland, R. W., van Baaren, R. B., & van Knippenberg, A. (2009). Finding comfort in a joke: Consolatory effects of humor through cognitive distraction. *Emotion, 9,* 574–578.

Sullivan, H. S. (1954). *The psychiatric interview.* New York: Norton.

Sullivan, P. F., Neale, M. C., & Kendler, K. S. (2000). Genetic epidemiology of major depression: Review and meta-analysis. *American Journal of Psychiatry, 157,* 1552–1562.

Susa, G., Mone, I. S., Salagean, D., Mihcala, L., Benga, O., & Friedlmeier, W. (2014). The relation between maternal perception of toddler emotion regulation abilities and emotion regulation abilities displayed by children in a frustration inducing task. *Procedia—Social and Behavioral Sciences, 128,* 493–497.

Sutter, M., & Kocher, M. G. (2007). Trust and trustworthiness across different age groups. *Games and Economic Behavior, 59,* 364–382.

Sweldens, S., Corneille, O., & Yzerbyt, V. (2014). The role of awareness in attitude formation through evaluative conditioning. *Personality and Social Psychology Review, 18*(2), 187–209.

Tamás, Z., Kovacs, M., Gentzler, A. L., Tepper, P., Gádoros, J., Kiss, E., . . . Vetró, Á. (2007). The relations of temperament and emotion self-regulation with suicidal behaviors in a clinical sample of depressed children in Hungary. *Journal of Abnormal Child Psychology, 35,* 640–652.

Tamir, M. (2009). What do people want to feel and why? Pleasure and utility in emotion regulation. *Current Directions in Psychological Science, 18,* 101–105.

Tamir, M. (2016). Why do people regulate their emotions? A taxonomy of motives in emotion regulation. *Personality and Social Psychology Review, 20*(3), 199–222.

Teasdale, J. D. (1988). Cognitive vulnerability to persistent depression. *Cognition and Emotion, 2,* 247–274.

Tennant, C. (2002). Life events, stress and depression: A review of recent findings. *Australian and New Zealand Journal of Psychiatry, 36,* 173–182.

Thayer, R. E., Newman, J. R., & McClain, T. M. (1994). Self-regulation of mood: Strategies for changing a bad mood, raising energy, and reducing tension. *Journal of Personality and Social Psychology, 67,* 910–925.

Theurel, A., & Gentaz, E. (2018). The regulation of emotions in adolescents: Age differences and emotion-specific patterns. *PLOS ONE, 13*(6), e0195501.

Thomas, J. C., Letourneau, N., Campbell, T. S., Tomfohr-Madsen, L., Giesbrecht, G. F., & APrON Study Team. (2017). Developmental origins of infant emotion regulation: Mediation by temperamental negativity and moderation by maternal sensitivity. *Developmental Psychology, 53*(4), 611–628.

Thompson, R. A. (1994). Emotion regulation: A theme in search of definition. *Monographs of the Society for Research in Child Development, 59*(2/3, Serial No. 240), 25–52.

Todd, R. D., Neuman, R., Geller, B., Fox, L. W., & Hickok, J. (1993). Genetic studies of affective disorders: Should we be starting with childhood onset probands? *Journal of the American Academy of Child and Adolescent Psychiatry, 32,* 1164–1171.

Tompson, M. C., Asarnow, J. R., Mintz, J., & Cantwell, D. P. (2015). Parental depression risk: Comparing youth with depression, attention deficit hyperactivity disorder and community controls. *Journal of Psychology and Psychotherapy, 5*(4), Article 1000193.

Tompson, M. C, Langer, D. A., & Asarnow, J. R. (2020). Development and efficacy of a family-focused treatment for depression in childhood. *Journal of Affective Disorders, 276,* 686–695.

Tompson, M. C., Sugar, C. A., Langer, D. A., & Asarnow, J. R. (2017). A randomized clinical trial comparing family-focused treatment and individual supportive therapy for depression in childhood and early adolescence. *Journal of the American Academy of Child and Adolescent Psychiatry, 56*(6), 515–523.

Trask, P. C., & Sigmon, S. T. (1999). Ruminating and distracting: The effects of sequential tasks on depressed mood. *Cognitive Therapy and Research, 23,* 231–246.

Trommsdorff, G., & Cole, P. M. (2011). Emotion, self-regulation, and social behavior in cultural contexts. In X. Chen & K. H. Rubin (Eds.), *Socioemotional development in cultural context* (pp. 131–163). New York: Guilford Press.

Trowell, J., Joffe, I., Campbell, J., Clemente, C., Almqvist, F., Soininen, M., . . . Tsiantis, J. (2007). Childhood depression: A place for psychotherapy. An outcome study comparing individual psychodynamic psychotherapy and family therapy. *European Child and Adolescent Psychiatry, 16,* 157–167.

Tsuno, N., Besset, A., & Ritchie, K. (2005). Sleep and depression. *Journal of Clinical Psychiatry, 66*(10), 1254–1269.

Tugade, M. M., & Fredrickson, B. L. (2004). Resilient individuals use positive emotions to bounce back from negative emotional experiences. *Journal of Personality and Social Psychology, 86,* 320–333.

Tuulari, J. J., Scheinin, N. M., Lehtola, S., Merisaari, H., Saunavaara, J., Parkkola, R., . . . Björnsdotter, M. (2019). Neural correlates of gentle skin stroking in early infancy. *Developmental Cognitive Neuroscience, 35,* 36–41.

Tymofiyeva, O., & Gaschler, R. (2021). Training-induced neural plasticity in youth: A systematic review of structural and functional MRI studies. *Frontiers in Human Neuroscience, 14,* Article 497245.

Uhl, K., Halpern, L. F., Tam, C., Fox, J. K., & Ryan, J. L. (2019). Relations of emotion regulation, negative and positive affect to anxiety and depression in middle childhood. *Journal of Child and Family Studies, 28,* 2988–2999.

Urano, Y., Ikeda, T., & Mearns, J. (2022). Receiving assistance in emotion regulation: A preliminary investigation. *Personality and Individual Differences, 188,* 111445.

Van Beveren, M.-L., Goossens, L., Volkaert, B., Grassmann, C., Wante, L., Vandeweghe, L., . . . Braet, C. (2019). How do I feel right now? Emotional awareness, emotion regulation, and depressive symptoms in youth. *European Child and Adolescent Psychiatry, 28*(3), 389–398.

Van Beveren, M.-L., Harding, K., Beyers, W., & Braet, C. (2018). Don't worry, be happy: The role of positive emotionality and adaptive emotion regulation strategies for youth depressive symptoms. *British Journal of Clinical Psychology, 57,* 18–41.

Van Beveren, M.-L., Kuppens, S., Hankin, B., & Braet, C. (2019). Because you had a bad day: General and daily relations between reactive temperament, emotion regulation, and depressive symptoms in youth. *PLOS ONE, 14*(10), e0224126.

van den Bos, W., Westenberg, M., van Dijk, E., & Crone, E. A. (2010). Development of trust and reciprocity in adolescence. *Cognitive Development, 25*(1), 90–102.

Van Dillen, L. F., & Koole, S. L. (2007). Clearing the mind: A working memory model of distraction from negative mood. *Emotion, 7,* 715–723.

Vanlessen, N., De Raedt, R., Koster, E. H. W., & Pourtois, G. (2016). Happy heart, smiling eyes: A systematic review of positive mood effects on broadening of visuospatial attention. *Neuroscience and Biobehavioral Reviews, 68,* 816–837.

Verdeli, H., Ferro, T., Wickramaratne, P., Greenwald, S., Blanco, C., & Weissman, M. M. (2004). Treatment of depressed mothers of depressed children: Pilot study of feasibility. *Depression and Anxiety, 19*(1), 51–58.

Visu-Petra, L., Cheie, L., Benga, O., & Miclea, M. (2012). The structure of executive functions in preschoolers: An investigation using the NEPSY battery. *Procedia—Social and Behavioral Sciences, 33,* 627–631.

Volkaert, B., Wante, L., Van Beveren, M.-L., Vervoort, L., & Braet, C. (2020). Training adaptive emotion regulation skills in early adolescents: The effects of distraction, acceptance, cognitive reappraisal, and problem solving. *Cognitive Therapy and Research, 44*(3), 678–696.

von Salisch, M., & Zeman, J. L. (2018). Pathways to reciprocated friendships: A cross-lagged panel study on young adolescents' anger regulation towards friends. *Journal of Youth and Adolescence, 47*(3), 673–687.

Vygotsky, L. S. (1962). *Thought and language.* Cambridge, MA: MIT Press.

Waller, J. M., Silk, J. S., Stone, L. B., & Dahl, R. E. (2014). Co-rumination and co-problem solving in the daily lives of adolescents with major depressive disorder. *Journal of the American Academy of Child and Adolescent Psychiatry, 53*(8), 869–878.

Wante, L. Van Beveren, M.-L., Theuwis, L., & Braet, C. (2018). The effects of emotion regulation strategies on positive and negative affect in early adolescents. *Cognition and Emotion, 32*(5), 988–1002.

Watanabe, N., Hunot, V., Omari, I. M., Churchill, R., & Furukawa, T. A. (2007). Psychotherapy for depression among children and adolescents: A systematic review. *Acta Psychiatrica Scandinavica, 116*(2), 84–95.

Waters, S. F., & Thompson, R. A. (2014). Children's perceptions of the effectiveness of strategies for regulating anger and sadness. *International Journal of Behavioral Development, 38*(2), 174–181.

Weersing, V. R., Jeffreys, M., Do, M.-C. T., Schwartz, K. T. G., & Bolano, C. (2017) Evidence-base update of psychosocial treatments for child and adolescent depression. *Journal of Clinical Child and Adolescent Psychology, 46*(1), 11–43.

Weersing, V. R., Rozenman, M., & Gonzalez, A. (2009). Core components of therapy in youth: Do we know what to disseminate? *Behavior Modification, 33,* 24–47.

Weiss, B., & Garber, J. (2003). Developmental differences in the phenomenology of depression. *Development and Psychopathology, 15,* 403–430.

Weiss, N. H., Bold, K. W., Sullivan, T. P., Armeli, S., & Tennen, H. (2016). Testing bidirectional associations among emotion regulation strategies and substance use: A daily diary study. *Addiction, 112*(4), 695–704.

Weiss, N. H., Kiefer, R., Goncharenko, S., Raudales, A. M., Forkus, S. R., Schick, M. R., & Contractor, A. A. (2022). Emotion regulation and substance use: A meta-analysis. *Drug and Alcohol Dependence, 230,* Article 109131.

Weissman, M. M., Wickramaratne, P., Pilowsky, D. J., Poh, E., Battern, L. A., Hernandez, M., . . . Stewart, J. W. (2015). Treatment of maternal depression in a medication clinical trial and its effect on children. *American Journal of Psychiatry, 172*(5), 450–459.

Weissman, M. M., Wolk, S., Goldstein, R. B., Moreau, D., Adams, P., Greenwald, S., . . . Wickramaratne, P. (1999a). Depressed adolescents grown up. *Journal of the American Medical Association, 281,* 1707–1713.

Weissman, M. M., Wolk, S., Wickramaratne, P., Goldstein, R. B., Adams, P., Greenwald, S., . . . Steinberg, D. (1999b). Children with prepubertal-onset major depressive disorder and anxiety grown up. *Archives of General Psychiatry, 56,* 794–801.

Weisz, J. R. (2004). Cognitive-behavioral therapies for child depression. In *Psychotherapy for children and adolescents: Evidence-based treatments and case examples* (pp. 104–128). Cambridge, UK: Cambridge University Press.

Weisz, J. R., Kuppens, S., Ng, M. Y., Vaughn-Coaxum, R. A., Ugueto, A. M., Eckshtain, D., & Corteselli, K. A. (2019). Are psychotherapies for young people growing stronger? Tracking trends over time for youth anxiety, depression, attention-deficit/hyperactivity disorder, and conduct problems. *Perspectives on Psychological Science, 14*(2), 216–237.

Weller, A., & Feldman, R. (2003). Emotion regulation and touch in infants: The role of cholecystokinin and opioids. *Peptides, 24*(5), 779–788.

Weller, R. A., Weller, E. B., Fristad, M. A., & Bowes, J. M. (1991). Depression in recently bereaved prepubertal children. *American Journal of Psychiatry, 148,* 1536–1540.

Werner-Seidler, A., Tan, L., & Dalgleish, T. (2017). The vicissitudes of positive autobiographical recollection as an emotion regulation strategy in depression. *Clinical Psychological Science, 5*(1), 26–36.

Wesselhoeft, R., Pedersen, C. B., Mortensen, P. B., Mors, O., & Bilenberg, N. (2015). Gender-age interaction in incidence rates of childhood emotional disorders. *Psychological Medicine, 45,* 829–839.

Westen, D. (1994). Toward an integrative model of affect regulation: Applications to social-psychological research. *Journal of Personality, 62,* 641–667.

Whiteside, U., Chen, E., Neighbors, C., Hunter, D., Lo, T., & Larimer, M. (2007). Difficulties regulating emotions: Do binge eaters have fewer strategies to modulate and tolerate negative affect? *Eating Behaviors, 8,* 162–169.

Wickramaratne, P. J., Greenwald, S., & Weissman, M. M. (2000). Psychiatric disorders in the relatives of probands with prepubertal-onset or adolescent-onset major depression. *Journal of the American Academy of Child and Adolescent Psychiatry, 39*(11), 1396–1405.

Wild, B., Erb, M., & Bartels, M. (2001). Are emotions contagious? Evoked emotions while viewing emotionally expressive faces: quality, quantity, time course and gender differences. *Psychiatry Research, 102,* 109–124.

Williams, W. C., Morelli, S. A., Ong, D. C., & Zaki, J. (2018). Interpersonal emotion regulation: Implications for affiliation, perceived support, relationships, and well-being. *Journal of Personality and Social Psychology, 115*(2), 224–254.

Williamson, D. E., Birmaher, B., Dahl, R. E., & Ryan, N. D. (2005). Stressful life events in anxious and depressed children. *Journal of Child and Adolescent Psychopharmacology, 15,* 571–580.

Wilson, S., Hicks, B. M., Foster, K. T., McGue, M., & Iacono, W. G. (2015). Age of onset and course of major depressive disorder: Associations with psychosocial functioning outcomes in adulthood. *Psychological Medicine, 45,* 505–514.

Winsler, A., Diaz, R. M., Atencio, D. J., McCarthy, E. M., & Chabay, L. A. (2000). Verbal self-regulation over time in preschool children at risk for attention and behavior problems. *Journal of Child Psychology and Psychiatry, 41,* 875–886.

Winsler, A., & Naglieri, J. (2003). Overt and covert verbal problem-solving strategies: Developmental trends in use, awareness, and relations with task performance in children aged 5 to 17. *Child Development, 74,* 659–678.

Wolff, J. C., & Ollendick, T. H. (2006). The comorbidity of conduct problems and depression in childhood and adolescence. *Clinical Child and Family Psychology Review, 9*(3/4), 201–220.

World Health Organization. (1992). *The ICD-10 classification of mental and behavioral disorders.* Geneva: Author.

Wray-Lake, L., & Flanagan, C. A. (2012). Parenting practices and the development of adolescents' social trust. *Journal of Adolescence, 35*(3), 549–560.

Xin, W., & Chan, J. R. (2020). Myelin plasticity: Sculpting circuits in learning and memory. *Nature Reviews Neuroscience, 21,* 682–694.

Xiu, L., Wu, J., Chang, L., & Zhou, R. (2018). Working memory training improves emotion regulation ability. *Scientific Reports, 8,* Article 15012.

Yang, L., Zhou, X., Zhou, C., Zhang, Y., Pu, J., Liu, L., . . . Xie, P. (2017). Efficacy and acceptability of cognitive behavioral therapy for depression in children: A systematic review and meta-analysis. *Academic Pediatrics, 17*(1), 9–16.

Young, K. S., Sandman, C. F., & Craske, M. G. (2019). Positive and negative emotion regulation in adolescence: Links to anxiety and depression. *Brain Sciences, 9*(4), 76.

Zaehringer, J., Falquez, R., Schubert, A.-L., Nees, F., & Barnow, S. (2018). Neural correlates of reappraisal considering working memory capacity and cognitive flexibility. *Brain Imaging and Behavior, 12*(6), 1529–1543.

Zaki, J., & Williams, W. C. (2013). Interpersonal emotion regulation. *Emotion, 13*(5), 803–810.

Zamora, E. V., Richards, M. M., Juric, L. C., Aydmune, Y., & Introzzi, I. (2020). Perceptual, cognitive and response inhibition in emotional contexts in children. *Psychology and Neuroscience, 13*(3), 257–272.

Zelazo, P. D., & Carlson, S. M. (2020). The neurodevelopment of executive function skills: Implications for academic achievement gaps. *Psychology and Neuroscience, 13*(3), 273–298.

Zhou, X., Hetrick, S. E., Cuijpers, P., Qin, B., Barth, J., Whittington, C. J., . . . Xie, P. (2015). Comparative efficacy and acceptability of psychotherapies for depression in children and adolescents: A systematic review and network meta-analysis. *World Psychiatry, 14,* 207–222.

Zhou, X., Teng, T., Zhang, Y., Del Giovane, C., Furukawa, T. A., Weisz, J. R., . . . Xie, P. (2020). Comparative efficacy and acceptability of antidepressants, psychotherapies, and their combination for acute treatment of children and adolescents with depressive disorder: A systematic review and network meta-analysis. *Lancet Psychiatry, 7,* 581–601.

Zimmer-Gembeck, M. J., Webb, H. J., Pepping, C. A., Swan, K., Merlo, O., Skinner, E. A., . . . Dunbar, M. (2017). Review: Is parent-child attachment a correlate of children's emotion regulation and coping? *International Journal of Behavioral Development, 41*(1), 74–93.

Zimmermann, L. K., & Stansbury, K. (2003). The influence of temperamental reactivity and situational context on the emotion-regulatory abilities of 3-year-old children. *Journal of Genetic Psychology, 164,* 389–409.

Zimmermann, P., & Iwanski, A. (2014). Development and timing of developmental changes in emotional reactivity and emotion regulation during adolescence. In P. M. Cole & T. Hollenstein (Eds.), *Emotion regulation: A matter of time* (pp. 117–139). New York: Routledge.

Zisook, S., Lesser, I., Stewart, J. W., Wisniewski, S. R., Balasubramani, G. K., Fava, M., & Gilmer, W. S. (2007). Effect of age at onset on the course of major depressive disorder. *American Journal of Psychiatry, 164,* 1539–1546.

Zlotnick, C., Donaldson, D., Spirito, A., & Pearlstein, T. (1997). Affect regulation and suicide attempts in adolescent inpatients. *Journal of the American Academy of Child and Adolescent Psychiatry, 36*(6), 793–798.

Index

Note. f or *t* following a page number indicates a figure or table.

D

E

F

J

K

L

M

Q

R

S

T